D0856517

Subacute and Transitional Care Handbook

Defining, Delivering, and Improving Care

Subacute and Transitional Care Handbook

Defining, Delivering, and Improving Care

Steven A. Levenson, M.D.

BCP ■Beverly Cracom Publications

St. Louis, MO   Wilton, CT   Pasadena, CA

A joint venture between Beverly Foundation and Cracom Publishing, Inc.

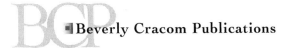

Beverly Cracom Publications

St. Louis, MO   Wilton, CT   Pasadena, CA

A joint venture between Beverly Foundation and Cracom Publishing, Inc.

Publisher & Editorial Director: Barbara Ellen Norwitz
Editor: Kate Aker
Production Editor: Chris Cook
Photography: Lightworks Photography & Design, Annapolis, MD, George Dodson

Notice: The author and publisher of this volume have attempted to offer easy-to-use information and assessment tools that are currently accepted and used by professionals in related fields. Nevertheless, new approaches are continually under development, which will expand the options available to the reader, and may alter some of the application concepts presented in this text. The publisher and author disclaim any liability, loss, injury, or damage incurred as a consequence, directly or indirectly, of the use and application of any of the contents of this volume.

Library of Congress Cataloging-in-Publication Data
Levenson, Steven A.
   Subacute and transitional care handbook : defining, delivering,
and improving care / Steven A. Levenson.
      p. cm.
   Includes bibliographical references and index.
   ISBN: 1-886657-08-4
   1. Subacute care facilities—Administration. 2. Hospitals—After
care—Administration. I. Title
   [DNLM: 1. Progressive Patient Care—organization & administration—
handbooks. W 49 L657s 1996]
RA975.C64L48 1996
362.1—dc20
DNLM/DLC
for Library of Congress   96-12509
                                                    CIP

Printed in the United States of America

10 9 8 7 6 5 4 3 2 1

INTRODUCTION

This book is about subacute care. However, it takes a different perspective from other references on the subject. Subacute care is currently being promoted as a significant business opportunity in a changing health care climate. Thus, there is abundant information about such things as negotiating managed care contracts, setting up and capitalizing subacute units, and obtaining adequate reimbursement. Some information is also available about specific services and programs, such as wound care and ventilator care, relevant to subacute patients. In contrast, comparatively little can be found about how to organize and implement a comprehensive system to appropriately select, admit, evaluate, manage, and transfer subacute patients, or how to evaluate the appropriateness and cost-effectiveness of care.

The late twentieth century is witnessing profound changes in the organization of health care delivery systems, including the roles of related practitioners and organizations. There are reasons for these upheavals, which go beyond commonly cited ones about needing to control costs. Those reasons are related largely to balance. As discussed in this book, nature has many built-in mechanisms to maintain balance and to forcibly restore it when excessive imbalances develop. Human beings are also subject to those natural mechanisms. Therefore, social systems that become too unbalanced suffer predictable consequences. Ironically, health care provision — which is supposed to be dedicated to maintaining essential balances and identifying and correcting imbalances in individuals affected by illness and injury — has itself suffered by neglecting these essential principles.

The underlying precept of this book is that subacute care requires a system to be successful. A systematic approach is needed whenever many different practitioners and patients, representing countless issues and variables, are involved. Subacute care should be viewed not only as needing a properly balanced environment to be maximally useful, but also as exemplifying the principles of proper balance.

Thus, this book approaches subacute care from the clinical systems perspective. That is, how should the programs be organized, and the practitioners organized, guided, trained, and supported, so that they can deliver consistently high-quality, cost-effective care, and why are those approaches most compatible with desirable business objectives?

Because subacute care must become part of integrated health care delivery systems, it cannot be discussed without also considering broader systems issues. Therefore, much of this book describes principles and practices of subacute care that have relevance to the whole health care system. For instance, Chapter 3 discusses the factors that influence service needs and placement of individuals at all levels of care, including subacute care. The book also considers steps that should be taken so that all components of the health care system—including direct care providers—can flourish and do the best possible job.

Therefore, this book is meant to complement, rather than repeat, much of what is found in other references. For example, instead of discussing in depth how to develop managed care contracts, this book emphasizes what programs and practitioners should know about managed care as it might influence their care decisions or create risks in caring for their patients. Although the book discusses many clinical issues, it is not about treating specific diseases or conditions, because that information can be found elsewhere.

The broader themes and items of interest to the reader that this book covers include the following:

- What subacute care is and is not
- How subacute care reflects major challenges and opportunities for health care providers

- Why subacute care has gained attention and has grown so much in a short time

- How subacute care fits into an integrated delivery system and managed care environment

- How subacute care relates to other programs throughout the continuum

- How the health care reimbursement system could be realigned to provide more appropriate incentives for creating a coordinated delivery system

- Why the right system for categorizing and placing patients is vital to an effective, efficient care delivery system

- How the health care system should revamp patient classification schemes to be more consistent with their real needs

- The desirable characteristics and behaviors of all players in subacute care, and the principles that should govern their actions

- The proper team approach, and why it is essential for successful service and care

- The essential processes of care throughout the health care continuum, especially in relation to subacute care

- The basis for coordinated service delivery and care management systems in relation to subacute care

- How health care networks and managed care organizations could develop more clinically relevant criteria to decide on lengths of stay and appropriate care objectives

- How physicians could become more constructive practitioners and performers in all programs and at all levels of care, especially those beyond their traditional acute and ambulatory care realms

- Factors that appear to influence risk and outcomes — including costs of care — of subacute patients, and how they can be taken into account in providing care

- The crucial difference between treating diagnoses and managing problems, and how this relates to successful care delivery

- Essential general organizational systems and support to facilitate complex care

- The vital importance of the natural principle of homeostasis in effective care delivery systems

- The components and principles of an effective quality management and improvement system for subacute care

- General public policy and educational, regulatory, and reimbursement issues that must be resolved to enable an effective health care system in which subacute care plays the most useful role possible

This book has been written for, and designed to be understood by and useful to, all those involved in the health care system including health care practitioners and clinical support staff, management, public policy and regulatory agencies, health care organizational governing bodies, corporate leadership, insurance companies, and even interested members of the public. Because of these many different disciplines and perspectives, readers should keep in mind that what seems obvious or simplistic to some may be unfamiliar to others. For example, geriatricians and members of other disciplines familiar with the care of the frail elderly will undoubtedly be acquainted with such concepts as the interdisciplinary team approach, the management of comorbidities, and the problem-oriented approach to care. For others—including many physicians and payers—the distinction between diagnoses and problems will be foreign.

The core clinical chapters (5 through 8) should be most relevant to those providing care, and to those providing or overseeing clinical support services. The outer chapters (1 through 3 and 10 through 13) should interest both practitioners and those who do not deliver direct care, because they cover relevant definitions and general health care systems issues, as well as issues related to quality improvement and patient risk and outcomes assessment. Chapters 4 and 9 are relevant for those planning, implementing, and operating subacute programs — and also for practitioners, who should understand how these processes relate to service delivery, even though they may not be involved in such processes. Chapter 11 offers actual case examples, which should be recognizable by those involved in subacute care. Those not familiar with subacute care may wish to start by reading Chapter 11 to get a sense of the scope of subacute patients and problems. Table 1, p. viii, describes the major items addressed in each chapter. Recognizing that many readers will approach this book in stages, some information is purposely repeated in several chapters, while other material is cross-referenced.

Finally, this book is written from the perspective of a physician who appreciates the outstanding work of so many health care practitioners and other dedicated, competent individuals, and who also recognizes the frustrations and problems that they must so often endure because of an unbalanced system that frequently rewards undesirable performance and impedes doing the right thing. It is dedicated to the perspective that these obstacles can and must be addressed, so that the health care system becomes one major component of a broad societal commitment to a better future. The knowledge we have gained in the twentieth century about health and illness includes many vital lessons for all human endeavors. The lessons of the twentieth century should be taken seriously and used prudently in refining health care in the next millennium.

ACKNOWLEDGMENTS

The author wishes to acknowledge the following individuals for their contributions and excellent suggestions during the writing of this book: Patricia Blanchette, M.D.; Larry Lawhorne, M.D.; Susan Levy, M.D.; Barbara Marte; Sally Rouses; George Taler, M.D.; Mary Tellis-Nayak, R.N.; and Debra Wertheimer, M.D. The author would also like to thank Kate Aker and Chris Cook of Beverly Cracom Publications for their excellent technical support and perseverance.

TABLE 1   MAJOR ITEMS COVERED IN EACH CHAPTER

Chapter	Issues Addressed
Chapter 1	What are the current challenges and opportunities for subacute care organizations and providers? What has stimulated the growth of this form of care?
Chapter 2	What is subacute care? What are the characteristics of subacute patients, compared to other patients throughout the care continuum? What factors define patient need across the continuum?
Chapter 3	What is the place of subacute care in an integrated delivery system? How does it relate to other components of the care continuum? How can this information be used to determine appropriate placement in a subacute program and after receiving subacute care?
Chapter 4	What are the steps to planning and implementing an effective subacute care program, both as a business and as a clinical service? How should practitioners be involved in these processes?
Chapter 5	What discrete clinical programs and services are typically offered in subacute care settings?
Chapter 6	What attitudes and philosophies are important for the players in subacute care? What are the roles of the various disciplines providing, supporting, and overseeing the care and the organizations and programs in which it is provided?
Chapter 7	What are the processes of care? What should occur during each of them, and by whom?
Chapter 8	How should the processes of care, and the performances of the various individuals involved in the care, be coordinated and optimized? What systems and processes are essential to providing consistently effective and efficient care? What are the elements of a care management system?
Chapter 9	What general support systems are important to enable organizations and individuals to provide consistently effective, efficient service and care?
Chapter 10	How can the risks of subacute patients be anticipated, and their outcomes evaluated? What factors appear to relate to risks and outcomes? How can knowledge of these factors be used to help provide the care? How can the care and the support systems help facilitate an effective quality improvement program?
Chapter 11	What are some actual case examples of patients cared for in subacute programs, and how do the principles discussed in this book relate to their care?
Chapter 12	What are the implications of subacute care for various public policy, regulatory, and reimbursement considerations? How do these external issues influence the role and successful performance of subacute programs?
Chapter 13	In a changing health care environment, how can the best possible framework for all patients and providers be achieved?

TABLE OF CONTENTS

7
THE PROCESSES OF CARE, 157

8
THE ORGANIZATION AND SUPPORT OF CARE AND PRACTITIONERS, 205

9

GENERAL SUPPORT SYSTEMS FOR SUBACUTE CARE, 253

10

ASSESSING AND IMPROVING PATIENT OUTCOMES AND SERVICE QUALITY, 309

11
SUBACUTE CARE PATIENT CASES, 353

12
PUBLIC POLICY, REIMBURSEMENT, AND REGULATORY IMPLICATIONS, 383

13
A FINAL WORD: THE CHALLENGES OF CHANGE, 399

INDEX, 405

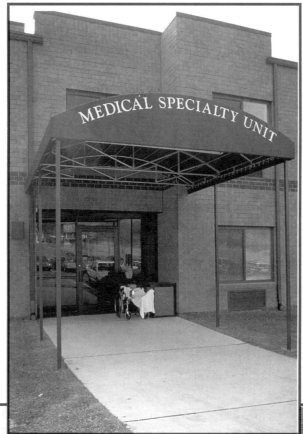

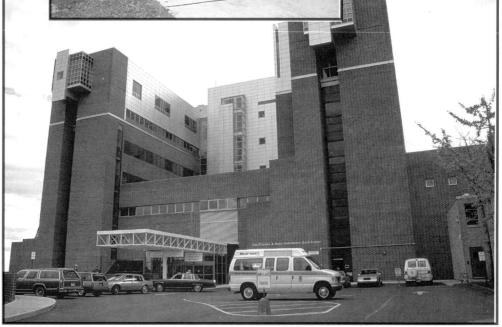

BACKGROUND AND ENVIRONMENT OF SUBACUTE CARE

*T*he future of health care holds major opportunities and significant challenges. The roles of various practitioners and care sites in the continuum of care are changing rapidly. In the future, all levels of service and care sites should be recognized as equally valuable. Succeeding in this environment will require some significant conceptual shifts. Practitioners and organizations must adjust their processes, attitudes, and systems accordingly. To do this effectively, it helps to understand how the health care environment sets certain boundaries for everyone's actions.

Successful subacute care requires an effective strategy. This includes understanding the circumstances within which the care is delivered, and providing that care in the proper context, at both the patient and programmatic levels.

The purpose of this chapter is to review the challenges and opportunities of a changing health care environment, and to show how those changes have influenced, and may be influenced by, the development of subacute care.

THE CHANGING FUTURE OF HEALTH CARE

All health care providers face both challenges and opportunities in the current and future health care environment. Table 1–1, p. 13, lists the essential steps to meet the challenges and take advantage of the opportunities.

Challenges

In this era of significant rapid change, health care reform means changed attitudes, systems, and processes, not just revamped reimbursement and improved access. The future demands both good quality and cost-effectiveness, not just one or the other. Reimbursement will tighten while expectations for quality service increase. Society has a major interest in streamlining and improving coordination of health care services.

Future care systems will differ markedly from those of the past. There will be a much greater focus on collections of providers who cooperate through alliances and networks to manage the problems and deliver the care for individuals with longitudinal needs. Fee-for-service reimbursement will be challenged by alternatives offering different incentives. Capitation and managed care should provide greater incentives for preventive care and should shift the care objectives away from providing services to maximize reimbursement, toward giving optimal (not maximum) service, for the lowest possible cost, for the shortest possible time, in the least restrictive setting.

In the workplace, a more diverse workforce will require extensive training and guidance to become a cohesive unit. Management of this workforce will be affected by the increased complexity of laws and regulations regarding care, employment practices, and oversight. Traditional roles and responsibilities will need to change to enable more effective use of relatively scarce, expensive personnel and practitioners. Creative use of available technologies will be important in maximizing the productivity and satisfaction of health care practitioners and support staff.

Practitioners and providers will need to develop more pertinent, empirically based standards and attain more consistent performance for individual disciplines. To reduce undesirable process variance, more protocols and practice guidelines will be used. There are also growing expectations for using more objective measurements and realistic comparisons among providers and practitioners to explain the benefits of their services and justify patient outcomes. For instance, there is a great need to measure outcomes in subacute patients, but it cannot be done just by using common traditional measures such as mortality, cost, or diagnoses. The common traditional approach of "quality by proclamation" ("We're good because we say so!") will also be unacceptable.

Thus, only some past attitudes and approaches will be relevant in the future. The challenge is to retain and improve upon the best of the past while adopting new approaches and systems to meet the requirements for quality and cost-effectiveness.

Opportunities

Health care providers also face unprecedented opportunities to apply knowledge and skills to improve individual lives. This is facilitated by the shift from high-technology acute care to a growing understanding and recognition of long-term and transitional care.

Another favorable trend is the shift in approaches to business management generally and to health care management specifically. The imbalances among various interest groups in health care are slowly being addressed. The old power structure of health care and the hierarchical/authoritarian approach to management are declining slowly. The value of attracting and retaining quality individuals to provide services, and the need to support those individuals adequately is more apparent.

Partly because of the interest in controlling costs, practitioners increasingly have been given flexibility to try new approaches. Rigidly defined care settings and reimbursement systems have begun to yield to vertically integrated approaches.

Over the past 30 years, a much larger knowledge base has developed and been used to resolve many significant health-related problems. There is an unprecedented opportunity to create standards and guidelines for effective practices and appropriate support systems and processes.

Because of their essential emphasis on effective problem management and on broad service coordination and interdisciplinary cooperation, long-term and subacute care should help lead the health care industry into the new century using different paradigms.

Shifts in Service Provision

Most service delivery is no longer strictly associated with a discrete care site. Until the mid- to late-1980s, each site was typically associated with specific services. Acute hospitals treated acute illness and injury, nursing homes and other similar facilities gave long-term care for those with chronic disabilities, and other care needs were met through a combination of outpatient, ambulatory, and home-based care.

However, these simple distinctions no longer apply. Care is now being delivered throughout a continuum of care sites. Gaps are being filled by new forms of service delivery and provider arrangements. Various levels of care are now given at the same site, and different sites now deliver similar levels of care.

For example, by 1994 more than half of all surgery in the United States was being performed on an outpatient basis. Some of that was being done in hospital-based ambulatory surgery units, and some in freestanding ambulatory units with no hospital connection. Many nursing facilities now manage some episodes of acute illness without transferring their residents to hospitals. A spectrum of rehabilitation services is being provided in every site from homes to hospitals, and hospitals are offering more long-term care and ambulatory health services. In-home treatments and care including rehabilitation therapies, hospice services, and ventilators are being offered. Providers are offering a spectrum of services through health alliances and networks.

Traditionally, hospitals have managed a broad spectrum of complex and simple illnesses. They were considered to be the only places with the staff, technology, and professional expertise to handle complex care, and the most convenient setting to assess and manage those with new but not necessarily complicated medical problems. For example, patients with a new-onset myocardial infarction would be admitted to the hospital's coronary care unit and would then remain in the hospital for weeks for recuperation. Someone with recurrent gastrointestinal bleeding or a fever of uncertain origin might stay in a hospital for several weeks until she was fully diagnosed and treated. A patient who suffered postoperative complications might stay for weeks or months until he became fully functional, died, or the decision was made that nothing further could be done.

Now, for various reasons—primarily economic—hospitals can no longer serve all their traditional functions. Having the essential personnel and spectrum of monitoring, diagnostic, and treatment modalities, they will specialize primarily as sites for the short-term evaluation and management of very complicated or life-threatening acute conditions.

Furthermore, hospitals and acute care practitioners have effectively managed only some aspects of complex illness. They have tended to focus on identifying and initiating management of the causes of acute illness and injury, with relatively less attention paid to addressing the consequences. They have generally only addressed coexisting problems (such as functional deficits, other active illnesses, and other non-life-threatening complications or conditions) that have a significant bearing on the primary problem.

But these other aspects of complex illness, including the consequences of partial treatment failures and residual disabilities, must be dealt with effectively and efficiently. A growing body of evidence suggests that they often influence patient outcomes as much as does the principal disease process. Thus, other care sites have assumed the management of both less complicated acute illness and these other aspects of complex care. This may include continuing treatment of partially resolved conditions, managing coexisting problems and illnesses, compensating for residual deficits left by the acute problem (including rehabilitative and restorative care), helping the patient or family cope with the psychosocial or economic consequences of the condition, and managing a progressive decline up to and including death.

For these and other reasons, it is no longer possible to strictly link discrete care sites with specific aspects of health care. Although hospitals will continue to treat high-acuity patients (see Chapter 2), a different approach can often meet the needs of individuals whose conditions are of moderate or low acuity. This is called transitional or subacute care, and the purpose of this book is to discuss such care in depth.

FACTORS INFLUENCING THE DEVELOPMENT OF SUBACUTE CARE

Several factors have contributed to the evolution of subacute care. These include the changing population, impact of technology, financing of care, and acceptance of alternative sites to provide care.

Changing Population

As in many other countries, the American population continues to increase in number and, on average, in age. More people have complex acute illnesses and long-term complications. High-risk populations include children who survive birth defects and birth-related complications such as prematurity; the frail elderly (especially those over age 75); those with bloodborne illnesses such as HIV infection; and those who survive serious injuries but have major residual disabilities. Such individuals may require lifelong care and support.

Technological Advances and Limits

Advances in medical knowledge and technology have had a significant impact on aspects of health and illness. Medical technologies have enhanced survival but not necessarily functional recovery. Technological advances have been especially successful at saving lives and improving the management of discrete, curable conditions. For example, new medical technologies have prevented many from dying of birth defects, infections, complicated illnesses, and trauma.

But survival does not ensure adequate function. Adequate social function requires a certain level of cognition and mobility, and the ability to perform various activities of daily living such as bathing, grooming, and dressing.

Medical technology cannot fix many problems and has created some new ones. It has had minimal impact on curing chronic conditions, but somewhat greater success in helping manage their consequences (for instance, cataract removal, joint replacement surgery, organ transplantation). Medical technology also has limited use in prevention. Effective preventive care consists mostly of low-technology social and personal activities such as appropriate diet and exercise, and vaccinations and other public health measures.

Financing of Care

The growing and changing population, advances in medical knowledge and technology, politics and public policy, and public expectations for care have combined to greatly affect the costs of health care. The number of health care service and treatment options has increased dramatically. The overall costs of the health care system have skyrocketed, as has the cost of treating individual episodes of illness and injury.

Both patients and providers now have more of a stake in overall system costs. In recent years, payers have forced a reduction in patient demand for services and required more providers to share greater financial risks of excessive service provision or excessively costly care.

Until 1983, hospitals were reimbursed retrospectively, based on their costs plus a markup. Then Medicare switched to a prospective payment system, which paid hospitals a fixed sum based on various diagnosis-related groups (DRGs). Until 1992, Medicare paid physicians under a "usual-and-customary" fee-for-service system. Starting in 1992, a different method was used to calculate physician payments based primarily on the "relative value" of various services reflected in associated workload and practice costs.

Several economic forces have driven the movement to subacute care. The Medicare skilled benefit for postacute care was limited to elderly beneficiaries. Because of the high cost of delivering services in hospitals, payers have sought less costly alternatives. As providers have had to share more of the financial risks of providing care, they have tried to lower their overhead. Both these goals have encouraged expansion of a setting that can manage moderately complex problems without requiring on-site availability of so many costly practitioners and support staff, and so much expensive high-technology equipment. Thus, subacute care also represents a merging of the goals of providers and payers.

Two factors, managed care and capitation, have increasingly become part of health care economics. Managed care may be defined as a system in which payers use stringent utilization criteria to influence the selection and duration of services. Capitation is a payment system by which a provider receives a fixed amount of money per person to provide all their care for a defined time. A provider who can give that care for less than the allocated amount may keep the difference, or must make up the difference if the cost of care exceeds it.

Managed care puts both providers and payers at risk, especially for excessive services and excessive capacity to provide service. This challenges providers to define the optimal (neither too much nor too little) quantity and duration of services, and to maintain the capacity to provide needed care in the face of controls on demand.

Managed care organizations are increasingly forging agreements with networks of providers who have demonstrated their ability to give good quality care at low cost. These networks are including subacute care among their programs so they can offer more affordable care for complex illness.

Recognition of Potential Alternatives

Slowly, the availability and appropriateness of alternatives to acute hospital care are being recognized. Certain factors have helped accelerate or have slowed such acceptance.

Accelerating Factors.   Typically, the movement to alternative care sites has been based on economics, followed by a recognition of the clinical advantages (for example, ambulatory surgery costs are less and often reduce the recuperative period; nonhospital sites often have a lower risk of nosocomial infection with virulent microorganisms). Subacute care follows a similar pattern. The primary factors have been payer demand and the willingness of payers to accept alternative sites that can achieve desired outcomes. The successful track record of health maintenance organizations (HMOs) in various states has helped patients become more familiar with receiving care at alternative sites.

The availability of alternative care sites has enabled quicker discharge of patients from hospitals. The wider availability and lower cost of sophisticated technologies has enabled sites other than hospitals to acquire and use them for patients. Although home-based care may often be desirable, it is not always feasible or as cost-effective as having a facility-based collection of services for a package price.

Inhibiting Factors.   Factors that have slowed the acceptance of alternative care sites include misunderstanding of the nature of transitional care, underdeveloped capabilities of alternative sites, and reimbursement and regulatory systems that still emphasize care sites rather than levels of care. Acceptance is also inhibited by inadequate public understanding of the limits of modern medicine, the realities and risks of hospital-based or high-technology care, the value of low-technology care in managing the consequences of illness and disability, and the scope of the capabilities of non-hospital-based providers.

Previously, hospital-based care has been considered to represent the pinnacle of modern medicine, with other care sites less valued. In the future care system, all those who help identify and manage both the causes and consequences of illness and disability must be considered valuable.

Physician attitudes have also inhibited development of subacute care. Many physicians have not practiced at inpatient sites other than hospitals. Some have equated subacute care with nursing home care and consider both the care and the care site inferior. Until very recently, physician reimbursement allowed un-limited daily visits in hospitals but had limited the frequency and value of vis-its at other sites.

Evolution of Levels of Care

Subacute care currently has two primary payment mechanisms: (1) government (Medicare and Medicaid) reimbursement and (2) managed care and private in-surers. The rules and incentives of these two sources are not yet synchronized, thus making it harder to establish consistent service categories and to modern-ize site definitions.

Traditional payer-established rules have shaped the care system and still in-fluence the evolution of new forms of care. Medicare's advent accelerated the evolution of skilled nursing facilities and specialty (long-term, psychiatric, can-cer, and rehabilitation) hospitals. However, qualifying for Medicare skilled ben-efits has required an initial 3-day hospitalization and the need for one or more skilled nursing services such as suctioning or injections. Facilities qualifying as long-stay or rehabilitation hospitals must maintain an average 25-day length of stay (LOS), which discourages transferring them to less expensive care sites.

Because subacute care combines health care and personal care services, the payment system must recognize the multiple services and practitioners in-volved in the care. Simultaneously it must avoid overstimulating supply or de-mand and thereby ultimately increasing costs too much.

THE OPPORTUNITIES AND CHALLENGES FOR SUBACUTE CARE IN A CHANGING ENVIRONMENT

Ultimately, health care systems should provide optimal, cost-effective service for the shortest amount of time to achieve defined care objectives. The existence of a subacute care option should help achieve that goal.

Current Delivery and Reimbursement of Subacute Care

Subacute care is being provided in various settings, including hospital-based units, freestanding skilled nursing facilities (SNFs), and long-term and specialty hospitals. Some sites specialize in one or more services. Some provide predom-inantly rehabilitation services, predominantly medical services, or a combina-tion. Chapter 5 discusses the diverse services offered in subacute programs.

Current Situation in Various States.   In 1996, efforts continued at the fed-eral and many state levels to redefine the care continuum and revamp payment systems to reflect the changing realities of service provision and the need for flex-ibility and cost containment. Most states had at least begun to consider regula-tory and payment issues relevant to nonacute care. Several states had established subacute reimbursement categories, and others were negotiating facility-specific rates. Some state Medicaid programs were looking closely at subacute care as part of their move toward a managed care orientation. In California, MediCal (the state Medicaid program) offered all-inclusive per-diem subacute rates for (1) hospital-based ventilator-dependent care, (2) hospital-based non-ventilator-dependent care, (3) freestanding ventilator-dependent care, and (4) freestanding non-ventilator-dependent care. In Virginia, Medicaid rates for adult or pediatric specialized care populations were all-inclusive except for physician and pharmacy costs. Minimum requirements included physician services at least weekly, 24-hour licensed nursing, a multidisciplinary team approach, and patient-specific medical and rehabilitative care. In New Jersey, the Medicaid program negotiated facility-specific rates for subacute care, including categories for ventilator, brain injury, AIDS, young adult, and pediatric care. Illinois started a subacute care hospital demonstration project in 1994, under which these units could be licensed as either a SNF or a hospital, and subacute care hospitals would be granted certificates of need. Maryland established special rates for ventilator care to be provided in nursing facilities. Other states, such as Pennsylvania, had established subacute study groups. Given the current health care environment, some of these programs may have already changed or will change soon.

Future Prospects for Subacute Care

Reactions to the expansion of subacute care have varied widely. They range from fully embracing the concept to skepticism that it is just a marketing tool of providers looking to replace lost revenues as the health care reimbursement system changes.

Another controversial area is what to call this kind of care. Alternative names for subacute units include transitional care, skilled medical/rehabilitation units, skilled nursing units, medical specialty units, subacute rehabilitation units, complex care units, intensive therapeutic care units, and step-down units. Hospital-based units appear to more often designate themselves as providing "transitional care," while freestanding facilities call themselves "subacute." Some providers feel that "transitional care" conveys more of a sense of care that is short-term and distinct from long-term care, while "subacute" conveys a sense of lower quality than acute care (BSCCR's Data Bank, 1995). Some insurance companies, regulatory agencies, and others recognize or will reimburse "transitional" care, but disdain the "subacute" care label. Still others spurn both labels and prefer to call the care "postacute."

As this book discusses, there is a population of patients with a combination of problems and service needs that falls into this category. Only some of these individuals receive postacute care, while others receive care for complex conditions not requiring initial hospitalization. Therefore, this category of care is legitimate, although the name may vary or change with time. This book will mostly use the term "subacute" to refer to the care as defined in Chapter 2, and will occasionally use the term "transitional" as a synonym. It will consider "postacute" care to be care that may sometimes be given in a formal subacute program and sometimes given in alternative settings.

Subacute care (or whatever else it may be called) is likely to survive, for several other clinical and business reasons. Compared to hospital care, it is slower paced and offers practitioners the opportunity to combine the best of technical proficiency and personal service. Practitioners have more time to manage all the aspects of complex care, including the psychosocial and ethical implications of illness.

Economics of Subacute Care.   Subacute revenues exceeded $1 billion in 1993 and are predicted to reach $5 to $10 billion annually by the year 2000, with annual growth estimates of as much as 50%. An estimated 1 to 5% of 30 million acute care patients do not go home after hospitalization, suggesting that about 3% could benefit from some form of subacute care (Thompson's Subacute Care Report, 1995). However, because the health care system is still developing many different alternative service packages, these estimates may change.

In many states, hospitals are still having trouble placing patients with postacute needs, suggesting that more subacute sites are needed. Many hospitals and some nursing facilities are just starting to develop subacute programs, and others are still sizing up the situation. Many physicians still hesitate to follow their patients into subacute settings, reimbursement is still inconsistent, and regulations and standards vary widely.

Subacute care will continue to evolve as an important part of a continuum of health care services and the managed care environment. Its further progress will be influenced by changes in regulations, reimbursement, and practitioner attitudes.

REFERENCES

BSCCR's Data Bank. Perception of subacute care. *Briefings Subacute Care Regs Reimburs*. August 1995:6–7.

Thompson's Subacute Care Rep. 1995; 1(3):1.

FOR FURTHER READING

Barnett AA. Subacute care: Passing fad or future of the nursing home industry? *Trends Health Business*. October 22, 1993:1–4.

Burk S. Subacute care. Defining the challenge. *Provider*. 1994; 20(2):37–38.

Burns J. Sorting out subacute care. Subspecialty's surge has Feds, States seeking proof of the product's promises. *Mod Healthcare*. April 25, 1994:28–30, 32.

Burns J. Subacute care feeds need to diversify. *Mod Healthcare*. December 13, 1993:34–36, 38.

Center for Health Services Research. *A Policy Study of the Cost-Effectiveness of Institutional Subacute Care Alternatives and Services: Project Summary*. Denver: Center for Health Services Research; 1994.

Coburn AF, Fortinsky RH, McGuire CA. The impact of Medicaid reimbursement policy on subacute care in hospitals. *Med Care*. January 1989: 25–33.

Deangelis PL. Hospital-based SNFs: An alternative to empty beds. *Healthcare Finan Manage*. August 1987: 60–68.

Falcone D, Bolda E, Leak SC. Waiting for placement: An exploratory analysis of determinants of delayed discharges of elderly hospital patients. *Health Sci Res*. 1991; 26:339–374.

Fowler FJ. Subacute care offers flexibility, revenue. *Mod Healthcare*. October 26, 1992: 50.

Fries BE, Schneider DP, Foley WJ, et al. Refining a case-mix measure for nursing homes: Resource utilization groups (RUGs-III). *Med Care*. 1994:668–685.

Gonzales C. Subacute care: Preparing for a new market. *Provider*. April 1994: 55–56.

Grim SA. Subacute care in urban hospitals: A case for urban swingbeds. *Henry Ford Hosp Med J.* 1990; 38(2&3):133–136.

Hartwell R. Subacute care: The LTC link. *Provider.* 1994; 20:21–22.

Hyatt L. *Subacute Care: Redefining Healthcare.* New York: Irwin; 1995.

Johnson DE. Integrated subacute care: 20% of your patient days. *Health Care Strategic Manage.* 1993; 11:2–3.

Joubert DW. Conversion from acute to subacute care beds. *Am J Health Syst Pharm.* 1995; 52(10):1042, 1048.

Kane RL, Kane RA. Long-term care. *JAMA.* 1995; 273(21):1690–1691.

Kelly M. Higher intensity specialization. Reach new heights through subacute care. *Contemp Long-Term Care.* November 1992:38–40.

Levenson SA. Subacute care: Why nursing home practitioners should take notice. *Nurs Home Med.* 1994; 2:23–34.

Lewin VHI. *Subacute Care: Review of the Literature.* Study prepared for the Office of the Assistant Secretary for Evaluation and Planning, Department of Health and Human Services, Washington, DC, December 1994.

Lumsdon K. Subacute care. Like ants to a picnic. *Hosp Health Netw.* 1995; 69(10):47.

Lutz S. Long-term hospitals do well, but face challenges. *Mod Healthcare.* March 28, 1994:43–44.

McDowell TN Jr. The subacute care patient: Hospital responses to the challenge. *J Health Hosp Law.* 1990; 23:289–294.

Micheletti JA, Shlala TJ. Understanding and operationalizing subacute services. *Nurs Manage.* 1995; 26(6):49,51–52,54–56.

Morrisey MA, Sloan FA, Valvona J. Medicare prospective payment and posthospital transfers to subacute care. *Med Care.* 1988; 7:685–698.

Morrow-Howell N, Proctor, E. Discharge destinations of Medicare patients receiving discharge planning: Who goes where? *Med Care.* 1994; 32: 486–497.

Stahl DA. Subacute care: The future of health care. *Nurs Manage.* 1994; 25(10):34,36,38–40.

Stateside: Illinois institutes a subacute demo project. *Briefings Subacute Care.* 1994; 1(4):3,5.

Subacute provider profile. *Contemp Long-Term Care.* October 1993: 35–38.

Taylor KS. Clamor over subacute care creates adversaries/new partners. *Hosp Health Netw.* 1994; 68(6):102.

Taylor KS. Poised for growth, subacute care gains a clearer identity. *Hosp Health Netw.* July 20, 1993:58.

Wilhelm ME, Wilhelm MA. Hospital development in a subacute care setting. *Hosp Progress.* 1984; 65(2):42–45,74.

TABLE 1–1	BASIC STEPS FOR PARTICIPANTS IN ALL HEALTH CARE PROGRAMS IN A CHANGING CLIMATE

- Identify the challenges and opportunities
- Appreciate common goals and objectives
- Recognize the need for change
- Identify obstacles to change and improvement
- Appreciate the common objectives
- Identify elements for optimal performance and service
- Implement ways to meet the challenges and make the most of opportunities

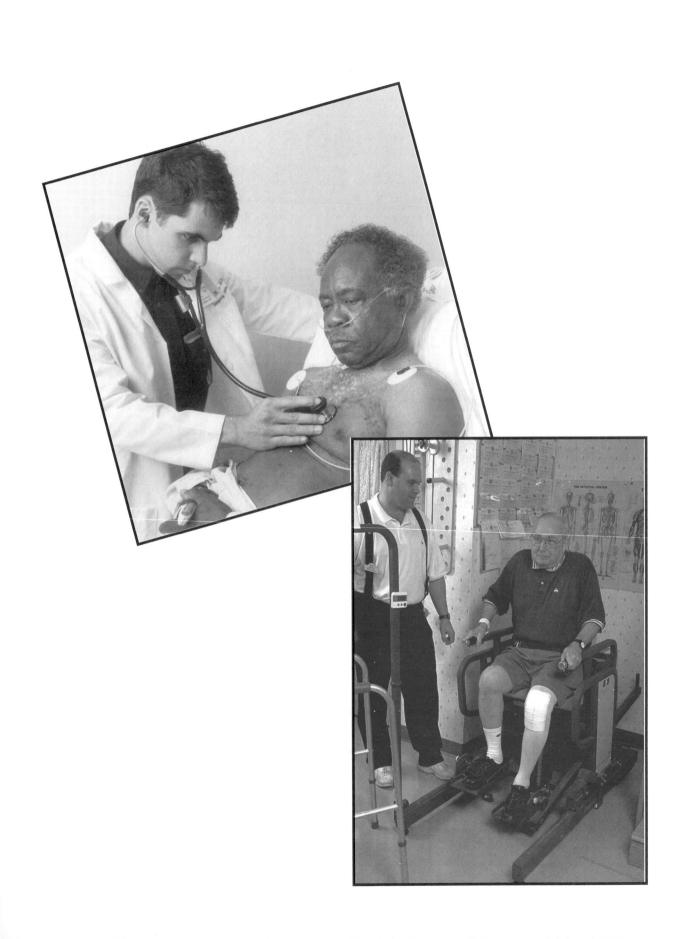

DEFINING THE SUBACUTE PATIENT POPULATION

*I*ndividuals with more than minor illness or injury often need some help to recover and to regain adequate personal comfort and social functioning. It is most helpful to look at the consequences rather than the causes of their condition in trying to clarify essential levels and sites of support and care.

Acute hospital care focuses mainly on identifying and initiating management of the causes of acute illness and injury. Other forms of care, including subacute care, must focus on refining the management of those causes and addressing the consequences. Subacute patients are usually in a different phase of their illness, or have a condition of different acuity, than those who need high-acuity care. Appropriate patients for subacute care share certain characteristics related to the intensity, complexity, scope, and frequency of the services they need.

Certain processes are associated with the care of those with acute illness and injury. Subacute care represents a packaging of these processes within a single program to try to provide more cost-effective care for individuals with conditions of moderate or low acuity.

The purpose of this chapter is to differentiate the management of causes and consequences of illness and injury, to define subacute care, to compare the characteristics of subacute patients to those requiring other levels of service in the care continuum, and to relate such information to the appropriate placement and management of these patients.

Defining Health-Related Service Needs

Many questions have been asked about subacute care. For example, is it a place, a program, or a level of care? How is it similar to, or different from, other kinds of care? What does it do that other programs or sites do not or cannot do? Answering such questions requires a step-wise approach (Table 2–1, p. 26).

The Many Facets of Acute Illness and Injury

All subacute care involves the management of some phase of an acute illness or injury. An acute illness is the rapid or sudden onset of a definable alteration in bodily structure or function that significantly disrupts personal comfort or psychosocial functioning. An injury is a significant disruption of bodily structure or function as a result of some external physical contact (for example, a fall, auto accident, or medical treatment) or the introduction of an external substance (such as medication, radiation, or poison) into the body. A subclinical illness (an asymptomatic infection, for example) exists without causing noticeable symptoms. A chronic illness occurs gradually over time and is irreversible, progressive, or both.

Many acute illnesses (upper respiratory infections or diarrhea, for example) or injuries (sprains, contusions, or the like) are self-limited and uncomplicated. Their management requires little or no professional care. Other acute illnesses or injuries cause so much disruption that the individual needs help to recover.

Additionally, a medical illness may cause other problems. Those other problems may resolve fully when the acute problem has been treated (respiratory distress may resolve when pneumonia is successfully treated). Or the acute problem may improve, but leave functional deficits (a stroke patient may have a residual speech deficit and left-sided weakness). The acute problem may improve but other problems may remain (despite curing an infection, an AIDS patient will continue to suffer other complications). Or the illness may improve but aggravate other coexisting conditions (an episode of acute congestive heart failure improves, but leaves the individual weaker and more confused). The acute condition may also improve partially but still need prolonged treatment to produce full resolution (endocarditis or osteomyelitis patients need lengthy antibiotic therapy; ventilatory failure may be stabilized quickly but the patient may need months of care before being able to breathe without ventilatory assistance).

Thus, the overall prognosis after initial treatment of an acute problem may be for full or partial improvement, stabilization (prevention of further decline), continued decline, or death. Compared to the initial condition, the residual problems may be more, less, or equally complex. Those problems may be medically related or may involve other dimensions (psychological, functional, or social) of a person's existence.

Identifying the Subacute Patient Population

Table 2–2, p. 26, lists options for classifying populations receiving health-related services, and gives examples of how each option has been used at times to organize health service delivery. The following considers how to best try to define subacute care and identify the population it serves.

Personal Characteristics.   Subacute patients span the age spectrum and may be of either sex. Many subacute providers find it convenient to divide their patients into pediatric, general adult, and geriatric categories. Each age group may have some unique needs, such as developmental deficits and educational needs in a pediatric population. However, many problems, needs, and risks are common to all age groups. Thus, personal characteristics are not the primary element to define the subacute population.

Diagnoses and Problems.   Hospital care focuses on identifying and initiating management of the causes of patient signs and symptoms. In those with an isolated acute illness or injury, treating the immediate cause often corrects their problems. But in many others, the problems persist despite trying to treat the underlying causes. This may be because of the severity of the acute illness or injury, because of the need for more prolonged treatment, or because of the effects of untreatable conditions, such as chronic illness or developmental disturbances. After the initial stages of management of illness and injury, the focus often must shift to managing the consequences, that is, the problems that result from, or are exacerbated by, the acute condition.

For example, an otherwise healthy skier may need surgery in a hospital to repair a leg fractured while skiing. Other than some outpatient rehabilitation, this individual does not need other postoperative care. But a frail older woman who falls and fractures a hip may have many other chronic conditions such as arteriosclerotic heart disease, dementia, diabetes, or hypertension, and many possible problems such as confusion, deficits in activities of daily living (ADL) performance, incontinence, or dizziness. For this individual, like others with chronic illnesses or disabilities, the acute condition influences the course and management of the chronic conditions and vice versa.

Subacute patients may have any diagnosis. They cannot be classified primarily by their diagnoses or problems because—even in otherwise healthy individuals—the same diagnosis may result in a range of possible functional deficits and service needs. For example, the condition of a patient with diagnoses of coronary atherosclerosis and a recent myocardial infarction could range from highly unstable or terminal because of severe heart failure to completely stable because of limited damage. Furthermore, subacute patient needs are rarely based on just one specific diagnosis, and their care needs are often significantly influenced by preexisting chronic conditions (for example, AIDS, alcoholism, or cancer), functional limitations, and behavioral and cognitive deficits. The cases in Chapter 11 illustrate some of these distinctions.

Some attempts have been made to indicate that those with certain diagnosis-related groups (DRGs) could receive treatment in subacute settings. However, this may not be true of all those with the same diagnosis or DRG because individuals with the same acute condition may have a markedly different overall medical stability and impact of their associated medical conditions (comorbidities).

Treatment Needs.   Subacute patients are often classified by their treatment needs, such as rehabilitation therapies or ventilator dependency. Although this approach may be convenient for organizing service delivery, it is not a primary determinant of patient need for this level of care. By itself, the need for treatments does not necessarily reflect the need for an overall package of services, including monitoring of stability and complications and adjustment of treatment regimens. Also, the same treatment may be rendered in various settings.

For instance, ventilator care may be given in hospitals, subacute units, nursing facilities, or as part of home care. On the other hand, complicated neurosurgery is feasible only in a hospital. However, some of the postsurgical nursing and rehabilitative care of neurosurgical and other patients, formerly only given in rehabilitation hospitals or hospital-based rehabilitation units, can be rendered elsewhere.

Service Sites.   Health care in the United States has traditionally been delivered at specific, identifiable care sites, defined primarily by reimbursement and reinforced by specific licensure and regulatory mechanisms. But these traditional classifications no longer apply. As noted, the entire health care delivery system is changing, familiar kinds of care are being delivered at various sites, and familiar sites are altering their scope of services. For example, tuberculosis patients are no longer put in separate hospitals. Many older patients with long-standing psychiatric problems have been shifted from psychiatric institutions into nursing facilities. Skilled nursing facilities (SNFs) and nursing facilities (NFs) provide many medical services to those with acute illnesses and injuries. About 10% of U.S. nursing facility residents are younger adults with chronic impairments. Rehabilitation services are now being given across the spectrum of care sites.

Additionally, where individuals receive initial assessment or treatment may not be where they need to be for ongoing care. A site or practitioner rendering the initial care may be able to do some, all, or none of the subsequent assessment and management. Alternatives for getting the necessary service may cost more or less and may also be more, less, or equally convenient and desirable for a patient or a practitioner.

For instance, many individuals are sent to a hospital to identify the causes of their acute condition changes, but only some of them need to be hospitalized to treat those causes or to manage their consequences. Table 2–3, p. 27, lists reasons why people may become hospitalized. Only a few of those reasons relate to legitimate clinical need while the rest result from systems problems. The processes and criteria for making such decisions have traditionally been very inconsistent and primarily practitioner-dependent. Any of several factors—convenience, comfort, cost, availability, and quality—may have been considered most important.

For instance, patients with acute onset of symptoms have often been assessed in the emergency room of a hospital where their personal physician has had admitting privileges. In the past, they were typically admitted if the hospital had a bed and it was convenient for their physician. But the same individual residing in a NF might be transferred to the hospital emergency room for evaluation and then subsequently returned to the nursing facility or admitted to the hospital for treatment, depending on available reimbursement for the care and the capabilities of the nursing staff in the NF.

Level of Care.   Another possibility for classifying subacute patients is by their level of care, based on needed services.

A collection of activities is associated with the care of people who become ill or dysfunctional (Table 2–4, p. 27). These processes involve determining the nature and causes of a patient's problems and possible courses to manage them, ascertaining the severity of the conditions, managing the problems and their causes and complications, monitoring for recurrences or exacerbations of a problem or the onset of new associated or unrelated problems, reviewing the efficacy and possible undesirable effects of the treatment, and deciding about the treatment course, duration, and site for continuation of the care. Assessing and managing the immediate effects of an illness or injury must be followed by assessing and managing the broader consequences.

Each of these steps involves various degrees of complexity, judgment, and skill. The frequency of the monitoring, assessment, and treatment may be continuous or intermittent. The services may need to be immediately available or simply accessible as needed.

Some patients need primarily individual services (for example, ventilator care or intravenous therapies via home care), and others require a package of services delivered by appropriate practitioners in a properly supportive setting. A systematic approach is needed to effectively match services to needs.

Defining Levels of Care. Of all the above options, the most systematic approach to classifying levels of service need appears to be based on identifying the consequences of illness and injury. As outlined in Table 2–5, pp. 28–30, each level of care may be defined by a combination of the medical instability (variance, course), needs for monitoring and assessment (frequency, skill level, availability), and treatment (complexity of judgment, availability). Because multiple factors are involved, there will inevitably be some overlap.

High-acuity patients have conditions that often may fluctuate widely and unpredictably. They need continuous or almost continuous monitoring or testing that requires a high degree of technical skill to perform or interpret. Frequent testing is needed to define the underlying diagnoses, or the extent of the consequences of the illness or injury. A high degree of judgment and skill are needed to select and implement appropriate treatments, or the therapeutic interventions carry a high risk of complications. The treatments must be immediately available on site, and could be needed promptly at any time.

Moderate-acuity patients may have one or more parameters (for example, electrolytes or blood gases) outside the normal range, but these do not fluctuate widely or frequently. They may need frequent but not continuous (for example, daily or less often) monitoring or testing. The monitoring and testing require moderate technical skill by the observer, either in performing the assessment or in interpreting the findings. Their major diagnoses are known or can be readily established. Managing their conditions may require the ready availability of specially trained personnel or special equipment or supplies for monitoring, evaluation, or treatment. Moderately complex judgment and skill are involved in selecting and implementing appropriate treatments, and any therapeutic interventions carry no more than a moderate risk of complications.

Low-acuity patients typically are stable or are infrequently unstable. Variance from normal is minimal or not immediately life-threatening. They need monitoring daily or less often. Monitoring requires moderate or minimal technical skill by the observer, both to perform the assessment and to interpret the findings. Any special monitoring or diagnostic equipment or personnel can be accessible routinely. Their major diagnoses are known or readily established, and complications are predictable or do not require a complex workup to establish. Moderate or minimally complex judgment and skill are involved in selecting and implementing appropriate treatment for their conditions and any therapeutic interventions carry a low or moderate risk of complications.

The care needs for different individuals with the same diagnosis, or receiving the same treatment, may differ markedly. For example, one ventilator patient may need substantial ADL support but not much medical or nursing care. Another ventilator patient may need little ADL support or nursing care. A third ventilator patient may need a lot of nursing assessment because of a new complication of uncertain cause. A fourth ventilator patient may be comatose and get frequent infections, and so need substantial ADL support and frequent nursing interventions, but may not require much medical workup because the source of the instability is known. Similarly, either an AIDS patient or a head injury patient may need (1) high-acuity care if vital signs are very unstable and there is continuous respiratory distress, (2) moderate or low-acuity care if the vital signs fluctuate only occasionally or there is occasional limited mild or moderate respiratory difficulty, or (3) only some extra nursing monitoring several times daily for several days if breathing and vital signs are stable.

Descriptions of Those of Various Acuity Levels.   Table 2–6, p. 30, summarizes and compares the characteristics of moderate and low-acuity patients, such as those in subacute programs, and those of the high-acuity patients typically found on acute care units. Ultimately, subacute patients (that is, those who may be properly cared for by subacute care programs) may therefore be considered to be those with conditions of moderate and low acuity. Even though subacute care does not introduce any new care components, it represents a different approach to providing care to those who require a specific package of medical, nursing, and related services. Although hospitals are still appropriate for treating high-acuity patients, other care sites can often meet the needs of individuals whose conditions are of moderate or low acuity.

OTHER LEVELS OF SERVICE NEEDS

Classification of Those With Predominantly Chronic Illnesses and Disabilities

Individuals with predominantly health-related needs often have other psychosocial and functional disturbances and personal care needs. For example, a stroke patient may be hospitalized initially while the diagnosis is made and vital signs are being stabilized, transferred to a subacute program for rehabilitation therapies, and then discharged to home, an assisted living facility, or a nursing facility depending on the individual's residual functional and cognitive deficits.

Those with chronic illnesses and disabilities also often have complex health-related problems and may have intermittent acute illnesses. But for these individuals, the problems caused by their chronic illnesses and disabilities predominate. Although medical care for acute illness may be given intermittently, it is not the primary focus of ongoing support and care. However, one or more chronic illnesses may need to be managed, monitored, or treated regularly.

Table 2–7, pp. 31–32, details the characteristics and service needs of those with various levels of chronic illness and disability. These needs may best be categorized according to

- Functional impairment (severity)
- Assessment and monitoring (frequency, skill level, availability)
- Treatment (complexity, availability)

Table 2–8, p. 33, summarizes the service needs of those with high, moderate, and low levels of chronic illness and disability, who have the following characteristics.

High chronic illness/disability individuals typically have significant residual functional, cognitive, or behavioral impairments as a consequence of some combination of major acute illness, chronic conditions, and developmental disabilities. They require regular daily assistance or supervision with most or all of their ADLs by trained individuals, and have health-related conditions that require trained health care practitioners (primarily nurses or physicians) to regularly assess them and initiate or adjust proper treatment. Their chronic conditions fluctuate sufficiently that they require frequent minor or occasional substantial changes in their plans of care, developed by a trained health care practitioner. They typically need substantial supervision or support to deal with acute illnesses. At least some of their medications and treatments are sufficiently complex or risky that they should be selected, rendered, and monitored by those with substantial skill in managing chronic illness and its complications.

Moderate chronic illness/disability individuals typically have moderate functional, cognitive, or behavioral impairments as a consequence of some combination of major acute illness, chronic conditions, and developmental disabilities. Although they may require some regular supervision or assistance with several ADLs or more substantial assistance with one activity almost daily, their chronic health-related conditions are usually stable. They require no more than intermittent monitoring of their chronic conditions, and occasional substantial changes in their plans of care, by a trained health care practitioner. They need only occasional supervision and support when they suffer acute illnesses. Only some of their medications and treatments are sufficiently complex or risky to require being rendered or monitored by those with substantial skill in managing chronic illness and its complications.

Low chronic illness/disability individuals typically have only minor residual functional, cognitive, or behavioral impairments as a result of either an acute illness or the complications of chronic conditions. They require minimal assistance either routinely with one or occasionally with several ADLs. Their chronic conditions are sufficiently stable that they require only occasional access to, rather than the routine availability of, trained individuals to monitor them or change their treatments and plans of care. Their care, supervision, and treatments can mostly be given by those with no special training in managing chronic or complex illness, and who themselves have little or no role in selecting or modifying those treatments.

Definition of Subacute Care

The past several years have seen many efforts to define subacute care (Continuum of care, 1995; Subacute care, 1994). These attempts have been hampered partially because the care spans a broad spectrum of programs and services, differs among various care sites using the same name, and involves care that incorporates the principles and methods of both acute and long-term care. The efforts have also been affected by the difficulties in recognizing the relevant common characteristics of the patients.

However, this variability in subacute care is in many ways similar to other levels of care. For instance, all hospitals may give acute care but they do not all offer the same programs and services or the same scope of similar services. Although they all have doctors and nurses, the number and specialties of medical staff and the roles and training of nurses vary within the same facility and among different hospitals.

In fact, efforts to define subacute care have also been inhibited somewhat by inadequate definitions of acute care—often defined as care given in hospitals. This is outmoded because of the changes in delivery of acute care and the uncoupling of service delivery from discrete care sites.

In many ways, subacute care used to be part of the care spectrum provided in hospitals but is now a discrete program, not necessarily requiring a hospital stay. Therefore, the definition of subacute care is influenced partially by the changing role of the hospital. Subacute care is not a new kind of care. Instead, it represents a different approach to delivering the multiple components of complex care to those with active medical illness or injury of no more than moderate acuity. It may best be defined by looking at several aspects: when it is given, why it is given, who renders it, and its frequency, intensity, and duration. Subacute care

- Is rendered immediately after, or instead of, acute hospitalization (**when given**)
- Treats one or more active, complex, or unstable medical conditions, or administers technically complex treatments in the context of the patient's general condition and overall care goals (**reason**)
- Requires the coordinated services of physicians, nurses, and other professionals who are trained and knowledgeable to assess and manage these conditions and perform the necessary procedures (**by whom**)
- Is given as part of a specifically defined program regardless of the site (**site**)
- Requires frequent (daily to weekly) recurrent patient assessment and review of the clinical course and treatment plan (**frequency**)
- Is at a level of service intensity somewhere between care of those with high chronic illness or disability and the care of those with high-acuity conditions (**intensity**)
- Is for a limited (several days to several months) time, or until a condition is stabilized or a predetermined treatment course is completed (**duration**)

Other Distinguishing Characteristics

As is true with many definitions of complex subjects, even this lengthy definition cannot fully clarify the care. Therefore, it is useful to explain further what subacute care is and is not.

Amount and Intensity of Care.   Generally, subacute patients require somewhere between 4 and 8 hours a day of nursing care. Another approach to defining this level of care is to consider the subacute patient to be one needing at least 5 hours of nursing care a day and a physician visit at least every 3 to 7 days, in contrast to the skilled nursing facility patient who needs 3 to 5 hours of nursing care a day and a physician visit every 7 to 30 days. However, there is overlap at the lower end between those patients and the traditional skilled Medicare patients, and at the higher end between the subacute patient and those in acute or specialty hospitals. Therefore, as the spectrum of subacute patients becomes clearer, it may be more appropriate to categorize subacute patients primarily by the scope, intensity, and complexity of their service needs rather than by the amount of care.

Practitioner Roles.   Understanding the practitioner roles in the subacute setting also helps distinguish the level of care. The need for practitioners, including physicians, to effectively manage both the acute problems and the chronic conditions and disabilities helps distinguish those situations that may be described as subacute care. Higher-acuity care emphasizes management of the causes of the acute condition, and longer-term care of chronically ill and disabled individuals emphasizes management of functional limitations caused by illness or injury with relatively little fluctuation in the management of the underlying disease processes.

Service Limitations.   To some extent, subacute care can also be distinguished by what it does *not* do. Subacute programs typically omit, as an integral part of the service, most or all of the following services: obstetrics, nuclear medicine, general surgery under anesthesia, intensive care units, coronary care units, emergency rooms, in-house laboratories, and invasive or high-technology radiology (such as arterial contrast studies or MRI scanners). However, some subacute programs may perform some of the functions associated with these various services; for example, subacute units monitoring high-risk pregnancies or providing a limited number of surgical procedures requiring general anesthesia. Subacute programs may provide limited or full cardiopulmonary resuscitation (CPR), may or may not have an in-house pharmacy, and usually transfer someone elsewhere for emergency or high-acuity care (for example, a fall with hip fracture or vigorous gastrointestinal bleeding with unstable vital signs). Subacute programs provide access to such services either elsewhere in the same facility or by referral to another setting.

The future continuum of care spans the spectrum from episodic services provided at home or in an ambulatory setting through high-acuity care provided in a high-technology setting (Figure 2–1). However, the most efficient use of these settings still awaits the proper alignment of levels of care designations, care sites, resource and staffing allocations, reimbursement methodologies, and licensure and accreditation categories. Chapter 3 discusses the implications of the factors outlined in this chapter for the selection and placement of subacute patients, and for the place of subacute care in the care continuum.

FIGURE 2–1 THE CONTINUUM OF SERVICE NEEDS AND CARE CATEGORIES

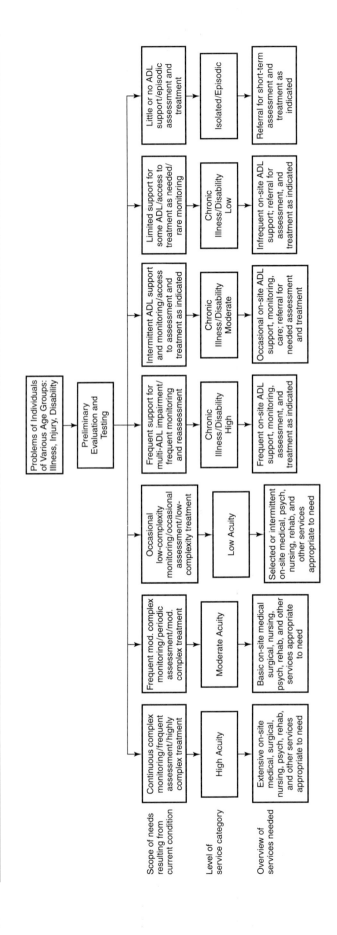

REFERENCES

Continuum of care . . . definition for subacute care [news]. *Hosp Health Netw.* 1995; 69(1):14.

Subacute care: the devil's in the definition [news]. *Hosp Health Netw.* 1994; 68(17):19.

FOR FURTHER READING

Joint Commission on Accreditation of Healthcare Organizations. *Survey Protocol for Subacute Programs.* Chicago: JCAHO; 1995.

Price MA. Case mix classification and health care of the elderly. *Med J Aust.* 1994; 161(suppl):S23–S26.

Walsh GG. How subacute care fills the gap. *Nursing.* 1995; 25(3):51.

Walsh GG. Myths & facts . . . about subacute care units. *Nursing.* 1994; 24(11):17.

| TABLE 2–1 | ELEMENTS IN DEFINING THE HEALTH-RELATED SERVICE NEEDS OF VARIOUS POPULATIONS |

Demographics
• Designate the population being served.

Problem Definition
• Define the scope of their significant problems and conditions.

Care Needs Assessment
• Categorize individuals based on a level of service need.
   Generic needs: Those common to all such individuals.
   Special needs: Those that might result from special situations or complications.

Service Delivery
• Determine what is required to meet those needs.
   Generic: Common to all categories.
   Care-specific: Those related to specific individuals and situations.
• Decide on required capabilities of those who propose to meet those needs.
   Generic: Common to all categories.
   Care-specific: Those specific to individual categories of needs.
• Determine how services should be delivered to accomplish care objectives.
• Decide how to evaluate the appropriateness of the quality of care.
   Establish quality criteria to assess service provision.
   Determine quality oversight methods and players.
• Decide implications of above for licensure, certification, and accreditation requirements.

Economics of Care
• Consider how services can be delivered most efficiently, consistent with quality expectations.
• Determine which services should be reimbursed, and who should be reimbursed to provide them.
• Decide on any reimbursement guidelines and limits.
• Decide how to evaluate the appropriateness of the charges for care actually provided.
   Establish utilization criteria.
   Determine utilization review methods and players.

| TABLE 2–2 | EXAMPLES OF POSSIBLE WAYS TO CLASSIFY PATIENTS |

Categorization Criterion	Examples of Use of These Categories
Personal characteristics (age, sex, etc.)	Nursing facilities traditionally have taken care of those over age 65
Diagnoses	TB hospitals for those with TB; coronary care units for those with myocardial infarctions
Syndromes	Rehabilitation programs for those with brain injury or spinal cord injury; special institutions for those with mental retardation
Treatment needs (e.g., surgery, rehabilitation therapies)	Dialysis units in hospitals; licensure and reimbursement based on hours of nursing care or hours of rehabilitation care
Service sites	Home care programs, outpatient centers, inpatient rehabilitation units
Care level	Hospitals for high-intensity care; Medicare SNFs for higher-intensity, longer-term nursing care; subacute units for moderate and low acuity care

TABLE 2–3	REASONS WHY INDIVIDUALS MAY BECOME HOSPITALIZED[a]

- **They are highly unstable medically and need a high level and frequency of monitoring.**
- They are not highly unstable and do not need a high level of monitoring, but they do need
  - **–Treatment that is not feasible elsewhere.**
  - –Treatment that is feasible but not available elsewhere.
  - –A diagnostic evaluation
    - **That cannot be readily obtained elsewhere.**
    - That could be obtained elsewhere but the physician, patient, family, or other party choose not to do so.
    - That could be obtained elsewhere but the physician, patient, or family are not aware of its availability.
- They came from home or another care setting to the emergency room or another hospital-based program for an assessment and were admitted.
- There were no other placement options available at the time of admission.
- There were no other placement options available after the admission and the initial evaluation.
- The physician does not practice at any other sites except the office and hospital.
- The insurance would only cover acute hospitalization.

[a]**Boldfaced** items reflect legitimate clinical needs; other items reflect systems issues that influence placement, often independent of need.

TABLE 2–4	PROCESSES INVOLVED IN CARING FOR THOSE WITH ACUTE ILLNESSES OR INJURIES

Assessment and Problem Definition
- Recognize presence of significant medical, psychosocial, and functional symptoms.
- Observe, interview, and examine the individual and review related information.
- Define the problems (nature, severity, scope, intensity, duration) correctly.
- Identify causes of the problems (including medical diagnoses).
- Define the consequences—including functional limitations—of the illness or injury.

Treatment of Primary and Secondary Problems
- Stabilize life-threatening conditions.
- Select appropriate treatments and associated management plan.
- Administer treatments.
- Determine scope and duration of treatment.
- Manage significant coexisting conditions.
- Address functional dependencies.
- Provide necessary support and supervision.

Monitoring
- Assess vital signs.
- Evaluate effects of illness.
- Monitor for exacerbations and complications of illness, treatments, or setting.
- Observe for recurrence of previous illness or onset of another illness.
- Assess effectiveness of treatments and problem management.

Prepare for Subsequent Care
- Define subsequent service needs.
- Arrange postcare placement or services.
- Coordinate continuation of appropriate treatments and support.
- Educate and train patient and family.

TABLE 2–5   RELATIVE PATIENT CHARACTERISTICS AND SERVICE NEEDS FOR THOSE WITH ACUTE ILLNESS OR INJURY

MEDICAL INSTABILITY

VARIANCE FROM NORMAL INTERNAL BALANCE

Level	Definition	Examples
++++	One or more parameters vary widely enough from normal range to be immediately life threatening	• Accident victim with head trauma may have frequent changes in vital signs and level of consciousness at any time soon after the accident • Patient with respiratory failure has severe hypoxia or CO_2 retention • Diabetic patient has blood glucose level over 800 and potassium level of 6.8
+++	Variance from normal range not immediately life threatening but requires prompt intervention	• Peritoneal dialysis patients may get hypotensive or have electrolyte imbalance • Respiratory failure patient on a ventilator has occasional dyspnea that can be managed by ventilator adjustment, or infections that can be managed by antibiotics
++	Variance from normal not likely to have significant short-term consequences and not presently causing symptoms	• Diabetic with blood glucose level consistently in 200 to 300 range
+	No significant variances from normal	

COURSE OF THE INSTABILITY

Level	Definition	Examples
++++	Condition fluctuates frequently	• Newly head injured patient may have constant fluctuations in level of consciousness and vital signs • Acute cardiopulmonary instability requiring ventilatory support and pressor or antiarrhythmic agents
+++	Condition fluctuates more than occasionally	• Cardiac patient has occasional symptoms requiring adjustment of antiarrhythmic or antianginal agents
++	Condition fluctuates occasionally	• COPD patient has an elevated but stable pCO_2 of 48 to 50
+	No clinically significant fluctuations	

MONITORING AND DIAGNOSIS

FREQUENCY

Level	Definition	Examples
++++	Continuous evaluation by observation and/or testing to assess for condition changes or complications	• Patient with a new-onset myocardial infarction needs continuous monitoring to detect significant arrhythmias • A newly head injured patient needs close observation and frequent testing as the condition fluctuates

TABLE 2–5	RELATIVE PATIENT CHARACTERISTICS AND SERVICE NEEDS FOR THOSE WITH ACUTE ILLNESS OR INJURY (CONTINUED)	

+++	Frequent (every 2 to 4 hours) monitoring needed to assess for condition changes or complications	• Dialysis patient with new-onset fever needs monitoring several times a shift to check for evidence of infection or development of septicemia
++	Routine or occasionally more focused monitoring needed at least every shift	• Vital signs and general observation of current condition of someone with potential for greater instability
+	Routine monitoring needed daily or less often	

SKILL LEVEL OF NECESSARY MONITORING

Level	Definition	Examples
+++	Monitoring requires extensive technical skill by the observer, either in performing the assessment or in interpreting the findings	• Swan-Ganz catheterization • Continuous cardiac monitoring of fluctuating cardiac rhythm
++	Monitoring requires moderate technical skill by the observer, either in performing the assessment or in interpreting the findings	• Evaluation of progress of weaning from a ventilator • Monitoring medically complex patient with multiple coexisting medical problems
+	Monitoring requires minimal technical skill by the observer, either in performing the assessment or in interpreting the findings	• Vital signs • Pulse oximetry • Progress of IV infusions • Laboratory chemistries

AVAILABILITY OF MONITORING/DIAGNOSTIC PERSONNEL OR INSTRUMENTS (EQUIPMENT, LAB, RADIOLOGY)

Level	Definition	Examples
+++	Immediate availability needed	• Cardiac monitoring for a new myocardial infarction patient with frequent arrhythmias
++	Urgent but not immediate availability needed (within 2 to 4 hours)	• STAT laboratory • Physician to assess a non-life-threatening complication in a postoperative patient
+	Timely access but not urgent availability (within 24 hours) needed	• Specialty consultation for non-emergency problems • Non-emergency ultrasound or CT scanning • Routine blood gases to check progress of a ventilator patient

TREATMENTS

COMPLEXITY OF JUDGMENT/SKILLS AND RISK INVOLVED IN TREATMENTS

Level	Definition	Examples
+++	High degree of complexity of decision making involved in selecting and implementing appropriate treatment; or high risk of complications of therapeutic intervention	• Initial management of trauma patient • Neurosurgical or cardiac surgical procedure

(continued)

TABLE 2–5   RELATIVE PATIENT CHARACTERISTICS AND SERVICE NEEDS FOR THOSE WITH ACUTE ILLNESS OR INJURY (CONTINUED)

++	Moderate degree of complexity of decision making involved in selecting and implementing appropriate treatment; or moderate risk of complications of therapeutic intervention	• New-onset fever in a ventilator patient • Electrolyte imbalance in a dialysis patient • Change in mental status in a demented patient • Cataract surgery
+	Minimal complexity of decision making involved in selecting and implementing appropriate treatment; or low risk of complications of therapeutic intervention	• Dressing changes • Parenteral therapies

AVAILABILITY OF TREATMENT

Level	Definition	Examples
++++	Treatment may be needed at any time and must be available immediately	• Myocardial infarction patient with a dangerous arrhythmia needs it recognized and action taken right away • Basic cardiopulmonary resuscitation
+++	Treatment should be available within 2 to 4 hours	• Intravenous antibiotics for a patient with a serious infection
++	Access to treatment should be possible within 24 hours	• Surgical placement of suprapubic catheter to relieve urinary obstruction
+	Treatment should be accessible on a routine basis	• Chemotherapy • Radiotherapy

TABLE 2–6   SUMMARY OF ACUITY CATEGORIES, BASED ON KEY CHARACTERISTICS AND SERVICE NEEDS

	Level of Care		
Criteria	High Acuity	Moderate Acuity	Low Acuity
Medical instability			
Variance	++++	+++	++/+
Course	++++	+++	++/+
Monitoring			
Frequency	++++	+++/++	++/+
Skill level	+++	++	+
Availability	+++	++/+	+
Treatment			
Complexity of judgment/risk	+++	++/+	+
Availability	++++	+++/++	+

TABLE 2–7   RELATIVE PATIENT CHARACTERISTICS AND SERVICE NEEDS FOR THOSE WITH CHRONIC ILLNESSES AND DISABILITIES

FUNCTIONAL IMPAIRMENTS

SEVERITY OF IMPAIRMENT

Level	Definition	Examples
++++	Totally impaired	• Must always be fed • Total dependency after traumatic brain injury • Comatose, bedbound, unable to perform any ADLs
+++	Moderately impaired	• Needs some assistance with dressing • Requires wheelchair for mobility
++	Mildly impaired	• Needs setup assistance with bathing or eating, and then can perform function
+	Minimal or no significant impairment	

ASSESSMENT AND MONITORING

FREQUENCY

Level	Definition	Examples
++++	Needs continuous direct or indirect assessment and monitoring of condition or change in condition	• COPD patient frequently has dyspnea requiring nursing evaluation for severity • Frequent faller needs to be checked after falls and intermittently for possible causes • Monitoring or supervision of behavior requiring prompt, specifically defined interventions
+++	Needs intermittent assessment and monitoring of status by trained individuals	• Monthly review needed of status of multiple chronic conditions and current medication regimen • Regular periodic review for general behavioral changes in demented individual
++	Needs intermittent access but not continuous assessment and monitoring	• Need for occasional assessment of stable chronic conditions or dementia
+	No need for significant monitoring	

SKILL LEVEL OF MONITORING/SUPERVISION

Level	Definition	Examples
+++	Monitoring or supervision requires substantial special training and skill by the observer, either in performing the assessment or in interpreting the findings	• Evaluation of fluctuating mental status, falling, incontinence to sort out multiple potential causes including medications • Monitoring and supervision of highly risky or threatening behavior

(continued)

TABLE 2–7   RELATIVE PATIENT CHARACTERISTICS AND SERVICE NEEDS FOR THOSE WITH CHRONIC ILLNESSES AND DISABILITIES (CONTINUED)

| ++ | Monitoring requires moderate technical skill by the observer, either in performing the assessment or in interpreting the findings | • Monitoring of response to medications (check pulse, blood pressure)
• Monitoring and supervision of unstable or problematic behavior of low or moderate risk or causing no imminent danger |
| + | Monitoring requires little or no special technical skill by the observer, either in performing the assessment or in interpreting the findings | • Occasional supervision or observation of behaviors
• Prevention of unsafe wandering |

TREATMENTS

COMPLEXITY OF JUDGMENT/SKILLS INVOLVED IN TREATMENTS/CARE

Level	Definition	Examples
+++	Moderate degree of complexity of judgment and skill involved in selecting and implementing appropriate treatment	• Oxygen administration • Suctioning • Relatively uncomplicated wound care and dressing changes • Inhaler treatment • Medication injections • Management of risky or threatening behavior
++	Minimal degree of complexity of judgment and skill involved in selecting and implementing appropriate care	• Range of motion exercises • Dispensing medications • ADL support greater than setup • Management of abnormal but not threatening behavior
+	No special skill or training involved in selecting and implementing appropriate care	• Setup or minimal assist with ADLs

AVAILABILITY OF TREATMENT/CARE

Level	Definition	Examples
++++	Availability of care needed on site	• Daily medication dispensing • Suctioning or inhaler treatment for COPD patient with chronic bronchitis
+++	Access to regular treatment at least weekly	• Dressing changes
++	Access to treatment monthly or less often	• Colostomy change • Tracheostomy tube change
+	Routine access to treatment only as needed	

TABLE 2–8   SUMMARY OF CATEGORIES FOR THOSE WITH CHRONIC ILLNESS/DISABILITY, BASED ON KEY CHARACTERISTICS AND SERVICE NEEDS

	Level of Care		
Criteria	High Chronic Illness/Disability	Moderate Chronic Illness/Disability	Low Chronic Illness/Disability
Functional Impairments			
Severity	++++	+++	++/+
Monitoring and Supervision			
Frequency	++++/+++	++	+
Skill level	+++	++	+
Treatment/Care			
Complexity of judgment/skill	+++	++	+
Availability	++++	+++	++/+

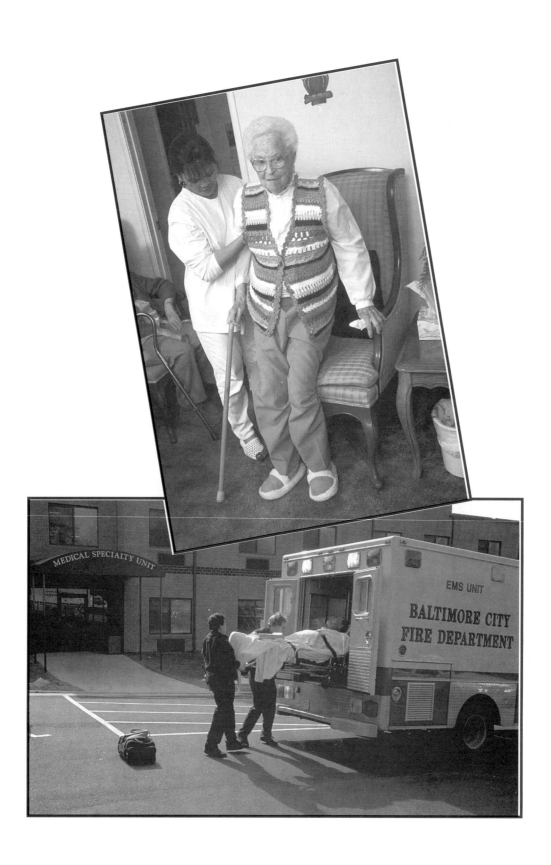

SUBACUTE CARE'S PLACE IN INTEGRATED CARE DELIVERY SYSTEMS

*S*o far, most subacute care has been provided as stand-alone programs—even when located in a multiprogram facility or organization. This will change as the health care system continues to evolve. Subacute programs are best viewed as a service package within a continuum of care.

Subacute care is right for an individual if its package of services is needed to achieve the essential goals of health care: optimal service to achieve defined objectives at the lowest possible cost for the shortest possible time, for someone with an active medical condition and related problems in multiple dimensions. If the patient's needs exceed the capabilities of a subacute environment, or if only some components of the package are needed, it may be more appropriate to provide the essential services elsewhere.

Practitioners should base placement and transfer decisions on matching patient needs and care objectives with the various options within the continuum. To do this, they must understand the alternatives.

The purpose of this chapter is to clarify those alternatives in relation to subacute care, and to relate this to the process of determining optimal patient placement.

A Shifting Framework

As discussed in Chapter 1, health care has traditionally been compartmentalized by site (for example, hospitals, nursing facilities, outpatient practices) and by practitioner (physician specialties, podiatrists, physical therapists, and so on) rather than based on individual care or service needs. Historically, facilities and practitioners have focused on gaining market share, and tended to view other providers as unrelated competitors. Those at each site have delivered care, but have not necessarily been much concerned about duplicating or conflicting with previously delivered service, or giving more service than necessary, or giving the care in a more expensive setting than might otherwise be required. Nor have they always considered seriously what happens to patients after their transfer elsewhere. For example, some practitioners have not deemed it their problem if tests were repeated elsewhere because they did not provide adequate hospital discharge information, or if the patient did not receive adequate follow-up or had to be rehospitalized shortly after discharge. Thus, health care has not been delivered within systems, but by countless independent entities who have made decisions and rendered treatments with relatively little attention to their broader impact.

Also, medical treatment has often been considered an end in itself; that is, it has been assumed to be beneficial by virtue of being given. For instance, many patients with end-stage respiratory failure have been placed on ventilators despite having no reasonable hope for recovery, because the ventilator could compensate for the respiratory failure. Care objectives (what is the treatment intended to accomplish, and is it realistic?) have often been vague.

Care outcomes have also been uneven. Some health care has been essential to survival or improved quality of life; some of it has been useful but not essential; some of it has been inconsequential; and some of it has been harmful. The interpretation of these results has often been left to providers, while patients and payers have rarely felt comfortable in understanding the results or challenging the interpretations. Even when defined objectives have not been achieved, some providers have assumed that their services were nevertheless both necessary and optimal, and that any untoward consequences or suboptimal results were unavoidable.

The problems of the traditional uncoordinated approach to service delivery have been well documented. They include unnecessary duplication of testing and treatment, higher costs, and preventable complications and iatrogenic illnesses. As the cost of health care has skyrocketed, both private payers and government have demanded change.

The health care system of the future requires a different approach. Table 3–1, pp. 48–49, compares the shifting philosophies of health services delivery under traditional and future approaches. These may be summarized as follows. Health care must be delivered systematically. In a genuine system, providers and practitioners all view the patient as a person with specified problems and needs. Before care is given, it is essential to define the objectives of care and consider how to meet them optimally. Other principles include the following.

- A shift from health care as an end in itself to care as a means to an end
- Determination of the value of care in part by relating results to objectives
- Yielding of the primary objectives of volume and utilization to objectives of minimizing use and reducing excess capacity

- Viewing beds and sites as cost centers rather than profit centers
- Sharing between providers and payers of financial risks and penalties for duplication and redundancy
- Coordination among providers during the same episode and between care episodes

Sometimes service delivery and site selection have been based on clinical necessity, but often they have been determined by reimbursement systems. In the future, service delivery and reimbursement must be determined primarily by assessment of the patient's condition and care objectives, secondarily by availability of necessary services, and only then by sites or practitioners. Increasingly, several forms of treatment can be given at more than one site, and the same provider can offer a spectrum of services.

Movement Toward Integrated Health Delivery Systems

Forms of Integration.   Health care provision is shifting toward recognizing the common interests of states and regions in having an integrated delivery system (IDS). An IDS may be defined as an organization, or group of affiliated organizations, offering a systematic approach to providing health care services, including access to various individual or packages of services through the continuum, such as subacute care, home health, hospice, skilled nursing, preventive medicine, mental health, rehabilitation, and long-term care.

In an effort to provide the continuum of services as efficiently as possible, providers are creating alliances and networks. Alliances are relationships of independent providers who agree to work together but who do not necessarily have common governance or shared accountability. Networks are relationships of providers who agree to common governance, goals, objectives, policies, and accountability. The partners agree to share risk to varying degrees.

Creation of alliances and integrated networks is often based on business considerations. But successful alliances and networks also employ philosophies and strategies that reflect an understanding of their patients' care needs and the appropriate roles of all players. Table 3–2, p. 50, lists roles and Table 3–3, p. 50, indicates operational strategies that are vital to successful integration.

Risks and Concerns.   Integration of health care delivery has both benefits and limitations. Many patients and practitioners are concerned about the loss of control and freedom of choice that might result from this shift. Emphasizing cost containment alone is likely to have a negative impact. But a systematic approach to providing health care can potentially address some major weaknesses of traditional health care delivery (duplication, inadequate follow-up, emphasis on giving service rather than achieving care objectives, relatively little attention to preventive care, inadequate coordination among practitioners, high incidence of preventable iatrogenic and facility-acquired illness), help maintain or improve care quality, and be more cost-effective. This approach emphasizes preventing illness and injury, providing optimal rather than maximal treatment based on realistic care objectives, optimizing function and quality of life, and helping manage the consequences of an unavoidable decline. Although financial viability obviously remains important, the primary focus shifts from revenue generation toward resource conservation. The primary determinant of the value of care is whether the care outcome achieves patient-focused, not provider-focused, objectives.

Subacute Care in Relation to These Principles

Currently, most subacute care programs are separate and nonintegrated, despite their location within another health care organization. They are often touted as a route to substantial revenues.

Subacute Care in a Managed Care Environment.   As with all facets of health care, subacute care programs should be seen as one component in a systems approach to care (Table 3–4, p. 51). Eventually they will become cost centers, not merely profit centers. Decisions about placement into, and transfer from, subacute care units must be based on matching a patient's care objectives and service needs to the availability and cost of those services. Therefore, practitioners and program and case managers should understand the relationships between subacute programs and other parts of the care continuum.

Subacute programs admit many of their patients from hospitals, but they may draw some patients from other sources, including the home and assisted living or nursing facilities. In the future, more patients with medical conditions who are not also highly unstable are likely to be admitted directly, bypassing acute care hospitals. Subacute programs may also discharge patients to any setting.

Although offering a less costly daily alternative to hospital care, subacute sites may not always be the most cost-effective alternative. Because a subacute patient may stay for weeks rather than days, the total cost of care can be considerable despite a lower per-diem rate than the acute care hospital. Many programs are currently reimbursed by several payment systems (Medicare and managed care) with substantially different incentives. Managed care payers expect providers to minimize the time spent at more costly care sites.

Some subacute programs will be part of a vertically integrated care network available to the patients enrolled in that system. Other subacute programs will provide care under contract to the patients of HMOs and other managed care organizations under a negotiated per-diem rate or other financial arrangement. In either case, pressure to restrain costs of care will be based on the fact that each service must be subtracted from a capitated payment, whether divided up within a network or paid to a subcontractor.

Subacute care should be provided when it offers the most cost-effective package of treatments and services to meet an individual's care objectives and needs. Those needing only some components—for example, treatments but relatively little monitoring—may be better served in other less costly settings, provided adequate support systems exist. When the subacute program has achieved the objectives of care, a decision must be made about transferring the patient to a less costly site or altering the reimbursement for continued stay in the subacute program.

To succeed in a highly competitive health care environment, subacute programs must be able to provide efficient, good quality care that achieves desirable objectives. In this climate, strength comes from within. Programs must successfully integrate the business and clinical components of care (Chapter 4);

provide the essential services according to well-defined care objectives (Chapter 5); understand and optimize the care processes (Chapter 7); optimize the efficiency and effectiveness of those giving the care (Chapter 8); provide effective, consistent support for the systems and process issues that directly or indirectly influence the care (Chapter 9); and use relevant criteria to evaluate and improve the care (Chapter 10).

OTHER SERVICE PACKAGES WITHIN THE CARE CONTINUUM

In Chapter 2, subacute care was categorized as a package of services for those with moderate or low-acuity conditions. The following sections describe the other levels of care and some of the existing sites or service packages.

In trying to select an optimal treatment plan and site, it is important to understand the essential functions and tasks needed to provide these levels of service within the care continuum (Table 3–5, pp. 51–52).

For example, a person who principally requires administration of medical or nursing treatments with little or no monitoring can receive those treatments in any of several settings. But someone who is also medically unstable may also need frequent testing and close monitoring, which may limit the site options.

High-Acuity Care

High-acuity services are for individuals who are highly unstable medically or who have some combination of need for intensive, rapid testing and monitoring to identify their major problems and their causes; frequent or continuous adjustment of their treatment regimen; and close or continuous observation and monitoring of the course of their condition and their response to treatment (see Table 2–6, p. 30). Short-term high-acuity services are typically provided through emergency services and as an inpatient in an acute hospital.

Emergency services are usually provided in a hospital emergency room, but may also be given in a freestanding emergency or urgent care setting. The sites are staffed by trained physicians and nurses, who may specialize in emergency care. Although there are some specialized emergency centers (children, major trauma, and others), most are equipped to handle a broad spectrum of illnesses and injuries.

Delivering this level of care requires the capability to rapidly identify and initiate management of primary causes of life-threatening instability. Once this is done, the individual can be transferred to a setting that can continue the required level of treatment and monitoring.

Emergency services have also often served as major providers of isolated, episodic care for individuals with minor problems or minimal medical instability. However, they may be an inefficient source of some such services. They may provide some forms of patient and family instruction, usually focused on the primary problem for which care was rendered, but they rarely address incidental abnormalities, coexisting problems, functional limitations, or personal care deficits.

More prolonged high-acuity care is most often provided in acute care hospitals. This level of service concentrates on managing individuals with significant medical instability because of illness or injury by providing frequent or continuous highly skilled monitoring and complex treatment (for example, major surgery) requiring extensive technical coordination or carrying a high risk of complications. A high-acuity provider must be able to identify the causes of a very broad spectrum of signs and symptoms, and to initiate any of a broad spectrum of treatments for medically correctable causes. They should be able to support rapid recognition and response to complications and condition changes. Providers should also be able to integrate the care of acute conditions with the management of coexisting chronic illnesses and recognize and prevent nosocomial and iatrogenic illnesses because of their relevance to outcomes.

Many of the treatments (for example, surgery) and some of the testing and monitoring formerly done almost exclusively in hospitals are now provided elsewhere. However, other sites are generally not equipped or staffed to provide the overall package of services (assessment, treatment, and monitoring) to the degree or with the frequency required by those with multiple complex problems and a high degree of medical instability.

Hospitals typically divide their care among intensive care units, surgical suites, and specialized medical, surgical, obstetrics, and pediatrics units. Because of the cost of maintaining a spectrum of staff, services, and diagnostic and treatment capabilities, hospital care is expensive.

In addition to providing high-acuity inpatient care, hospitals are increasingly joining together and with other providers in networks of services including outpatient centers, specialty clinics, long-term and subacute care, and community outreach centers.

High Chronic Illness/Disability Care

High chronic illness/disability (CID) care providers must be able to assess and manage the various medical, psychosocial, behavioral, and functional consequences of complex chronic conditions and occasional acute episodes of illness. These providers must also be able to manage illnesses in the context of a person's psychosocial needs and overall condition; modify treatment regimens for the chronic conditions in response to frequent minor or occasional substantial changes in status; rapidly assess condition changes and judge the likely sources and potential severity of the condition; provide or rapidly access those who are skilled at managing chronic illness and can select, render, and monitor the effects of medications and treatments; and determine when temporary transfer to another setting is indicated to better manage or monitor acute condition changes. High CID care providers should also be able to routinely address personal care and quality of life issues by involving patients and families in care decisions, and handle those with a progressive condition decline or terminal illness.

To manage these diverse problems, high CID care providers should be able to provide at least some skilled nursing care on a 24-hour basis. "Skilled nursing" refers to treatment and continuing observation and assessment of the medically stable and unstable chronically ill. Licensed physicians must direct or supervise the services, and licensed nursing personnel must either deliver the services or supervise trained nonlicensed nursing personnel 24 hours per day.

This level of care is most often provided by freestanding or hospital-based skilled nursing facilities (SNFs) and nursing facilities. Most high CID care facilities offer around-the-clock nursing and ancillary services to a mixture of frail impaired elderly and some younger chronically ill and impaired adults. Services may also include specialized dementia units, convalescent stays, dentistry, dialysis, geropsychiatry, home health, hospice care, hyperalimentation, intermediate care, rehabilitation therapies, pastoral care, podiatry, postoperative care, recreation, respiratory therapy, respite care (short-term stays), sheltered care, and social services.

High CID care providers may have limited capacity to assess and manage new onset illnesses and condition changes on site, to monitor widely or frequently fluctuating conditions, to quickly access diagnostic and treatment services, and to respond promptly to emergencies.

Moderate and Low Chronic Illness/Disability Care

Moderate CID care providers must be able to manage the care of individuals with moderate functional, cognitive, or behavioral impairments with relative medical and functional stability. They must be able to provide some regular assistance with personal care and ADLs, and may need to monitor relatively stable chronic health-related conditions and administer predetermined uncomplicated treatments. They should be able to respond to the onset of acute illness with basic triage of the problems and the ability to access off-site practitioners.

Low CID care providers typically support and supervise individuals with stable functional, cognitive, or behavioral impairments. Their direct care and support staff have variable training in managing chronic illness and dysfunction and usually play little role in selecting or adjusting those treatments.

More sophisticated sites can potentially provide more observation, assessment, and problem identification—including the management of some uncomplicated acute condition changes and complications—as well as the more controlled initiation of some medications and treatments. They can also potentially modify the course of chronic conditions through early detection and prevention.

Low and moderate CID care is given either in formal residential or in outpatient settings. Formal residential settings include nursing facilities (NFs) and assisted living programs. Assisted living (AL) programs (also called "board and care," "domiciliary," and "personal care") are organized programs of housing that include other packages of personal supervision, support, and psychosocial services. They may also administer medications, offer regular meals, and provide counseling and pastoral care, supervised activities, and health and psychosocial assessments. Their primary emphasis is on residential living with access to other service components depending on need. Some NFs and many varieties of housing communities provide some form of assisted living.

The costs of these programs vary depending on the scope of an individual's functional limitations and need for nursing support. They are limited in the staff's ability to recognize new-onset medical conditions and to monitor for the complications of illnesses and treatments. They are also limited in the speed of accessing testing, equipment, medications, supplies, and services and in their ability to ensure that those with problems are transferred to the most appropriate, least costly site for subsequent care.

The outpatient versions of moderate and low CID care may be given in day care, home care, day treatment, and outpatient settings. However, the scope and consistency of such services vary widely, partially because there are fewer mechanisms for overseeing and influencing the performance of the practitioners and other care providers.

Home Care.   Home care programs may provide personal care, health-related services, or both in the home setting. The care may be either episodic or more prolonged for those with low or moderate CID. Typical care providers include nurses, rehabilitation therapists, physicians, social workers, and home health aides. Personal care services may include assistance with activities of daily living (bathing, dressing, grooming, continence, and so on) and instrumental activities of daily living (meal preparation, light housekeeping, grocery shopping, and similar tasks). Health-related services may include initial evaluation of the individual and family in the home, intermittent direct nursing care, evaluation of the patient and family's abilities and limitations, monitoring of the patient's progress and complications, instruction and supervision of patient and family, and communication with other disciplines and agencies. The services may be given after inpatient care, or instead of such care if the individual primarily needs intermittent treatment or personal care without more extensive monitoring.

Day Care.   Adult day care programs offer various social, personal care, and health services in a supervised ambulatory group setting to individuals who are transported to and from home, usually 3 to 5 days per week. Several levels of day care service have been identified. Level 1 service provides socialization, some supervision, supportive service, and minimal ADL assistance to a stable individual not requiring nursing observation or intervention. Level 2 service provides moderate (30 to 60% of the time) assistance and some health assessment, oversight, or monitoring by a nurse, plus maintenance therapy services and moderate assistance with one to three ADLs. Level 3 service provides regular monitoring or intervention by a nurse of no more than moderately unstable chronic medical or behavioral conditions, rehabilitative or restorative therapy services, and total care in one or more ADLs or moderate assistance with more than three ADLs. Other services for any level may include medication administration, nutritional assessment, meals, activities, social services, and screening.

Day Treatment.   Day treatment programs are provided to those individuals whose conditions require more complex care plans and more aggressive initiation and adjustment of medications and treatments than day care or other outpatient settings can manage, but who do not require continuous daily care or an overnight stay. A significant advantage of these programs is their capacity to offer the care with few of the "hotel" costs that apply in inpatient settings. These patients are usually no more than mildly medically or psychiatrically unstable. Their care is delivered by an interdisciplinary team including physicians, nurses, social workers, dietitians, activities therapists, and physical and occupational therapists.

For example, psychiatric day treatment centers continue monitoring the progress and adjusting the medications of individuals recently discharged from inpatient psychiatric programs. The patients may participate in activities, group therapies, and receive their medications from nurses and a periodic reassessment from an on-site physician. After a predetermined period, or when the rate of improvement has leveled off, these individuals would switch back to receiving their usual care and monitoring in their inpatient (for example, nursing facility) or residential (for example, home care or doctor's office) setting. Those who become more medically or behaviorally unstable are likely to be transferred out of the program to an inpatient setting able to provide more extensive monitoring and problem management.

Isolated/Episodic Care

Isolated or episodic care is provided to individuals requiring occasional treatment or support, but who are otherwise stable or functional even though they may have chronic illness or disabilities. It is typically provided in outpatient centers, physicians' offices, and in the home. These individuals need only intermittent medical management, adjustment of their medications and treatments, or monitoring.

This approach is relatively inexpensive because the costs of care are principally related to the practitioner's service and not to the overhead of the site. There are limits to the capacity to monitor or manage more widely or frequently fluctuating conditions, the speed with which tests can be obtained and the treatment plan changed in response to those results, and the coordination and communication among various practitioners giving different aspects of care.

Outpatient Centers.   Outpatient centers span a spectrum of practitioners and services, ranging from multispecialty groups to hospital-based rehabilitation programs. Individuals come from outside for a defined assessment and/or treatment and then return home. These settings offer one-stop access to multiple practitioners, treatments, and testing, and internal coordination of referrals, treatments, and orders. However, they are usually limited in their capacity to monitor or manage unstable medical conditions and to coordinate the care with other care sites and practitioners.

Table 3–5, pp. 51–52, compares the desired capabilities of service providers at each level of the health care continuum. For instance, both acute care hospitals and subacute care sites must be capable of determining severity of illness; hospitals must be able to initiate comprehensive treatment to stabilize emergent conditions; and subacute care sites must be able to define a patient's functional limitations caused by illness or disability.

THE PROCESSES OF MATCHING NEEDS TO SERVICES

Placement decisions may involve subacute care programs in one of two ways: (1) decisions about whether someone needs that level of care and (2) decisions about where to transfer someone after they have received subacute care. To optimize such placement, practitioners, facilities, and payers should follow the steps outlined in Table 3–6, p. 52.

Appropriate assessment enables more complete problem identification and definition, which permits accurate identification of service needs and clarification of care objectives. Awareness of the costs and the options for packaging and providing those services then enables optimal placement. Effective follow-up after placement allows individuals and programs to refine their abilities to manage care effectively and place individuals appropriately.

The primary determinant of placement should be stability because the management of medical instability requires a level of monitoring and assessment capabilities only available in some settings. Secondary determinants relate to problem definition and initiation of medical treatment. Some patients require rapid or intensive testing to define the scope of the problem, identify the causes, and select and initiate the appropriate treatments to begin to address the problem satisfactorily.

Once problems are defined and the appropriate treatments initiated, the third phase of patient management is to continue to deliver the treatments, to evaluate the course of the illness and the response to treatments, and to monitor and identify new problems or complications that might arise. Thus, a third-level determinant of placement is the level and complexity of problem management and the complexity and availability of ongoing monitoring. If the major problems and their causes have been defined already, then the treatments might proceed in a less intensive setting depending on the complexity and risk of those treatments and the frequency with which the patient's progress must be assessed.

For instance, a 32-year-old auto accident victim with probable head injury, likely multiple internal injuries, and rapidly fluctuating vital signs needs close monitoring, rapid multiple diagnostic testing, frequent lab tests, and frequent skilled reassessment by physicians and nurses. The problems, including the extent of damage, have not yet been fully identified. The need for stabilization and rapid identification of problems requires a high frequency of monitoring and skill level of assessment.

A fourth-level determinant is the individual's level of overall personal and social functioning and the availability of social support systems to compensate for deficits. For example, the same individual needing postacute care after hospitalization for respiratory failure could wind up in a nursing facility, assisted living residence, or at home, depending on the availability of family or other support systems to help with personal care, shopping, cooking, taking medications, and monitoring for fluctuations in condition.

Figure 3–1 represents a systematic approach to determining patient placement based on the considerations discussed above. It distinguishes the processes and decisions involved in dealing with the causes of illness and injury from those involved in managing their consequences. For example, as discussed further in Chapters 5 and 12, rehabilitation services are primarily directed toward managing consequences, not dealing with causes, of illness and injury. Therefore, for purposes of determining proper patient placement, rehabilitation services should be viewed as a treatment package, not a treatable condition. The intensity and complexity of medical therapies are related to managing the causes of a person's medical instability, whereas the intensity and complexity of their rehabilitation needs are related to the consequences of their conditions. Their ability to tolerate more rehabilitation therapies is related to the degree of their medical stability. A comprehensive rehabilitation program can be given in several different settings, its scope being limited principally by reimbursement. Therefore, the principal determinant of placement of all individuals with active medical and rehabilitative needs should be their level of medical service need rather than the amount or intensity of their rehabilitation program.

Choosing Subacute Care.   When a condition is not immediately life-threatening or has been stabilized so that it is no longer life-threatening, and the major problems and complications have been identified and at least some treatment initiated, then the focus of care shifts to ongoing problem management, including the consequences as well as the causes of those conditions.

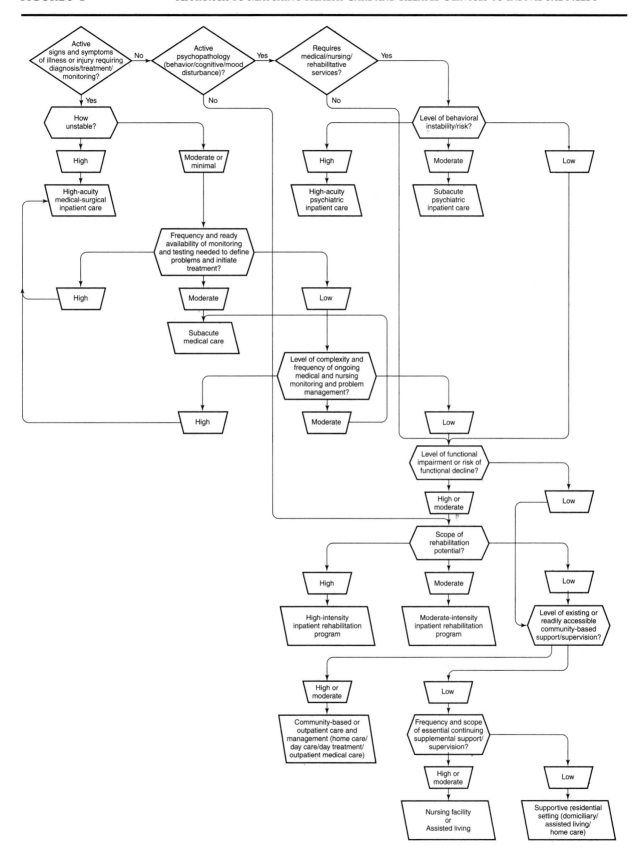

For example, after the above patient is stabilized, her problems might include potential for injury, infection, potential skin impairment, inability to take adequate nutrition, activity intolerance, altered breathing pattern, impaired mobility, self-care deficit, and depression. Her service needs might include blood transfusions, management of a chest tube because of a partially collapsed lung, medication titration, laboratory monitoring, physical and occupational therapy, and suctioning. In addition, she could need lumbar puncture for sudden change in neurological signs or feeding tube care if she were unable to eat for a prolonged period. Although her initial care would most likely require a high-acuity care setting, the subsequent care could be given in a subacute setting. When some of the more significant consequences are stabilized or resolved (lungs reexpanded, bleeding stopped, vital signs more stable, depression partially improved), the care might then be provided at home or in a less costly and restrictive inpatient setting. Table 3–7, p. 53, gives examples of patients and their possible placement related to the level of intensity, complexity, and frequency of their need for problem identification, monitoring, and problem management.

Facilities and practitioners must be aware of the capabilities of potential transfer sites, and clarify an individual's service needs (for example, frequent monitoring, ventilator support, catheter care, or infusions) and other deficits such as fecal incontinence, confusion, undernutrition, or immobility. Practitioners and programs should be as concerned about the subsequent care as they are about the current care. The cases in Chapter 11 are presented in a format that might serve as a discharge report containing relevant information for those needing to provide follow-up care.

It is also important to distinguish availability and access in determining need and placement. That is, not all services (lab testing, dialysis, radiological testing, physician evaluation, and so on) needed by an individual necessarily have to be on-site at all times. It may be possible to send the patient to the practitioner or service (for example, transfer to a local hospital temporarily for a surgical procedure or MRI scan) or have the practitioner or service come to the patient (for example, portable X-ray or contract lab service).

Ultimately, all providers in a health care continuum must clarify their capabilities and recognize their limitations. A provider with only some of the capacity to deliver a certain level of service must be able to supplement the missing components appropriately. For instance, many subacute patients do not need frequent physician visits but they need some periodic physician assessment. Therefore, the site must at least be able to determine when physician intervention is indicated (including the onset of a significant condition change) and access medical services. Or, a potential care site may claim it can change dressings or provide wound care, yet may not be able to handle complex wound care or may not have those who can recognize complications such as infection or excessive bleeding.

Additionally, all care sites must be able to identify and manage certain core problems of their patients. These conditions—discussed at more length in Chapters 7 and 10—include undernutrition, skin breakdown, altered mental status, and medication-related complications. They can occur at any site in any patient with any diagnosis or other conditions. They are major contributors to mortality and morbidity, as well as increasing the costs of care.

The appropriate settings for meeting patient needs are likely to shift further as their capabilities develop further, and regulations and reimbursement methodologies evolve. The most important goal should be to efficiently match needs to services to achieve desired care objectives, regardless of what programs or sites call themselves.

For Further Reading

Hudson P. Legal aspects of managed care. *Transitions*. November/December 1993:1–4.

Lumsdon K. Beyond four walls: Case management evolves into management of a continuum of care. *Hosp Health Netw*. March 5, 1994:44–45.

Masso AR. The next generation of managed care. *J Subacute Care*. 1994; 1(1):7–8.

Montague J. Eroding empires. *Hosp Health Netw*. April 5, 1995:56–58.

Stahl DA. The changing managed care arena: Impact on subacute care. *Nurs Manage*. 1995; 26(8):16, 18.

Stahl DA. Managed care and subacute care: A partnership of choice. *Nurs Manage*. 1995; 26(1):17–19.

Stahl DA. The phases of managed care: Where does subacute care fit? *Nurs Manage*. 1995; 26(5):16–17.

TABLE 3–1   COMPARISON OF PAST, PRESENT, AND FUTURE HEALTH SERVICES DELIVERY

Item	Past and Present	Future
Objectives of care	Treat illness with little regard to ultimate impact of the treatment; care of individuals	Prevention; maintain maximal function; care for populations, not just individuals; consider care objectives in choosing care plan and care site
Systems capacity	Growth and maximum occupancy	Consolidation; downsizing; empty beds
Means of services delivery	Independent practitioners and care sites; autonomously functioning institutions	Coordinated delivery systems
Sites	Independently operating profit centers (clinics, office practices, pharmacies, nursing facilities, etc.); partners and groups	Practitioners and institutions as part of delivery systems
	Either inpatient or outpatient, with little in between	Full care continuum
	Hospitals are profit centers, driven by volume; primary customer is physician; emphasize financial benefits of physician referrals; competition for physicians drives up costs	Hospitals are cost centers, where growth in revenue takes resources from the system; patients are hospitals' primary customer; both hospitals and physicians have a major stake in reducing utilization and costs
Facility/program leadership skills, objectives	Skills: someone with strong entrepreneurial and marketing skills	Skills: someone with strong operational and re-engineering skills
	Objectives: expand physical plant, more beds, larger staffs, increased revenues	Objectives: attention to detail, preparation for major change, focus on collaborative instead of competitive efforts, link resource utilization and quality
Reimbursement	Cost-based reimbursement shifting to discounted fees and prospective payment; based on delivering service; payment and profits based on volume, technical complexity; no penalty for redundancy	Capitation and risk sharing; reward for optimal care based on fulfilling care objectives and effective resource utilization, not volume
Patient risk	Minimal incentive for patient to be cost-conscious	Patients share financial risk of care choices
Provider risk	Little or none	Risk sharing among providers and payers
Information systems	Focused primarily on costs and charges	Focused on helping those delivering patient care, facilitating care processes, assessing and improving quality, determining costs of care, managing outcomes

TABLE 3–1   COMPARISON OF PAST, PRESENT, AND FUTURE HEALTH SERVICES DELIVERY (CONTINUED)

Item	Past and Present	Future
Practitioners	Some disciplines or individuals are considered more "important" than others; the scope of a discipline's role is confused with their value to the outcome	Each individual and discipline is considered valuable to the outcome, even though not all play the same role or to the same degree
Physicians	Emphasis on specialists and procedures; physicians as fiercely independent practitioners fighting outside "interference" with care decisions	Recognition that health care is not solely a physician domain; emphasis on primary care; physicians as components of delivery system
Consistency of care	Care is often delivered inconsistently among providers, from one episode to the next in the same person, or even by different practitioners during the same episode	Coordination of care among providers, from one episode to another, and between practitioners during the same episode
Accountability	Unrelated teams of providers are rarely held accountable for either quality or costs of care	All providers share a stake in outcomes and costs
	Quality by declaration or perception	Quality based on relevant outcome indicators
Utilization	Managed by physicians or hospitals, and by insurers Goal of expansion and high occupancy	Managed by an integrated system in conjunction with payers Goal to eliminate excess capacity and duplicate services; lowest possible occupancy
	Use of high-cost sites, linking cost and complexity to quality	Using the entire continuum, avoiding the high-cost sites whenever possible

Adapted with permission from Creative Healthcare Solutions, Minneapolis, MN.

TABLE 3–2   PARTIES ESSENTIAL TO SUCCESSFUL INTEGRATION

Parties	Function
Practitioners	Select appropriate care settings based on relevant criteria (quality, care objectives, and cost-effectiveness); recognize that resource utilization and quality of care are not necessarily directly related; address problems that could lead to poorer outcomes or more costly care
Management/ownership	Reduce pressures for occupancy and market share; recognize shift in thinking from entrepreneurial to resource conservation
Patients	Have better understanding of the continuum and what various sites can offer; recognize the benefits and the limitations of medical care; be more active participants in decision making; understand better how to judge quality care and better distinguish appearance from substance
Payers	Provide proper reimbursement incentives to minimize duplication and high cost utilization; find lowest-cost alternatives that can meet the objectives of care; reward prevention

TABLE 3–3   OPERATIONAL STRATEGIES ESSENTIAL TO SUCCESSFUL INTEGRATION

Strategy	Description
Strategic plan	Must emphasize balance of interests of all parties; must consider service provision and consolidation in relation to the defined community
Facilities plan	Should consider each party's existing physical plants, major equipment, and other assets; identify unnecessary resources and facilities for closure or divestiture
Financial	Plans to address short- and long-term financial needs of system; sources of capital and methods of repayment; include all essential expenditures including facilities, staff, technology, and information management systems
Information systems	Creation of a core patient database; efficient management of patient care and other service-related documentation; establishment of effective, efficient means of conveying information among providers and across care sites; effective use of data to assess and improve quality
Programmatic	Understand how proper coordination of systems and processes both directly and indirectly influences the care
Human resources/staffing	Identify essential human resources/staffing needs, including work areas, equipment, and physical locations; identify roles, functions, job descriptions based on their relevance to the care and its support systems
Relationships	Identify necessary and desirable external contractual relationships to support an integrated system and continuum of care

TABLE 3–4   PRINCIPLES OF AN EFFECTIVE CARE CONTINUUM RELEVANT TO A SUBACUTE PROGRAM

- Provide realistic expectations.
- Be patient-centered.
- Focus on care objectives and outcomes, using appropriate indicators and measurements.
- Discharge patients to less costly sites as soon as possible.
- Provide essential information to other individuals and sites.
- Coordinate closely with follow-up care sites and practitioners.
- Emphasize patient education and patient and family responsibility.
- Emphasize primary care and care continuity.
- Use clinical guidelines and critical pathways across the continuum.

TABLE 3–5   ESSENTIAL PERFORMANCE CAPABILITIES NEEDED AT VARIOUS LEVELS OF CARE IN THE CONTINUUM[a]

Function/Task	Level of Care						
	High Acuity	Moderate Acuity	Low Acuity	High CID[b]	Moderate CID	Low CID	Outpatient
Assessment/Problem Definition							
Perform a detailed assessment of medical status and stability	+++	+++	+++	++	+	+	++
Identify and correctly define individual's health-related problems	+++	+++	++	++	+	+	++
Define causes of those problems	+++	+++	++	++	++	+	++
Identify and correctly define functional deficits and chronic conditions	++	+++	+++	+++	+++	++	++
Monitoring							
Unstable vital signs	+++	+++	++	++	+	0	+
Routine vital signs	+++	+++	+++	+++	+	+	+
Response to care and treatment	+++	+++	+++	+++	++	+	+++
Recognize onset of exacerbations and complications of illness	+++	+++	+++	+++	++	+	++
Detect complications of treatments and care	+++	+++	+++	+++	++	+	+++
Detect onset of another illness	+++	+++	++	++	+	+	++

(continued)

TABLE 3–5   ESSENTIAL PERFORMANCE CAPABILITIES NEEDED AT VARIOUS LEVELS OF CARE IN THE CONTINUUM[a] (CONTINUED)

Function/Task	Level of Care						
	High Acuity	Moderate Acuity	Low Acuity	High CID[b]	Moderate CID	Low CID	Outpatient
Problem Management							
Stabilize life-threatening conditions	+++	++	+	+	0	0	+
Select correct treatments	+++	+++	+++	+++	+	+	+++
Administer a spectrum of treatments	+++	++	++	++	+	+	+
Instruct patient and family effectively	+++	+++	+++	+++	++	+	+++
Coordinate complex or multifaceted treatment plan	+++	+++	++	+++	++	+	+
Effectively manage coexisting chronic conditions	++	+++	+++	+++	++	+	++

[a]*Use of this table.* As discussed in this book, various tasks are associated with the care of those with illness, injuries, and disabilities. Those providing each level of care must be able to perform the tasks associated with those needs to accommodate the needs of those served. Care sites have different levels of capability in performing those tasks. For each task (left-hand column), +++ represents the greatest required capability and 0 denotes essentially no need. Proper service placement may then be ascertained by matching the service needs of individuals with various levels of illness and disability to providers' capabilities. See Chapter 2 for discussion of levels of care.
[b]CID = chronic illness/disability.

TABLE 3–6   STEPS IN DETERMINING PROPER PLACEMENT

- Perform relevant patient assessment.
- Gather appropriate information.
- Define individual's active problems and potential high-risk areas.
- Identify the objectives of care.
- Determine service needs based on those objectives.
- Define options for service packages and placement.
- Discuss options with patient and family.
- Match service needs with available options.
- Communicate with the prospective care site.
- Carry out transfer.
- Follow-up to assess eventual outcome.

TABLE 3-7 EXAMPLES OF PLACEMENT DECISIONS BASED ON EVALUATION OF PATIENT NEEDS

Case Example	Assess/Problem Identification	Monitoring	Problem Management	Appropriate Placement
32 y.o. auto accident victim with probable head injury; likely multiple internal injuries; rapidly fluctuating vital signs. Needs: Close monitoring, rapid multiple diagnostic testing, frequent lab tests, frequent physician reassessment	+++	+++	+++	Intensive care unit in acute hospital
Same individual has recovered partially, vital signs are stable, and has no further internal bleeding; now tube fed, gets occasional aspiration pneumonia. Needs: Suctioning, physical therapy, occasional monitoring and testing, periodic routine physician reevaluation, support for all ADLs	+	++	+++	Subacute care unit while receiving rehabilitation services monitoring, multiple problem management provided daily, and while medical problems need periodic physician evaluation
85 y.o. nursing facility resident transferred to hospital after fall. Needs: Surgery to repair hip fracture, management of postoperative functional limitations, rehabilitation	+	++	+++	Subacute care unit after hospital stay if daily participation in rehabilitation is possible or recovery period is complicated by multiple medical problems and self-care deficits
68 y.o. COPD patient with progressive respiratory failure recently hospitalized on ventilator	+	+++	++	Subacute care unit for attempt to wean off ventilator

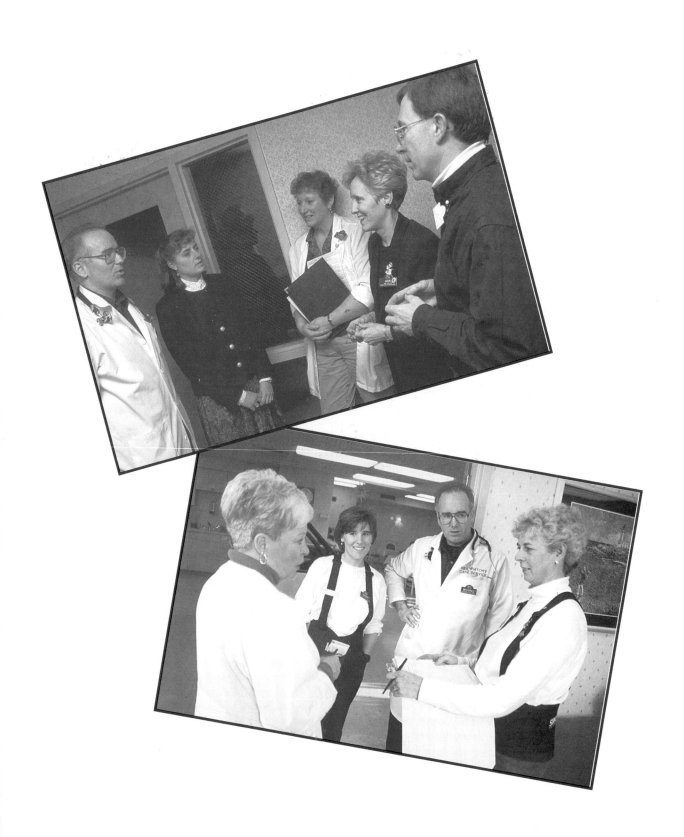

STEPS TO PLANNING AND IMPLEMENTING SUBACUTE CARE PROGRAMS AND UNITS

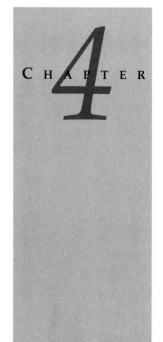

CHAPTER 4

A subacute unit can be implemented and managed more successfully when certain steps are followed. Although this book's primary focus is the delivery of care rather than the business aspects, the two are necessarily intertwined. Any organization must be well prepared from both the business and the clinical perspectives.

The time needed for planning and implementation of a program and unit will depend partially on the degree of existing successful systems and processes. Because some practitioners and other care providers will be involved in planning, implementing, and operating subacute programs, they should be aware of relevant issues and concerns.

This chapter addresses the specific steps in planning and implementing a subacute program, and the issues that must be faced in the process. Frequent reference is made to other chapters that expand upon the tasks involved in performing these steps.

GENERAL RECOMMENDATIONS

Time Frames for Development

Developing or expanding a good quality subacute program takes time and must be done properly. It requires adequate clinical and business preparation. For various reasons, some of those interested in starting a subacute unit may want to do so quickly. However, acting too hastily may increase the risk of inadequate care, which would in turn undermine the program's attractiveness to patients and insurers.

EXAMPLE

A multistate corporate owner of long-term care facilities decided to start a large subacute unit in a renovated former community hospital. Although the unit marketed extensively, it opened too many beds, did not select patients carefully, lacked a proper quality oversight or risk management program, did not have relevant policies and procedures, and did not staff effectively. Staff turned over frequently, many managers left, problems developed with patient care, and eventually the state licensure agency forced the unit to close down.

A series of processes is involved in planning and implementing a subacute program (Table 4–1, p. 70). Regardless of their existing programs and services, both hospitals and nursing facilities (NFs) must do certain things to create an effective program. The timetables for each organization will depend on several factors. These include the current scope and capabilities of existing programs, adequacy of existing support systems, availability of appropriate practitioners, and availability and roles of current management. Also, the local health care delivery environment may influence the urgency of developing a program or the feasibility of being able to have enough patients to justify the development costs.

A series of steps concerning the planning and implementation of a subacute program are discussed below. They should all occur, although not necessarily in the order discussed. Although the decision to proceed should not necessarily hinge on the results of any one step, ignoring the red flags raised at any point can lead to later complications.

STEPS FOR PROGRAM PLANNING

Assess Opportunities and Risks

Although both hospitals and nursing facilities may view subacute programs as attractive because of the potential revenues, these programs present both opportunities and risks (Table 4–2, p. 70). Those contemplating such units must prudently consider both.

Hospitals.   Many hospitals have converted, or are considering converting, acute care beds to subacute care as a way to keep their patients while bypassing prospective payment reimbursement rates, preserving their market share, and utilizing their excess bed capacity. They may consider the conversion to be fairly easy because they already have skilled physicians and nurses and high-technology diagnostic and treatment resources and staff.

However, like long-term care, transitional care differs fundamentally from acute care in its requirements, perspectives, and care objectives. It is not simply downsized acute care. Acute care hospital administrators and staff must understand these differences and adjust accordingly. Considerable culture and attitude adjustment may be needed, the lack of which may cause many problems.

The hospital-based subacute unit should establish a separate identity from the acute program. Management, support staff, and practitioners must be educated about the unit's philosophies and purposes. Hospital boards, administration, and management must understand what they are getting into so they can establish the appropriate systems and teach the proper attitudes.

Subacute units need comparatively low overhead and must minimize the use of expensive technologies that are of questionable value to the care objectives. But achieving both effective and efficient care requires not just cost cutting but also systems that optimize the care and enhance the efficient performance of care processes.

At least presently, subacute units using skilled nursing facility (SNF) beds must operate under the Medicare rules for long-term care facilities, which are substantially different from those for acute care hospitals. Therefore, the hospital must be flexible enough to adapt its charges and billing, management, policies and procedures, and staff functions. Medicare skilled facilities—even those only providing short-stay, medically oriented care—must comply with the federal regulations for Medicare and Medicaid participation. The staff must familiarize themselves with these requirements and must balance both personal and health-related care. They must do a mandated comprehensive assessment for those staying longer than 14 days, and must comply with requirements concerning restraints, psychoactive medications, catheter use, and resident rights, among other things.

Nursing Facilities.   Nursing facilities also have incentives for offering subacute care. Mostly reimbursed through personal funds and state Medicaid programs, NFs view subacute care as a way to bring in Medicare and managed care patients.

NF-based subacute units can potentially offer, often less expensively, many medical, nursing, and rehabilitative services traditionally given in acute care hospitals. These cost advantages are based upon (1) the experience of NFs in providing a comprehensive package of service for relatively low cost; (2) lower capital costs for skilled nursing beds; (3) absence of costly laboratories and high-technology diagnostics, surgical facilities, emergency rooms, and obstetrical services; and (4) experience using less costly staff such as nurses and others to extend the services of more expensive providers such as physicians, respiratory therapists, and rehabilitation therapists.

Some NFs are discovering unanticipated benefits of subacute units. These include enhancing their staffs' professional and leadership skills, allowing them to use their existing skills of providing comprehensive care for the traditional long-term care patient, and offering career advancements. Subacute programs may have a spillover effect into the rest of the facility. The presence of the unit can create a more sophisticated care environment and a more diverse service base. Those with skills essential to the care of subacute patients, such as assessment of acute condition changes and provision of more complex treatments, can help other staff provide better care for traditional long-term care patients.

To succeed at subacute care, NFs must create an environment and culture that will provide high-quality services and convince both patients and insurers of the service quality. Hospitals may have a credibility advantage, because they have better developed systems for managing complex acute illness, and because much of the public is unaware of the capabilities of nonhospital settings or of hospitals' historical problems in effectively managing those with chronic illnesses and disabilities.

A NF must decide how much it wishes to broaden the age range of its traditional population. Some facilities decide to provide subacute care only to those over a certain age, although others include a younger patient population. Although the market shrinks somewhat with a narrower age range, the elderly constitute the bulk of those who need the kinds of services offered in subacute care programs.

Caring for a younger population also introduces a different, more diverse range of health and personal care issues. Most older subacute patients have major acute illnesses and coexisting chronic problems. But many younger subacute patients have had trauma due to accidents, injuries, or violence sometimes associated with drug and other substance abuse. To care for younger patients, the NF may have to adjust its environment, systems, staffing, activities programs, and food service, among other things.

Perform a Market Analysis

Subacute care's high start-up costs, and the growing competition to provide it, demand an appropriate market analysis and feasibility study. As of 1995, there were approximately 63 potential providers for every 6 existing subacute units (Lumsdon, 1995).

Depending on the community, perhaps 1 to 5% of acute hospital admissions are good candidates for admission to a transitional care unit. As managed care evolves and reimbursement patterns shift, another potential market is for the direct admission and short-term evaluation and care management of elderly and other chronically ill or impaired individuals currently living in assisted living, group home, or independent living facilities, or in the community, who need assessment and management of condition changes or new problems but are not highly unstable.

Subacute program planners should check with referral sites (especially local hospitals) to help determine needed services such as postoperative care, physical therapy, and ventilator care. Insurance companies, managed care companies, and health maintenance organizations (HMOs) should also be asked about those patients that cost them the most money. The program may want to prioritize those services for moving these problem patients out of the hospital.

A subacute care program should also decide on the scope of its services. It is risky to try to be too many things to too many people, without being able to deliver the care effectively and efficiently. For example, the potential liability for the extended monitoring and management of medically complex patients or of high-risk obstetric patients may be too great for the marginally prepared facility, despite the potential market.

Review Reimbursement Opportunities and Limits

Each subacute program, and the practitioners working in it, should understand the various payment methodologies, which are likely to change with time. Traditionally, health care has been reimbursed by site and by provider, rather than by level of service. This approach is less relevant to a changing situation where different sites offer similar levels of service and the same site may offer multiple levels.

Subacute reimbursement methodologies vary by payer source, and also may vary based on a facility-specific contract or on a case-by-case basis. The payment sources for a case may be mixed or they may shift during the stay. Presently, these various reimbursement methodologies offer different incentives. The primary payers for subacute care are Medicare, Medicaid, private insurance companies, HMOs, and preferred provider organizations (PPOs). Alternatives for payment include fee-for-service, straight discount, per diem (either all-inclusive or partly exclusive rate), fixed per-case rate, and capitation rate. Of these, fee-for-service represents the lowest risk to providers and capitation the highest risk. Managed care payers tend to prefer all-inclusive per diems, which cover room and board, nursing, medications, psychosocial support, therapies, and discharge planning. Additional payments may be negotiated for special medications, special beds, intravenous (IV) therapies, total parenteral nutrition (TPN), and other special supplies. Table 4–3, p. 71, summarizes the various forms of payment.

Attracting managed care patients requires keeping costs down, and maximizing Medicare reimbursement has required keeping costs up because—using complex formulas—Medicare reimburses many ancillary costs. Additionally, the rates paid for managed care subacute patients even under per-diem or negotiated per-case rates may still reflect the lack of competition for such patients or the lack of a satisfactory way to calculate a realistic cost of care.

Medicare Issues.   Under Medicare, hospitals are reimbursed according to diagnosis-related groups (DRGs), which give them a fixed payment for the care of any patient in a diagnosis category, regardless of the duration of the care. DRG-exempt settings providing acute and subacute care (long-term, psychiatric, and rehabilitation hospitals) have received cost-plus reimbursement based on rules for cost calculations, and additional reimbursement for ancillary services (physical therapy, respiratory therapy, and so on).

Medicare SNF beds are subject to the same general rules as hospital beds for Medicare payment. Medicare reimburses for routine SNF care by applying a limitation to routine costs based on the average cost in a geographic region. Reasonable provider costs may not exceed what the Health Care Financing Administration estimates is necessary to efficiently deliver needed health care services. Ancillary services are reimbursed separately from routine costs and generally are not subject to limitations.

Medicare does not recognize a subacute category, but does have an exception process which recognizes actual costs for high-acuity services. Exceptions may be based on either "new providers" or "atypical services" (Table 4–4, p. 71). SNFs may request an exception from the routine cost limitations (RCLs) if they can demonstrate that they are providing "atypical services;" that is, the patients' special needs or circumstances require a broader nature and scope of services and items than the typical SNF patient.

By developing transitional care units in relicensed hospital beds as "new" skilled nursing beds, hospital-based transitional care units have been eligible for the exemption from RCLs. Freestanding NFs most often convert an existing wing of skilled nursing beds into a transitional care unit. Therefore, they may only apply for the exception to RCLs, not the exemption.

However, federal budget pressures are likely to accelerate the movement away from a cost-based reimbursement system. In the near future, Medicare may shift more to the use of prospective payment, based on case mix (see Chapter 12). Also, the number of individuals in cost-based, fee-for-service Medicare plans is likely to decline as more are shifted into Medicare managed care plans.

Other Medicare rules have influenced the location of services and the ability of alternative sites to lower the costs of care. For example, at least through 1995 Medicare regulations required NFs to obtain respiratory therapy services only through a hospital with whom they had a transfer agreement. SNFs could not be reimbursed by Medicare for ancillary services provided by either on-staff or contract respiratory therapists. Therefore, subacute units could directly serve private patients, but not Medicare patients, needing respiratory therapy. This limited the financial feasibility of a subacute program trying to lower costs by providing its own respiratory therapists.

Medicaid Issues. The Medicaid program has not required states to pay for subacute care services. Most states have not developed a specific licensure or reimbursement category for subacute care, and only some states have offered special or enhanced rates for clearly defined higher-acuity patients. Chapter 1 presented some examples of approaches in various states.

Capitation Issues. Under a capitation system, providers are paid a flat fee to serve all enrollees in a managed care health plan, regardless of whether the members of the health plan actually use the services. The payment is typically monthly (for example, $30 per enrollee per month). Providers accept the financial risks, and are responsible for every aspect of the care of enrolled patients. They must either provide the care directly or contract for it. In either case, they will seek the least costly alternative to achieve the desired goals. More expensive forms of care represent a failure of preventive care and case management instead of a revenue source.

Facility Reimbursement Strategies. Even though subacute programs may not be reimbursed directly under capitation, they must increasingly deal with the managed care environment in which they may share a fixed amount of money with physicians, hospitals, and others. Subacute programs that are part of integrated networks may be providing care to patients within the network, either by being allocated a portion of the network's reimbursement for that patient's care, or under contract to another organization or insurer. They must also consider the relative division of payments among themselves and the physicians and others involved in the care. For example, under capitated arrangements in Southern California, hospitals receive about 36% and physicians about 43% of the reimbursement for non-Medicare patients, and about 43% and 35%, respectively, for Medicare patients (Cerne, 1994).

Any provider considering capitation must recognize the risk that the capitated rate may not cover provider costs or unanticipated increases in utilization. Until the costs of caring for those with multidimensional problems are better defined and more predictable, subacute programs may be prudent not to take on prepaid (capitated) contracts. Per-case or per-diem rates are more favorable for individual providers within the care continuum.

Subacute care programs need enough information to accurately determine patients' needs. Managed care contracting requires rapid negotiation because managed care organizations typically want to transfer a patient within 1 to 2 days of referral. Each subacute program must be able to predict accurately the full cost of providing subacute care, including both routine and ancillary costs. This requires understanding the cost of providing each category or type of care, and tracking the overall facility and per-patient costs. Three suggested steps include determining (1) the facility-wide cost of providing 1 day of routine inpatient care; (2) the average number of nursing hours provided facility-wide by each category of nursing personnel, and the average hourly wage for each category; and (3) the amount of nursing care and ancillary services needed by a prospective patient, based on a detailed assessment of their nursing needs (Froisness, 1994). One key to successful cost accounting lies in detailed understanding and analysis of care processes (see Chapter 7). Some costs of care are problem-independent (for example, assessment and patient education) and others are problem-specific (for example, wound dressing changes). Certain predictable tasks are associated with managing those problems and giving treatments.

The costs of care represent a combination of program-specific, patient-specific, support services, and capital costs. An accounting system must be flexible enough to calculate these costs accurately, and a billing system must be capable of billing different payers with different ways of calculating rates and various billing and payment cycles. To do this, effective computerized cost accounting systems are important tools.

Physician Reimbursement.   There are also various alternatives for physician reimbursement. Physicians must be aware of how they are to be reimbursed for the care of each subacute patient, as it may vary. Managed care organizations (MCOs) may pay them on a fee-for-service basis, or may negotiate a capitation rate with physician-hospital organizations (PHOs) or independent practice associations (IPAs) which will then pay the physician. Or, the physician may bill Medicare or another insurer on a fee-for-service or discounted rate.

Although there are no specific physician billing codes for subacute patients, there are ample hospital and SNF-based service codes to allow for appropriate billing under Medicare. Physicians must be aware of how the facility's subacute beds are licensed so that they can select the correct billing codes. In most cases, they should use SNF billing codes. Many physicians are unaware of the reimbursement opportunities in subacute care, whether in a hospital-based or SNF-based setting. Additionally, older rules limiting the number of SNF physician visits per month have been eliminated, enabling physicians to bill for visits for managing acute illnesses in both the hospital and the SNF as long as these are medically necessary. Table 4–5, p. 72, summarizes the various billing codes relevant to physician SNF-based subacute patient visits. In July 1993, the Health Care Financing Administration (HCFA) also adopted "prolonged visit" codes for intensive visits resulting from higher patient acuity. These codes (99356 and

99357) can be used only to bill for actual patient care contact and the visit must exceed the typical time for a NF visit code by at least 30 minutes.

Review the Regulatory and Certificate of Need (CON) Framework

Bed Conversion Issues.   Subacute beds are being established primarily in hospital-based or freestanding SNFs or NFs or in converted acute care beds. Some state regulations require those wishing to convert beds to another level of care to follow a formal certificate-of-need (CON) process. Certificate-of-need requirements also vary by state. Whether a facility must go through a CON process depends on whether it is converting existing beds or adding new ones for its subacute program, and on how its state handles bed allocation and conversion. Some states count subacute beds separately, while others include them with their acute or long-term care bed inventories. Each program should check local CON requirements carefully and at least inform the state of its actions, even if it is just converting rather than adding beds.

State Licensure.   Most subacute care is being provided under existing state licensure requirements for either hospitals or NFs. In 1995, Illinois included a separate licensure category as part of a pilot program. Other states have created special or supplemental requirements for providers offering certain kinds of care, for example, special regulations for NFs wishing to provide ventilator care. Facilities should check with their state health licensure agency regarding any additional requirements for providing subacute care.

Federal Requirements.   Currently, there are no federal regulations for subacute care. However, SNF- or NF-based subacute care is subject to the same federal regulatory requirements as long-term care. These regulations are based on portions of the 1987 Omnibus Budget Reconciliation Act (OBRA), and hence are referred to as the OBRA '87 requirements. They emphasize the rights of residents and patients in long-term care settings, regardless of the level of care they are receiving. They require facilities to competently manage numerous clinical problems common to institutionalized chronically ill individuals (for example, pressure sores, functional and behavioral problems, use of catheters and feeding tubes, and adequate nutrition and hydration). Thus, although oriented toward the care of the frail elderly, they apply to a large extent to any individual with multiple comorbidities and significant chronic illnesses and disabilities, characteristics common to many of those receiving subacute care. Other references provide more detail about the background (Institute of Medicine, 1986) and content (Medicare and Medicaid requirements for long-term care facilities, 1989) of these requirements, and their implications for practitioners (Levenson, 1993).

Chapter 12 discusses some of the implications of subacute care for the regulatory and licensure process.

Determine Available Resources and Need for Additional Ones

Whether adding beds or using existing ones, creating a subacute unit requires a considerable capital outlay, especially for facilities not accustomed to providing more intensive medical care. A substantial portion of the implementation costs relates to needed physical plant modifications. Such expenses may range between one-half million and several million dollars, depending on the extent of needed renovations and the desired scope of the program and size of the unit.

Facilities must assess their capital available for renovations, for hiring staff, for other start-up costs, and to tide them over while waiting for cash flow as they bill for the services. At least a $500,000 cash reserve is recommended for a facility to be able to make improvements and pay its bills before payments start coming in.

Facilities can raise capital for such projects in several ways. For-profit organizations may do so through investor cash infusions (stock sales), nonprofits through fund-raising, and either may do so by using cash on hand or by deficit financing (revenue bonds).

Joint Hospital–Nursing Facility Ventures.   Hospitals and NFs can develop subacute units separately or jointly. Under managed care, stand-alone programs are less viable. Payments for an episode of care, or for care across a continuum, are likely to dominate. Also, NFs may have the expertise, but not the capital, to develop such units. Therefore, more hospitals and NFs are joining forces (Fisher, 1995). Table 4–6, p. 73, lists the various options for these joint endeavors.

Determine Location, Size, and Physical Aspects of a Unit

Whether part of a hospital, SNF, or NF, subacute units will differ from other parts of the facilities in which they are placed.

NFs must decide whether to create a separate unit for subacute care, or to try to provide the care with the patients scattered among existing long-term care patients. Most observers recommend a separate unit, but sometimes—for instance, in rural facilities—the care has been provided successfully without extensive physical renovations and a dedicated unit. Most freestanding NFs try to locate their units in areas of the building separate from the long-term residents and near a separate entrance. An alternative to a separate outside entrance is having doors that separate the subacute unit from the rest of the facility. A discrete unit may also offer advantages in staffing, staff training, appearance, and cost accounting.

Hospitals should separate subacute from acute care units. Because hospitals giving subacute care under Medicare must follow the requirements for SNFs, they may need such renovations as making bathroom facilities handicapped accessible to be consistent with regulatory requirements.

Whether or not the unit is separate, the program should be distinct in goals, management, and staffing. The program must recognize the general and specific problems and characteristics of patients needing this level of care, as discussed throughout this book. It must have appropriate systems and processes, emphasizing an effective interdisciplinary approach. Regardless of location, the unit's atmosphere should be more relaxed and home-like than the acute hospital, with extensive visiting hours.

Facility/Unit Size.   The size of transitional care units varies. Twenty beds is often cited as the minimum number for financial viability but some successful subacute programs operate with fewer. Most units range from 20 to 50 beds. Facility size does not appear to be a major barrier to establishing subacute services, and many subacute units are in medium-sized (101 to 149 bed) NFs.

Depending on the services offered, the unit may need to be large enough to include a rehabilitation therapy area, respiratory therapy utility room, patient dining room/day room, social services office, administrator's and director of nursing's office, examination or procedure area, reception/admitting area, and family room. Units providing physical rehabilitation programs should have dedicated space for physical and occupational therapy services. There should also be adequate space for activities programs, perhaps in conjunction with the occupational therapy space.

Rooms and Room Size.   The unit should have both semiprivate and private patient rooms. Existing rooms may need to be reconfigured to accommodate special beds and equipment. For example, rooms with ventilators should ordinarily not have more than two beds. It is useful to install custom cabinets in or outside each room so that specialized equipment and supplies will be readily available. Room and over-bed lighting should be bright enough to allow physical assessment and to enhance the environment. Many patients want in-room telephones and televisions, necessitating the wiring and space.

Equipment and Supplies.   Equipment and supplies should be of sufficient quality and quantity to enable both effective and efficient care. A regular preventive maintenance program is essential. Because of the higher acuity level of patients in transitional units, electric beds and a nurse call system are essential. For units giving ventilator care, central suction and piped-in oxygen may be more convenient, although they are not essential. Physical plant modifications to install these features may involve major costly construction and electrical work.

Electrical Capacity.   The unit's electrical capacity must be evaluated. It may need to be upgraded for any of the following: ventilator care, generator capacity, suctioning equipment, defibrillators, cardiac monitors, additional electrical outlets, or better air conditioning. A reliable backup system is needed to handle peak loads and additional demands. Some facilities wire each ventilator unit and power source directly to the generator. Wiring should also accommodate computers, printers, faxes, and other items essential to an efficient computer-based information system.

Ventilation System.   The unit's ventilation system must accommodate patients admitted who require special isolation for tuberculosis (TB) or other airborne pathogens. Existing systems should be evaluated for possible modifications.

The Centers for Disease Control (CDC) recommends that health care facilities assess the risk of TB transmission throughout the facility. The facility should place itself in one of five risk categories (high, intermediate, low, very low, or minimal risk). Patients who are isolated because of TB should remain in their rooms with the doors closed. For isolation, single-patient rooms should be used and the ventilation system maintained under negative pressure. The air should be exhausted to the outside. If that is impossible, special filters should be installed in the exhaust duct leading from the room to the general ventilation system. On a given subacute unit, the number of such rooms will depend on the risk of TB transmission in the facility, geographic region, or occupational groups from which patients are derived (Centers for Disease Control, 1994).

Transportation.   Subacute patients may need to be transported to other sites for testing or ancillary services. The facility may need to upgrade transportation services for the subacute patients, or may need a different kind of vehicle to accommodate those with portable ventilators, oxygen equipment, or other equipment.

Establish Program Goals and Objectives

Each program should establish its goals and objectives (Table 4–7, p. 74). These should provide a broad overview of its intended market, how it proposes to meet the market's needs, the scope of programs and services, and how the program relates to other parts of the organization and care continuum. These goals and objectives should be created via an interdisciplinary discussion including governance, management, practitioners, support staff, and the community. The board and/or owners should also review and approve the goals and objectives.

STEPS FOR PROGRAM IMPLEMENTATION

Review Strengths and Weaknesses of Current Clinical Programs

Each program should review its current programs and services and see how it can build upon them in developing its subacute program. It may help to categorize subacute programs as basic and more advanced. Basic subacute programs can more readily build on existing facility programs and services. For example, a NF that had already been offering skilled rehabilitation could use its staffing and systems as the basis for a broader rehabilitation program for those with more intensive or complex rehabilitation needs. Similarly, a facility already giving intravenous fluids for some patients could expand on this to offer infusion therapies. These services would require relatively modest capital investments.

For these reasons, many NFs start their subacute programs with rehabilitation, infusion therapies, and wound care services. These programs can be set up in about 4 months. Because many NFs already provide rehabilitation services, just operating a subacute rehabilitation program may be simpler than developing an entirely new level of care, such as medical subacute care.

More advanced subacute programs—which might include dialysis, ventilator care, or pain management—usually take at least 6 months to plan and market and another 6 months to implement. They typically require more numerous and more highly trained staff, physical plant renovations, and additional equipment and supplies. Even after implementation, a more advanced subacute program requires at least 12 to 18 months to provide a return on the initial investment.

Design and Implement a Care Management and Delivery System

Every program needs an organized approach to care that operates effectively 7 days a week. This must involve close collaboration among all parties including practitioners, support staff, patients, management, and ownership.

The foundations of such a system should be in place by the time the program starts. Existing systems and processes may need to be modified to meet the needs of the subacute program. Table 4–8, p. 74, lists the steps in creating a care management and delivery system, and the chapters in which related discussions can be found.

Find, Train, and Retain Practitioners and Other Staff

Subacute programs must coordinate many different individuals from diverse backgrounds (see Table 6–10, p. 151). They need competent, dependable practitioners and support staff who can appreciate the characteristics of this level of care and the needs of the patients, and who can thrive under an interdisciplinary approach in a managed care environment. But relatively few skilled practitioners and capable managers enjoy and understand transitional care and are willing to conform with its essential attitudes and processes. Recognizing the competition for such individuals and their great value, facilities must strive to select, hire, and retain experienced direct care, management, and support staff. To help retain their staff, they must appreciate and support the challenges of providing transitional care. Because the work is often difficult and complex, staff will be influenced by how they are treated and the support they receive. Salary adjustments and enhanced employee benefits are attractions, but they also must be accompanied by a good work environment and effective systems support.

Determining the appropriate level and scope of practitioner and staff support must be based on analyzing the programs and services to be offered, which in turn results from anticipating the likely needs and problems of the patients who are to be admitted and the essential processes of care. For instance, the problems and risk areas for patients receiving various services, and the roles of the different players, can be defined and anticipated (see Tables 5–3 to 5–17, pp. 94–119). This knowledge can help a program better refine its staffing needs.

Subacute programs should emphasize those aspects of care that might appeal to their staff. For example, some nurses who would formerly have worked only in hospitals may be attracted by the greater variety and medical orientation of subacute patients compared to the traditional NF. Some NF staff may be attracted by the opportunity to broaden their skills and experience. Diverse practitioners may also appreciate the opportunity to give more personal as well as technical care to their patients, because the patients stay longer and need their psychosocial and functional, as well as medical, problems managed jointly.

Define Quality Indicators and Performance Standards

Despite the current scarcity of national standards for subacute care, the programs still have civil and administrative liabilities. The facility is always under the duty of due care. Subacute providers can be found negligent for failing to meet commonly accepted national standards and for not following their own policies and procedures (Miles, 1994). They must ensure the availability of appropriate staff and resources. Competitive pressures to admit patients must be weighed against available resources to provide the care (Infante, 1994).

One way to reduce risk is by complying with existing standards and regulations, such as state licensure laws and federal regulations regarding NFs. Many subacute programs are becoming accredited by organizations such as the Joint Commission on Accreditation of Healthcare Organizations (JCAHO), which has developed specific subacute standards.

Subacute programs must establish and use quality programs. As discussed in Chapters 9 and 10, this includes imparting appropriate attitudes, using relevant quality indicators, establishing performance monitoring mechanisms, assessing patient-care-related data, and providing feedback to the various players.

Practice guidelines and protocols may come from government agencies, independent organizations, and other sources. The medical and nursing literature contains substantial information about appropriate practices despite the fact that much of this may not be widely standardized. Therefore, programs and practitioners have ample resources to help them find the basis for quality indicators and practice guidelines. However, they may find it time consuming to track these down and confusing as to which ones they should employ.

SNF- and NF-based subacute programs must pay particular attention to federal requirements (for example, resident rights, Minimum Data Set, and quality of life). The relevance of these requirements has been challenged because they were developed for a residential long-term care population. However, much of subacute care includes management of comparable problems and requires some similar assessments. Eventually, they might be revised to be more flexible for different levels of care delivered at the same site.

Establish Training and Education Programs

Chapters 5 through 8 consider knowledge and skills relevant to the various programs, players, and processes. Effective performance requires a formal system and informal approach to education and training, which address both knowledge and performance. This is discussed in more detail in Chapter 9.

Market Programs

Each program should develop a marketing plan to promote the services. Facilities contemplating subacute programs should perform appropriate market analyses (Table 4–9, p. 75). When managed care payers and hospitals need placement, they expect decisions to be made within 24 to 48 hours. However, contractual agreements with payers do not ensure referrals to the subacute program. A program's marketing team must still actively encourage referrals and ensure timely placement when discharge is imminent.

Matching Reality to Promises.   The literature about subacute care contains many discussions about selling subacute programs—that is, how to maintain high occupancy, how to attract referral sources, and how to convince patients and families to want to come. However, marketing activities must be closely coordinated with the staff's capacity to *provide* the care. Providers cannot just establish a unit and claim to deliver subacute care.

As discussed in Chapter 5, each subacute category (pulmonary care, rehabilitation, cardiac care, and so on) covers a broad spectrum of medical conditions, problems, and service needs. For instance, a ventilator patient's needs could range from short-term support to the care of catastrophic, irreversible ventilatory failure. Thus, the subacute program cannot say "We give subacute care" or "We have a ventilator service" without further qualifying the levels or complexity of the services.

In any program, one of the highest-risk areas is that of the perceptions and assumptions of patients and families who enter the program. They often come to a subacute unit after a major episode of acute illness or injury with little detailed understanding of what has happened, what will happen next, or realistic care objectives. Because many care outcomes are less than curative, and because complications often arise in this patient population, the credibility of the program and its staff strongly influences how patients and families react to problems and complications. The same result can elicit appreciation or anger depending on expectations.

Although the management and marketing staff want to present the brightest possible picture, they must understand the realities of care and the limitations of their program. They should not promise things that the staff cannot deliver, and should try not to admit patients that the staff cannot care for and the facility cannot support. One or several disasters can cause major legal complications and can quickly inhibit referrals. Therefore, key clinical leadership should review the marketing plan and the contents of any written or verbal information to be presented to referral sources.

EXAMPLE

Determined to fill the beds and expand capacity, a subacute program administrator continually overrode the concerns and objections of his staff, and told his marketing staff to assure referral sources that the program could handle any patients they could send. Unfortunately, the program was understaffed because of the administrator's budget demands and the support services and staff could not keep up with the patient turnover. Several serious complications arose because of gaps in care and support. The administrator attributed all of these to staff incompetence despite the pleas of key clinical leadership. The administrator refused to acknowledge any responsibility for contributing to the problems, saying repeatedly, "We've got to keep those beds filled."

Marketing staff must be trained about subacute care and the relevant aspects of the facility's program so that they can answer specific questions likely to be posed by managed care organizations and other payers. Marketing staff should shift from selling the program based on generalities and be prepared to show objectively how the program can help achieve desirable care objectives (optimal service, lowest cost, shortest time, measurable outcomes), especially under a managed care approach.

Physicians and Marketing.   Physicians have a unique position in the subacute program. They are needed to define and manage the medical causes of a patient's problems and to diagnose and treat complications and other fluctuations in condition. But they are often not the major decision makers, may have a limited role in implementing the care plan, and may only occasionally be on site. Care outcomes are the result of the efforts of many other individuals as well.

Subacute programs are likely to be more successful if their physicians understand and are interested in the care and the facility's programs. But some physicians may not understand subacute care and may be reluctant to admit their patients or to attend on a subacute unit. A subacute program must get physicians to recognize that the care is relevant, that they have a vital role which is different than in other settings, and that they can get reimbursed for their care.

Therefore, marketing to physicians must be educational as well as promotional. It may help to get the participation of various physician groups in the community while developing the program. For example, ventilator programs might be developed with the participation of pulmonologists.

The program medical director is a natural candidate for such efforts. However, programs that just use their medical directors to sell the unit to outside physicians may overlook the various ongoing systems and process issues that a physician leader must address. They should not confuse the clinical participation of specialists with true medical direction.

Eventually, as medical care shifts more from the hospital to alternative settings and care is provided as part of a continuum, more physicians may appreciate alternatives such as subacute care. Also, the placement of subacute patients depends increasingly on payers and discharge planners rather than on physician preferences.

REFERENCES

Centers for Disease Control. Draft guidelines for isolation precautions in hospitals. *Federal Register*. 1994; 59(214):55552–55570.

Cerne F. Shaping up for capitation. *Hosp Health Netw.* 1994; 68(7):28–37.

Fisher C. Facilities, hospitals, working together. *Provider*. 1995; 21(7):43–45.

Froisness R. The financial path to managed care. *Provider*. April 1994; 47–48.

Infante M. Subacute units need to be aware of standards. *Contemp Long-Term Care*. 1994; 17(4):64.

Institute of Medicine (Committee on Nursing Home Regulations). *Improving the Quality of Care in Nursing Homes*. Washington, DC: National Academy Press; 1986.

Levenson S. *Medical Direction in Long-term Care*. 2nd ed. Durham, NC: Carolina Academic Press; 1993.

Lumsdon K. Subacute care. Like ants to a picnic. *Hosp Health Netw*. 1995; 69(10):47.

Medicare and Medicaid requirements for long-term care facilities. *Federal Register*. 1989; 54(21):5316–5373.

Miles F. Subacute and civil liability. *Provider*. 1994; 20(9):63–64.

FOR FURTHER READING

AHCA (American Health Care Association). *Medical and Rehabilitation Definition and Guide to Business Development*. Washington, DC: AHCA; 1994.

Anders KT. Is subacute care right for you? *Contemp Long-Term Care*. June 1994:32–42.

Buss DD. As the staff turns. *Contemp Long-Term Care*. 1994; 17(8):61–66.

Micheletti JA, Shlala TJ. Understanding and operationalizing subacute services. *Nurs Manage*. 1995; 26(6):49, 51–52, 54–56.

Nichols D. California project would pay subacute facilities for acute care. *Contemp Long-Term Care*. June 1994; 22.

Stahl DA. Maximizing reimbursement for subacute care. *Nurs Manage*. 1995; 26(4):16–17, 19.

Stahl DA. Development of subacute care services. *Nurs Manage*. 1994; 25(11):32–34.

Tokarski C. Riding the express. Is your subacute strategy on track? *Hosp Health Netw*. 1995; 69(13):20–23.

TABLE 4–1	STEPS TO ESTABLISHING A SUBACUTE PROGRAM

Planning
- Assess opportunities and risks.
- Perform a market analysis.
- Review reimbursement opportunities and limits.
- Review regulatory and CON framework.
- Determine available resources and need for additional ones.
- Determine location, size, and physical aspects of a unit.
- Establish program goals and objectives.

Implementation
- Review current clinical programs and strengths.
- Design and implement a care management and delivery system.
- Find, train, and retain practitioners and other staff.
- Establish quality and performance standards.
- Establish training and education programs.
- Market programs.

TABLE 4–2	CHALLENGES FOR HOSPITALS AND NURSING FACILITIES ESTABLISHING SUBACUTE PROGRAMS

	Hospitals	Nursing Facilities
Business		
• Dealing with managed care organizations	✓	✓
• Calculating care costs effectively to enable appropriate managed care contract negotiations	✓	✓
• Asserting tight control over supplies, recovery of reimbursement, and control of waste	✓	✓
• Reducing overhead	✓	
• Expanding potential referral sources	✓	✓
• Creating an effective, pertinent marketing program	✓	✓
Clinical		
• Shifting mindset from resident care to patient care		✓
• Shifting from care of diseases to problem management approach	✓	
• Handling much more rapid patient turnover and multiple daily admissions		✓
• Learning to emphasize early intervention, prevention, and risk-management activities	✓	✓
• Augmenting current preventive maintenance program		✓
• Improving staff assessment, documentation, and problem analytic skills	✓	✓
• Establishing appropriate staffing and management for the unit	✓	✓
• Creating effective, pertinent clinical systems and processes	✓	✓
• Ensuring appropriate clinical and general support systems	✓	✓
• Reorienting staff used to aggressive, procedure-oriented, high-acuity care	✓	
• Learning to create appropriate patient and family expectations	✓	✓

TABLE 4–3   REIMBURSEMENT ALTERNATIVES FOR SUBACUTE CARE PROGRAMS

Methodology	Description	Impact on Providers	Impact on Payers
Fee-for-service	Reimburses provider based on lesser of booked costs or the usual and customary charges	Least risk to provider	Usually greatest exposure to payer; little incentive to limit services
Straight discount	Provider receives fee-for-service rate minus negotiated discounted amount	Provider can still bill for costs at lower rate; volume can make up for discount	Also relatively little incentive to limit services
Per diem (all-inclusive rate)	Provider receives a pre-determined amount per patient day without any adjustment for the type, amount, or frequency of actual services provided	Provider can anticipate payment without having to itemize charges	Shifts substantial financial risk to provider
Per diem (partly exclusive rate)	Same as above, except provider receives separate re-imbursement for specified services such as physical therapies and pharmaceuticals	Provider at lower risk than with all-inclusive per diem	Ancillaries can add substantially to cost of care overall
Fixed per-case rate	Provider receives pre-determined amount per patient stay based on diagnosis or condition, similar to the hospital diagnosis-related group (DRG) payment	Provider at high level of financial risk Provider knows amount of reimbursement in advance	Shifts most of risk to provider
Capitation rate	Provider receives flat fee for all enrollees in a managed care health plan regardless of whether the members of the health plan actually use the services	Greatest financial risk for the provider Incentive to reduce quantity and duration of expensive services	Unclear if capitated approach can work with complex care of those with multiple comorbidities and fluctuating conditions

TABLE 4–4   ISSUES RELATED TO COST EXCEPTIONS FOR DEVELOPING SUBACUTE CARE UNITS
                                            UNDER MEDICARE

Requirements (Must Meet at Least One)
- Provision of atypical services
- Extraordinary circumstances—floods, earthquakes, strikes
- Unusual labor costs represent a high percentage of total costs
- Providing services in areas with fluctuating populations

Steps in Obtaining an Atypical Services Exception
- Calculate atypical service costs
- Show reasonableness of individual cost centers when compared to peer group
- Demonstrate higher case mix
- Submit package for intermediary/Health Care Financing Administration review

TABLE 4–5   MOST RELEVANT BILLING CODES FOR PHYSICIAN PATIENT VISITS IN SNF-BASED SUBACUTE UNITS

Code	Description	Examples
99303	**Initial admission or readmission** • Comprehensive history, comprehensive examination, and medical decision making of moderate to high complexity • Medical plan of care must be created in conjunction with the facility requirement to perform a comprehensive initial assessment • Time spent (approximately 50 minutes at the bedside and on the patient's floor or unit) may include counseling and/or coordination of care with other providers or agencies depending on the problems and needs of the patient and family	Admission or readmission of a subacute patient
99311	**Subsequent evaluation and management of a new or established patient** including at least two of the following: a problem-focused interval history, a problem-focused examination, and medical decision making that is straightforward or of low complexity • Time spent at the bedside and on the unit would be about 15 minutes	Routine visit to a subacute patient who has been mostly stable medically and functionally
99312	**Subsequent evaluation and management of a new or established patient** including at least two of the following: an expanded problem-focused interval history, an expanded problem-focused examination, and medical decision making that is straightforward or of low complexity • Time spent at the bedside and on the unit would be about 25 minutes	Visit to a patient who needs adjustment of medications and medical care plan, has some fluctuations in condition, requires examination of several organ systems, has developed a minor complication of an existing problem, or who has a fairly uncomplicated new problem that needs medical evaluation or follow-up
99313	**Subsequent evaluation and management of a new or established patient** including at least two of the following: a detailed interval history, a detailed examination, and medical decision making of moderate to high complexity • Time spent at the bedside and on the unit would be about 35 minutes	Patient who has developed a significant complication or new problem that requires an extensive differential diagnosis, a detailed history and physical, test ordering, and new medications

TABLE 4–6   OPTIONS FOR HOSPITAL–NURSING FACILITY COLLABORATION IN SUBACUTE CARE

Option	Description	Implications for Partners
Joint ownership	• Hospital and nursing facility form third legal entity with shared capital. • Facility is separately licensed and has own Medicare/Medicaid provider number.	• Governance and management, profits and losses shared between hospital and nursing facility.
Leasing	• Separately licensed subacute provider takes revenues, but makes lease payments to hospital. • Subacute provider governs facility and revenues, but can contract to share day-to-day management with hospital.	• NF saves on capital costs of development; hospital provides predictable patient source, personnel, and resources. • Hospital expands access to care; its only revenue sources are lease payments and shared services contract.
Management	• Hospital owns licensed subacute unit on site; NF manages unit.	• Hospital keeps profits, pays NF management fee. • NF avoids capital outlays, gets hospital referrals. • Hospital expands access to care; able to scrutinize operation and performance more closely than under leasing arrangement.
Shared services	• Hospital and NF do not share ownership. • Fees determined by services provided. • Can use existing space at either hospital or NF.	• Management, governance, and licensing arrangements may vary. • Both partners have flexibility.
Bed reserve and priority	• Hospital contracts with licensed NF for reserved beds or priority patient placement.	• Used when access to NF beds is difficult or hospital unable to develop its own subacute program. • NF has guaranteed source of income and secure patient referral source. • Hospital has low-cost, low-risk option for placing subacute patients that would otherwise have to stay in hospital.

Adapted with permission from Fisher C. Facilities, hospitals, working together. *Provider.* 1995; 21(7):43–45. Washington DC: American Healthcare Association.

TABLE 4–7	EXAMPLES OF GOALS AND OBJECTIVES FOR A SUBACUTE PROGRAM[a]

- **Deliver optimal, cost-effective care to individuals who need a package of services including management of some phase of an acute illness.**
  Offer a spectrum of programs and services.
  Ensure that the care meets appropriate quality standards.
  Provide care efficiently and in a fiscally responsible fashion.
  Individualize care based on careful assessment and problem identification.
  Employ an internal case management system to promote interdisciplinary collaboration and efficient care.
  Serve as part of an effective health care continuum.

- **Strive for optimum levels of patient independence.**
  Assess each individual's strengths and limitations.
  Emphasize rehabilitative and restorative care.

- **Support physical and psychological adjustments to long-term physical and functional impairments.**
  Educate patients and families about the short- and long-range outcomes of conditions and treatments.
  Provide programs and services that can help individuals cope with the implications of limited recovery or decline.

[a]Goals are shown in bold type, objectives in regular type.

TABLE 4–8	STEPS IN ESTABLISHING AN EFFECTIVE CARE MANAGEMENT AND DELIVERY SYSTEM

- Identify the services to be provided within the program (Chapter 5).
- Define and implement a process for appropriate patient identification and selection (Chapters 2, 3, 7).
- Identify roles and responsibilities of all players, consistent with an effective team approach (Chapter 6).
- Identify processes of care, and roles of various players in those processes (Chapter 7).
- Define and implement a system to assess patient needs and problems, and match them to available services (Chapter 7).
- Create a system to coordinate care delivery (Chapter 8).
- Create and implement a system to support those delivering the care (Chapter 8).
- Create and implement general support systems for all processes and players (Chapter 9).
- Create and implement a process to oversee the care (Chapter 9) and assess outcomes (Chapter 10).

TABLE 4–9   STEPS INVOLVED IN A MARKETING ANALYSIS FOR SUBACUTE CARE

- Identify potential or actual competitors.
- Assess referral patterns of insurance case managers and hospital discharge planners.
- Discuss with referral sources the types of patients they find most difficult to place.
- Investigate physician practices and physician/hospital referral patterns.
- Compare competitors' charges.
- Discuss managed care expectations.
- Review regulatory, licensure, and CON issues.
- Review area hospital statistics on patient care types and DRGs.
- Define patient populations to be served.

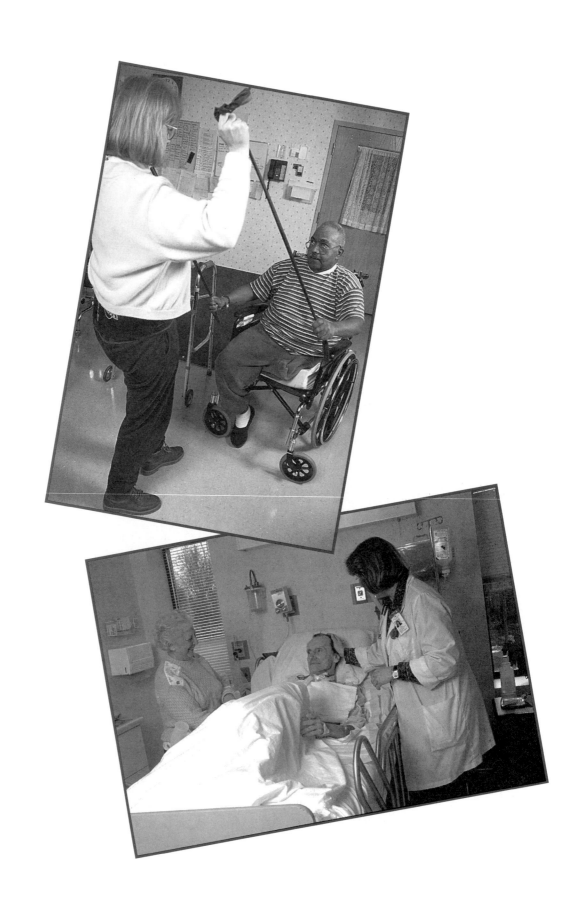

CLINICAL PROGRAMS AND SERVICES

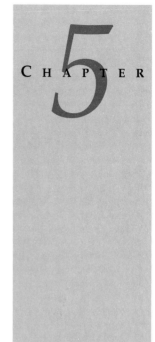

CHAPTER 5

Chapters 2 and 3 identified the common characteristics of subacute patients and the place of subacute services in the care continuum. Understanding patient characteristics and problems and knowing what is needed to manage those problems helps clarify essential service needs. By knowing the components involved in delivering those services and how they might best be organized it is possible to define specific programs and services for the subacute patient.

This chapter will identify the various subacute programs and the relevant roles and functions of the practitioners and others who provide the care. Subsequent chapters will address other related issues: integration of the various disciplines and individuals involved in delivering and overseeing the services (Chapter 6), the processes involved in delivering the care and the roles of the disciplines in those processes (Chapter 7), the organization of those individuals and disciplines into effective clinical services and support systems (Chapter 8), and the general support systems needed by all players in the program (Chapter 9). It is then possible to create and use relevant quality indicators and quality management systems (Chapter 10) to assess the success of the care and the systems supporting it.

Subacute care is commonly discussed and marketed by reference to its clinical programs (Table 5–1, p. 92). Clinical programs are identifiable packages of care involving certain discrete activities or functions by collections of individuals. For example, a wound management program is a collection of processes of assessment, monitoring, management, and follow-up for individuals with complicated or extensive acute or chronic wounds resulting from causes such as amputation, malignancy, surgery, vascular insufficiency, and chronic infection. The processes are performed by physicians, nurses, and others.

Some patient care needs are condition-specific, many are problem-specific, and some are generic. Condition-specific needs relate to a particular circumstance. For example, a knee-replacement patient has needs related to the surgery (braces, splints, physical therapy of the leg) that a cardiac rehabilitation patient would not have. Problem-specific needs cut across conditions. As discussed in Chapter 7, some common situations and problems (for example, depression, altered cognitive function, volume deficit) could occur in any patient regardless of admission reason. Therefore, the care plan for all subacute patients must be defined not only by the treatments they receive for their most prominent condition but by the overall care they require for their existing or potential secondary problems. Generic needs are the core group of services including assessment, monitoring, treatment, and follow-up that are provided in various combinations for each subacute patient regardless of his/her diagnosis or primary reason for receiving the care.

Treatments and Procedures

Subacute patients commonly undergo certain treatments and procedures (catheter insertion, drainage tubes, and the like). Most major procedures are done in the hospital before transfer. Others may be done on the unit (Table 5–2, pp. 92–93).

The program's staffing must distinguish (1) care needs resulting from previously performed procedures, (2) the time and skills involved in performing procedures, and (3) the time and skills involved in monitoring for the results and complications of the procedures. Each one of these uses staff time differently. For example, a chest tube may have been placed in the hospital. On the subacute unit, the chest tube drainage must be monitored, the dressings changed, and the patient observed for local complications such as bleeding and infection. Adequate support staff, supplies, and equipment are essential to enable appropriate practitioners to perform essential procedures quickly and easily on the unit. The equipment should be maintained effectively. Problems reported by staff or physicians related to procedures, equipment, or supplies should be logged and tended to promptly. Any supply or equipment problems that could have contributed to morbidity or wasted staff time should be referred to the quality management program for review and follow-up.

Quality Oversight.   A mechanism is needed to ensure that procedures are done correctly. A checklist should detail the steps for each procedure. Specific, detailed protocols should exist for performing each procedure and for the subsequent care of the devices or items (catheters, tubes, implantable devices) inserted during the procedure. These protocols should be developed collaboratively by relevant disciplines, including the medical staff. They should be used on each unit by all shifts.

In most subacute programs, relatively few medical procedures are done but there are many nursing procedures. Sometimes, physicians will perform procedures on the unit; at other times they will transfer patients elsewhere to perform the procedure. As part of the credentialing process (see Chapter 8), physicians should be appropriately qualified to do these procedures.

Additionally, other nonphysicians who perform procedures should demonstrate their competence, which may require direct observation and confirmation by a supervisor or manager. The quality assessment program should review the results and complications of these procedures.

COMMON CLINICAL PROGRAMS

The common subacute care programs are discussed in more detail in the sections that follow. Each discussion is accompanied by a table that addresses the program objectives and components. Inevitably, there is a certain amount of overlap among these services and the patients they treat. For example, patients in many service categories receive some rehabilitation therapies, and a pediatric service might provide elements of head injury care, postoperative care, and ventilator care. A predominant or primary service need for one individual may be a secondary need for another. Thus, different programs may well treat comparable patients in programs or services of different names. This does not matter as long as there is the flexibility to provide essential components of care and service to individuals based on their needs.

For the purposes of this book, some of the services are considered to be subsets of a larger program (for example, stroke rehabilitation is included as part of rehabilitation even though it may have some unique associated issues). Others (for example, cardiac recovery) have been split out because they are commonly found as discrete programs in subacute settings. However, this in no way suggests that various programs could not or should not arrange services differently.

Table 5–17 at the end of the chapter, pp. 114–119, notes the principal roles and functions of the main clinical disciplines involved in each program. It is consolidated, because many of these roles are similar in the various programs. Also, it does not include all possible individuals, some of whom are noted in the program-related tables and others of whom (for example, clergy) are discussed in Chapter 6. This separation is not meant to imply that their roles and participation are less valuable.

AIDS Patient Care

An AIDS service (Table 5–3, p. 94) is intended for the evaluation and management of HIV-positive individuals and those with AIDS who have significant complications and instability as a result of their illness, or who need follow-up treatment after a recent hospitalization. A typical patient is a young HIV-positive male who has had recurrent hospitalizations for infections.

Infections are the most prominent and serious of these patients' problems. Because many AIDS patients choose to receive home-based services for as long as possible, they usually do not require subacute care unless they have pain or other major medical complications such as a significant opportunistic infection. These latter are typically caused either by common organisms with more severe consequences than in non-HIV patients or by opportunistic parasitic, fungal, and viral infections. There may also be other medical, functional, and psychosocial problems associated with this major immune system disorder.

Treating these patients presents several conspicuous issues, including infection control and ethical and social concerns. Subacute AIDS care programs need a strong infection control program to ensure that proper precautions, including isolation when needed, are taken. Decisions must be made about when to isolate AIDS patients from others for the protection of one or the other. The immunocompromised status of these patients makes them susceptible to serious consequences of infections from organisms carried by others, and makes the patients susceptible to carrying tuberculosis or other infectious agents that may put others at risk. Expensive, relatively uncommon intravenous and oral medications are often needed to treat the infections.

Equipment, supplies, and staff training to handle isolation patients are needed. The program must be able to start and maintain intravenous infusions, and depend on pharmacy support to obtain and prepare the medications properly. Also, the nurses and physicians must be able to recognize the onset, course, and complications of these infections and other conditions.

Another essential component is a well-developed system for managing ethical issues and documenting patient treatment choices. Many of these individuals are at different stages in the dying process and require appropriate support and counseling. Although some of them will continue to have recurrent illnesses, they may be discharge candidates despite expected recurrence of their problems. Some patients may be candidates for long-term care or home care fairly soon after admission. Subsequent decisions must be made regularly about when to send them back to the hospital and how aggressive to be if their overall condition declines.

AIDS patients may also present certain social and behavioral issues more often than other subacute patient categories. These may include the absence of an effective family support system, a history of drug or other substance abuse, highly manipulative behaviors, and the management of an often terminal illness in a young individual. The psychosocial problems may influence subsequent placement as much as the medical ones do.

Cardiac Recovery

A cardiac recovery program (Table 5–4, pp. 95–96) is intended for individuals who have complications of heart disease or who need continuing management after surgery or other treatment for heart disease. This typically combines both medical management and rehabilitation therapies. Case examples include recent valve replacement or bypass surgery, recent acute myocardial infarction, continuing management of endocarditis, and continued management and rehabilitation after severe heart failure or cardiogenic shock.

Cardiac patients require substantial observation and may have sudden condition changes requiring rapid assessment and intervention. The program must have explicit guidelines for what it can manage and when patients should be considered for transfer. Patient and family expectations about monitoring and intervention capabilities must be clarified. For example, the subacute unit is not an intensive care unit and only rarely provides continuous cardiac monitoring. The program may offer only basic cardiopulmonary resuscitation (CPR). Some staff training in assessing symptoms and recognizing significant arrhythmias and other condition changes is important.

Cardiac Rehabilitation. The objectives of cardiac rehabilitation are to improve functional and physical work capacity, better control risk factors, provide education about cardiovascular disease and its management, offer psychosocial support and reassurance, reduce anxiety and depression, increase a person's sense of well-being, and help the individual return to customary routines. Typical patients are those who have had an acute myocardial infarction (MI), those with problematic but currently stable congestive heart failure, and those who have undergone a heart transplant, percutaneous transluminal coronary angioplasty (PTCA), or heart valve surgery.

The need for a supervised program often depends on function and complications. Generally, the trend toward more aggressive inpatient management of acute MI has led to a much better prognosis and functional capacity. The effects of cardiac rehabilitation on prolonging life and preventing recurrence following MI remain unproven. Two meta-analyses of studies on exercise-based programs in the years immediately following MI suggest improved survival, but the studies do not clarify the relative impact of the nonexercise and exercise components of the programs (Amsterdam et al, 1994). One nonrandomized study suggests that participation in cardiac rehabilitation may lower cardiac rehospitalization costs in the 3 years following a coronary event, but it does not exclude the possibility that those going into a rehab program had healthier behaviors initially (Ades et al, 1992).

Physical inactivity is an independent risk factor for heart disease and relates to cardiovascular mortality. Therefore, exercise is a key component of cardiac rehabilitation programs. Another important component is psychological support to help the patient deal with any concerns about the effects of chronic illness, limits on personal and work-related functioning, family roles, body image, and sexual activity. Depression and delirium—both risk factors for increased morbidity and mortality—may occur after acute MI (Frasure-Smith et al, 1993). Anxiety accompanied by denial is also common. Any medications used to treat psychological disturbances should be selected carefully to try to minimize their impact on cardiovascular functioning. Other components include dietary interventions, help in smoking cessation, and group therapy and other peer support. Services in each case should be based on the patient's overall condition, presence of risk factors, pulmonary reserve capacity, comorbidities (associated medical problems), and treatment goals.

Dialysis/Renal Failure

A renal program (Table 5–5, pp. 96–97) is for the management of individuals who have recent acute renal failure or decompensated chronic renal failure. This often—but not necessarily—includes either peritoneal dialysis or hemodialysis. However, because dialysis can be given at home or in an outpatient setting, the subacute renal failure patient should be unstable enough to require close monitoring and treatment adjustments that cannot be provided elsewhere. Some additional problems needing the attention of a more intensive setting might include pain, complications of dialysis, or more severe or complicated fluid and electrolyte imbalances. Depending on the degree and reversibility of their renal failure, some of these patients may also potentially be candidates for a hospice program.

For those receiving dialysis, a potential obstacle to discharge may be the difficulty in placing them in a community-based dialysis program. Inquiries about such arrangements should be initiated soon after admission to try to ensure essential postdischarge support.

Medically Complex Care

A medically complex care service (Table 5–6, pp. 98–99) covers a multitude of conditions and needs. Its major purpose is to provide either (1) continuing care of patients with multiple medical and functional problems and complications prolonging their recuperative period or (2) short-stay assessment and management of relatively uncomplicated acute conditions that require a moderate degree of monitoring and some treatment but are not accompanied by high instability.

Medically complex patients tend to need not only management of a principal condition or diagnosis but also monitoring and management of comorbidities and potential complications. Like others with complex chronic or acute conditions, they are periodically prone to suffer adverse clinical events—episodic recurrences or exacerbations of their underlying illnesses or the onset of a new condition (Bernardini et al, 1993).

There are several varieties of medically complex care, including infusion therapy, oncology/cancer care, pain management, and hospice/terminal care.

Infusion Therapy (Including Transfusions).   Infusion therapy is a service for individuals who require infusions of fluids and nutrients and who have additional needs for monitoring and assessment that cannot be provided in an alternate setting. The need for infusion alone is rarely enough justification for subacute care because infusions may be handled in other settings such as home or a nursing facility. Those requiring additional monitoring and more intensive treatment might include patients who have become more confused and debilitated because of significant dehydration and electrolyte imbalance, those with active illness causing bleeding and hypotension, and those with severe pain requiring frequent medication adjustments and supplementation to arrive at an appropriate dose.

Common infusions include fluids and potassium supplements, antibiotics, blood and blood products, chemotherapies, and other medications. The program needs appropriate supplies and equipment, including infusion pumps. It requires individuals who can calculate proper dosages; who are skilled in starting, monitoring, and adjusting these infusions; who can manage the various lines and devices; and who can help adjust the medications and treatments based on assessing a patient's fluctuating condition (Nicholson, 1993).

Oncology/Cancer Care.   An oncology program (Table 5–7, pp. 99–100) provides continuing care for patients who have undergone surgery, chemotherapy, radiation, immunotherapy, or hormone therapy as a result of cancer. The subacute unit is more likely to deal with the complications of the illness or the treatment along with other factors such as infection, nutritional deficit, and pain management.

The staff should be able to recognize and manage these problems and complications. They may also need to administer chemotherapy in some cases, but patients are often transported elsewhere for their radiation or chemotherapy treatments.

Patients with cancer may arrive in the program at any stage, from newly diagnosed to terminal. Because of the rapid treatment and discharge in hospitals, these patients and their families may not have received a clear indication of the prognosis, care plan, or potential complications. As with many other patients, the program may need to take the time to educate the patients and families about these issues so that they will have more realistic expectations. The staff also must deal with terminal illness and ethical decision-making challenges.

Pain Management.   A pain management service (Table 5–8, p. 101) is intended for the care of individuals with pain requiring comprehensive management, including frequent titration of medications and the possible use of other pain relief modalities. Typical patients are those with severe or prolonged pain postoperatively or from chronic conditions, cancer, or neurological or musculoskeletal disorders. The service's major objectives are to relieve pain, to address medical and psychosocial issues that may be influencing or causing the pain, and to allow the individual to function more effectively in social, family, and work situations. The service typically combines medical, nursing, and rehabilitative approaches. Various measures may include medications, mechanical devices, rehabilitative therapies, and psychosocial and recreational interventions to address underlying causes.

Hospice/Terminal Care.   Two categories of terminal care (Table 5–9, pp. 102–103) may be identified, one where the individual has specifically chosen to receive terminal care only, and the other where continued decline or death is highly likely but a formal hospice program may not have been chosen. Typical conditions that may involve terminal care include the end stages of cancer, Alzheimer's disease, renal failure, congestive heart failure, stroke, AIDS, Parkinsonism, and emphysema.

Subacute programs may provide formal hospice services, or they may arrange for an outside hospice service to support the patient during or after the subacute stay. Even without a formal hospice program, the care of the dying patient should focus on comfort measures and pain relief, as desired by the patient's direct wishes or previous advance directives. Whether or not advance directives exist, substantial discussions should occur regarding comfort measures, pain relief, and specific limitations on care (Do Not Resuscitate, Do Not Hospitalize, and the like). Grief and bereavement services for patients and families are an important part of the care. Pain management should be aggressive, as there is a tendency to undertreat such individuals. Staff should be trained in the management of intravenous lines and infusion equipment.

Orthopedic Care

Orthopedic care (Table 5–10, pp. 103–104) is intended to manage individuals with musculoskeletal problems or those who have recently undergone an orthopedic surgical procedure. Examples include those with a recent total hip replacement or other prosthesis, open reduction of hip fracture, or surgery for multiple injuries received in an accident.

The care focuses on the orthopedic problem, the postoperative course, rehabilitation, and associated medical, functional, and psychosocial problems.

The patients must learn to use appropriate assistive devices and other alternatives to help manage their activities of daily living (ADLs) and instrumental activities of daily living (IADLs) either temporarily until the condition resolves, or permanently if the condition is likely to result in enduring impairment.

Pediatric Care

Pediatric subacute programs (Table 5–11, pp. 104–105) manage the care of children with multidimensional medical and nursing needs. Examples of relevant problems of children include tracheostomy and ventilator dependency, need for supplemental oxygen, traumatic brain and spinal cord injury, cystic fibrosis, malignancy, bronchopulmonary dysplasia, and reactive airway disease.

Children have several significant care requirements not relevant to adults. Pediatric subacute programs should accommodate their developmental, educational, psychological, and recreational needs, and requirements for immunization and physical therapies. Equipment and supplies (for example, cribs, highchairs, infant seats, and changing tables), medications and infusion equipment, and food and dietary care plans should all be compatible with the needs of this younger age group. The environment must be modified to include safety latches, locks on storage cabinets, electric outlet covers, and corner padding on furniture. Decision making will almost always center on the parents, but the child should be included to the extent permitted by the level of emotional and cognitive maturity. Families therefore need extensive support and education.

Pediatric programs require pediatricians and other specialists in childhood diseases and surgery as attending and consulting physicians. A pediatrician may be the medical director or principal consultant on the unit. Nurses should have experience in the care of children. Typical staffing ratios are between 1:5 and 1:3 for licensed nursing staff, and 1:5 for certified nursing assistants. A typical 25-bed unit requires 48 hours of RN coverage daily (Swensen, 1995). These programs may also use the skills of a developmentalist or child life specialist, especially for brain-injured children.

Pediatric Rehabilitation.   Rehabilitation space, equipment, furniture, and other materials should be designed specifically for children. There should also be specific measures to assess changes in the functional status of children over time. Rehabilitation teams serving children may need specialists who help assess and manage educational and developmental needs. It is also often necessary to begin to prepare children with disabilities for school reentry on admission to the rehabilitation program. These services, which may be coordinated with local school districts and public agencies, may include transportation; special education; speech, occupational, physical, and recreational therapies; counseling; and social work.

Postoperative Care

Postoperative care (Table 5–12, pp. 105–106) is intended for individuals whose needs for monitoring and treatment after surgery are too complex for outpatient management but not complex enough to require the intensity of an acute hospital. The care needs typically result from both the surgery and other coexisting or complicating factors, such as pain, nutritional and hydration deficits, associated medical conditions, infections, bleeding, or complex or nonhealing wounds.

Resolving the problems of the postoperative patient requires effective coordination between the surgeon, a medical physician, and therapists and others providing the care. Each physician may be able to handle some part of the care, but may be less comfortable with another aspect. This is a good illustration of the need for physicians to understand their varying roles in the care of subacute patients.

Psychiatric Care

Subacute psychiatric care (Table 5–13, pp. 107–108) is intended for individuals requiring comprehensive medical, nursing, and rehabilitative/restorative services to manage significant behavioral, emotional, or mood disturbances. Examples are major depression, dementia with additional psychotic features, and recent escalation of aggressive or socially inappropriate behaviors. These individuals have often already undergone some interventions, with varying degrees of success, in outpatient or day treatment settings or in a nursing facility. However, the subacute program would be appropriate when the individual needs more frequent adjustment of medications and treatments, is significantly (but not dangerously) unstable, is significantly impaired functionally and socially as a result of the unstable condition, or requires an intensive multidimensional program to address the problems. Overtly suicidal or physically violent individuals would not be appropriate for the subacute setting.

The care in such a program would be delivered by a team including a generalist physician and a psychiatrist, activities therapists, rehabilitation therapists, nurses, nursing assistants, social workers, dietitians, and possibly a psychologist. The program would also include activities, group therapies, medications, and periodic psychiatric reassessment. Typical goals of care are sufficient behavioral and mood stabilization to enable a return to the previous living situation, with follow-up at that site or in another program such as psychiatric day treatment or day care.

Pulmonary Care

Hospitals treat new or recurrent acute respiratory failure. Many pulmonary and ventilator-dependent patients with complicated respiratory conditions need initiation or continuation of care for low- or moderate-acuity conditions, but do not necessarily require an acute hospital stay (Table 5–14, pp. 108–110).

Prior to the advent of transitional care ventilator programs, many difficult-to-wean patients spent months or years in hospitals at enormous cost. In 1991, over 11,000 chronic ventilator-dependent individuals were estimated to be receiving care each day in acute hospitals. Approximately 5% were under age 18, 56% between 18 and 64, and 39% over age 64. About 70% were hospitalized for medical reasons, and many of those remained in the hospital either because of limited reimbursement for alternatives or while awaiting postacute placement. About half of the chronic ventilator patients were discharged to skilled nursing facilities (SNFs), 40% to another long-term care facility, and about 10% to home (Milligan, 1991).

The American Association of Respiratory Care (AARC) defines a chronic ventilator patient as one needing mechanical ventilatory support for at least 6 hours of each 24-hour period and who has been receiving mechanical ventilation for 30 days or more. A mechanical ventilator is any device used to help a patient breathe.

Appropriate patient selection is important. Despite their common problem of respiratory compromise, the different causes of these problems may require different levels of monitoring and treatment. For example, some pulmonary patients have stable blood gases and need occasional inhalation therapies or chest physiotherapy; others may need frequent suctioning and pulse oximetry or blood gases. For a subacute ventilator-dependent patient care unit to be cost-effective, the patient's medical needs should be met within the unit to avoid repeated acute hospital transfers for further medical interventions.

Pulmonary and ventilator programs must have dependable, well-maintained equipment and a supportive physical plant. To reduce patient risk, there should be adequate electrical backup and oxygen delivery systems and a consistent system to ensure that medical gases are delivered and replenished in a timely fashion.

Ventilators like those used in the home use less power and are generally less complicated to operate. More extensive physical plant modifications will be needed if the program accepts patients needing more high-powered ventilators. A spare ventilator should be available in case of a catastrophic equipment failure. The power supply must be adequate to avoid overloads, and there should be an emergency generator in case of a general power failure. Ventilators should plug into receptacles with direct access to the emergency generator.

Typical staffing for pulmonary care programs includes 3 to 5 nursing hours per patient day (typical nurse-to-patient ratio between 1:4 and 1:6), 1 to 3 respiratory therapy hours per patient day, and 1 to 3 hours per patient day for other care providers.

Because of the many tasks involved in giving pulmonary care, programs should carefully identify the roles of various practitioners and support staff and try to help simplify and consolidate their workload. For example, recent evidence suggests that a simple once-daily ventilator weaning program is more effective than either intermittent mandatory ventilation or pressure-support ventilation (Esteban et al, 1995), both of which are more time consuming and complicated.

Pulmonary Rehabilitation.   Pulmonary rehabilitation provides rehabilitation therapies, emotional support, medical and nursing care, and education and training for those with significantly compromised ventilatory status. The essential elements are respiratory therapy, physical therapy, exercise conditioning, education, and social services. Psychological, psychiatric, and vocational evaluations may also be provided. Most individuals participating in pulmonary rehabilitation programs have chronic obstructive pulmonary disease (COPD). Generally, those with very mild or very severe underlying illness do not receive as intensive and comprehensive a rehabilitation program as those with mild to moderately severe disease. The frequency and length of these programs varies among providers. Services may be provided from 1 to 8 hours per day, and from 1 to 7 days per week.

Rehabilitation

Many individuals have functional deficits resulting from their illnesses or injuries (Table 5–15, pp. 110–111). Because many subacute rehabilitation patients have coexisting medical conditions requiring active management, they may also receive medical and surgical consultations and other related services. The same illness in different individuals may produce widely varying damage and deficits. Different illnesses may produce common problems. Therefore, a patient may be receiving rehabilitation therapies as the primary service during the subacute stay, or as one among several major care components.

Rehabilitation services thus constitute a significant part of either general, specialized, or mixed medical/rehabilitation subacute care programs. They may be short-term, leading to community discharge, or longer-term for those such as ventilator-dependent and brain-injured individuals who also need considerable nursing and medical support. The medical component of subacute rehabilitation services is often overseen by a physiatrist or another physician with substantial experience in rehabilitation who may visit the unit several times weekly.

Several major types of specialized rehab programs, in addition to those already mentioned in conjunction with other programs, include brain and spinal cord injury, burns, and stroke. Rehabilitation services may also be given along with medical care to individuals after joint replacement surgery or repair of fractures (especially hips), and those with general medical deconditioning.

The goals of rehabilitation services are to improve functional and psychological status, maximize quality of life, reduce risk through secondary and tertiary prevention, and reintegrate patients into their families, communities, and jobs. Where complete recovery is not possible, patients should be helped to adapt to an altered lifestyle required to cope with the effects of their injury or illness.

As with other services and programs, a rehabilitation treatment plan should consider essential issues, such as measurable rehabilitation goals and objectives, described in functional or behavioral terms; relevant time frames for achieving the objectives; discussion of factors that may help or inhibit reaching the goals; and identification of pertinent rehabilitation interventions.

Although a rehabilitation program must also manage its patients' medical problems, the principal purpose of rehabilitation therapies is to manage the consequences rather than the causes of illness and injury. Although reimbursement has often limited the number of hours of rehabilitation that are provided in a subacute program, nothing about subacute settings inherently limits them from offering more. Because an individual's tolerance for rehabilitation therapies is roughly inversely related to their medical instability and the severity of their underlying causes, those who can tolerate more rehabilitation may often benefit from being in a nonhospital setting.

The benefits of formal rehabilitation programs may include closer medical supervision and trained staff to assist with exercises, patient education, and psychosocial support and services. However, the relative contributions of the therapies or of the additional and alternative interventions—for example, nutritional management, lifestyle and behavioral counseling, management of comorbidities, supervised exercise training, and risk factor reduction—to outcomes associated with these programs remain unclear.

Brain and Spinal Cord Injury Rehabilitation.   These patients are primarily individuals with traumatically acquired brain or spinal cord damage.

Other types of brain injury may be included based on age, disability profile, and complexity of deficits. Programs usually distinguish between brain injury and stroke rehabilitation, as recovery from traumatic brain injury tends to be more prolonged and unpredictable than from nontraumatic brain disease.

Brain-injured individuals frequently have fluctuations or substantial alterations in levels of consciousness, intellectual function, and mood. Their rehabilitation includes sensory stimulation programs involving both structured stimulation to comatose patients and stimulation by nurses and therapists during general care. Spinal cord injury patients have functional and mobility problems related to the level of their spinal cord injury. Their programs typically include rehabilitation nursing, respiratory therapy, physical and occupational therapy, and intermittent catheterization. For both categories of patients, major components of patient and family education, psychosocial support, and counseling are essential.

Burn Rehabilitation.   Comprehensive rehabilitation services are part of the overall care of those who have suffered serious or widespread burns. These services begin during acute care and continue after discharge. These patients often have complex nutritional, psychological, and surgical problems and complications. Pain management is a prominent need. They are likely to face permanent disfigurement and disability, and possibly major alterations in their social, family, and job roles.

Stroke Rehabilitation.   The principal goals of stroke rehabilitation include maximizing level of independent functioning, preventing and managing complications, facilitating reentry into the community, and optimizing psychosocial adaptation. The overall objectives are to improve quality of life by enhancing functional capacity and to facilitate discharge to a less rehabilitation-intensive setting (Alter et al, 1995).

Many factors influence the need for rehabilitation and the potential for benefit. These include overall health status, comorbidities, functional and psychosocial status before and after the stroke, willingness and capability of caregivers, and social and economic considerations. Because strokes vary widely in their severity and residual damage, not all stroke patients need or can benefit from extensive rehabilitation.

Stroke patients are often divided into three groups. Those with mild strokes resulting in few or no motor deficits usually return to normal function within a few days or weeks and do not require extensive rehabilitation. Those with clinically significant hemiparesis or quadriparesis who were conscious at the beginning (about one quarter to one third of acute stroke patients) have a substantial likelihood of improvement in rehabilitation. Those who are comatose after the onset of the stroke, with hemiplegia or quadriplegia and additional neurological deficits and medical complications, are often too medically unstable or unable to undergo intensive rehabilitation. Stroke patients who remain semicomatose or completely dependent weeks afterward are more likely to deteriorate or die and are very unlikely to achieve functional independence. Those with very low functional scores on admission have a high probability of discharge to an institution.

Stroke rehabilitation programs should include assessments of disability and function, psychosocial and environmental factors, mental status and mood, activity tolerance, and endurance. Depression following stroke is common, and its possible presence should be anticipated and managed vigorously with antidepressants, patient and family therapies, and treatment of contributing medical factors. Common concurrent medical problems include active cardiovascular disease and urinary tract and pulmonary infections. Secondary and tertiary prevention should be a major care component, including control of blood pressure and prevention of the complications of immobility such as skin breakdown, venous thrombosis, and contractures. Early mobilization, bed positioning, and range-of-motion exercises are all important.

Stroke rehabilitation appears to result in more functional recovery than spontaneous improvement alone. This additional function may make the difference between eventual institutional placement and community discharge. Early initiation of rehabilitation interventions, and active patient and family participation, may be more important influences on ultimate recovery than the amount and duration of treatment. Designated stroke units appear to achieve greater levels of functional independence in specific self-care skills than general medical wards (Smith et al, 1982; Indredavik et al, 1991). Stroke units can reduce intermediate-term (3 to 12 months) mortality (Langhorne et al, 1993). Other studies suggest that the benefits of inpatient rehabilitation are maintained for at least one year (Davidoff et al, 1992).

Trauma Rehabilitation. Rehabilitative efforts may benefit those who have suffered major trauma. The program commonly begins during the acute phase of care, even in intensive care units. However, significant medical instability may substantially limit the individual's participation in the therapeutic program. This service combines components of general rehabilitation, head or spinal cord injury, and orthopedic rehabilitation programs.

Wound Care

A wound care service (Table 5–16, pp. 112–113) is directed toward managing and preventing wounds of various kinds. The patient population requiring wound care has expanded. In addition to the traditional patients with pressure-related, circulatory, and diabetic ulcers, there are also those with poorly healing wounds due to surgery, cancer, or immune disorders such as AIDS. New treatments have become available, and are increasing the healing rates and the pace of improvement.

A wound care service requires a large patient volume to be cost-effective. Basic equipment includes special beds and mattresses, most of which may be rented. At least under current reimbursement systems, the costs of these beds can be billed to Medicare or other third-party payers. Many different and expensive kinds of topical medications and treatments must be available for handling the different kinds of wounds. For example, categories of wound care products that might be used at different times include alginates, composite dressings, exudate absorbers (pastes, contact layers, beads, powders), carbon-impregnated dressings, foams, gauze dressings (impregnated and nonimpregnated, adherent and nonadherent), hydrocolloids, hydrogels, skin sealants, transparent film dressings, wound cleansers, wound pouches, debriding agents, leg ulcer wraps, topical sprays, and other miscellaneous items. Other commonly recommended approaches to total patient management include attention to nutrition, hydration, and environmental manipulation.

Correct identification of the type and cause of wounds is important to their successful management. The program needs an individual (such as a physician or clinical nurse specialist) who is skilled in correctly defining wounds, selecting the appropriate treatments, and identifying progress and obstacles to progress. Protocols are very valuable because there are so many different options for treating these conditions. The physicians who attend these patients should agree to use the protocols, yet still be able to modify them for special circumstances.

Additionally, staff training in assessing and documenting various aspects of wounds is important. Important elements of assessment and documentation include the history of wound development, causative factors such as dehydration and circulatory impairment, an assessment of the wound's characteristics (including drainage, location, size, tissue disruption, and circulatory status), the goals of the treatment (healing, reduction of risk factor, surgical preparation, and so on), and the periodic progress in healing.

Wound care requires a clean but not sterile environment. Universal precautions should be followed. The program also needs consistent and timely support for infectious waste supplies and disposal from central supply and housekeeping.

REFERENCES

Ades PA, Huang D, Weaver SO. Cardiac rehabilitation participation predicts lower rehospitalization costs. *Am Heart J*. 1992; 123:916–921.

Alter M, Rothe E, Stiens SA, et al. Stroke rehab. *Patient Care*. 1995; 29(17):14–37.

Amsterdam EA, Cadieux RJ, Debusk RF, et al. Cardiac rehab: Still a good idea? *Patient Care*. October 30, 1994:24–40.

Bernardini B, Meinecke C, Zaccarini C, et al. Adverse clinical events in dependent long-term nursing home residents. *J Am Geriatr Soc*. 1993; 41:105–111.

Davidoff GN, Keren O, Ring H, et al. Who goes home after stroke: A case-control study. *Neurorehabilitation*. 1992; 2:53–62.

Esteban A, Frutos F, Tobin MJ, et al. A comparison of four methods of weaning patients from mechanical ventilation. *N Engl J Med*. 1995; 332:345–350.

Frasure-Smith N, Lesprance F, Talajic M. Depression following myocardial infarction: Impact on six-month survival. *JAMA*. 1993; 270:1819–1825.

Indredavik B, Bakke F, Solberg R, et al. Benefit of a stroke unit: A randomized controlled trial. *Stroke*. 1991; 22:1026–1031.

Langhorne P, Williams BO, Gilchrist W, et al. Do stroke units save lives? *Lancet*. 1993; 342:395–398.

Milligan S. AARC and Gallup estimate numbers and costs of caring for chronic ventilator patients. *AARC Times*. May 1991:6.

Nicholson SH. Infusion therapy program requires nursing skill and knowledge. *Provider*. 1993; 19(4):38–39.

Smith ME, Garraway WM, Smith DL. Therapy impact on functional outcomes in a controlled trial of stroke rehabilitation. *Arch Phys Med Rehabil*. 1982; 63:21–24.

Swensen C. Challenges of staffing a pediatric subacute care facility. *Transitions*. 1995; 2(3):7–8.

FOR FURTHER READING

Anders KT. Ventilator care. *Contemp Long-Term Care*. January 1994:54–55.

Cornish K. Post-acute pulmonary units offer specialized care. *AARC Times* May 1993:54–56.

Elpern EH, Larson R, Douglass P, et al. Long-term outcomes for elderly survivors of prolonged ventilator assistance. *Chest*. 1989; 96:1120–1124.

Greenland P. Efficacy of supervised cardiac rehabilitation programs for coronary patients: Update 1986 to 1990. *J Cardiopulm Rehabil*. 1991; 11:197–203.

Oberman A. Does cardiac rehabilitation increase long-term survival after myocardial infarction? *Circulation*. 1989; 80:416–418.

O'Connor GT, Buring JE, Yusuf S, et al. An overview of randomized trials of rehabilitation with exercise after myocardial infarction. *Circulation*. 1989; 80:234–244.

Oldridge NB, Guyatt GH, Fischer ME, et al. Cardiac rehabilitation after myocardial infarction: Combined experience of randomized clinical trials. *JAMA*. 1988; 260:945–950.

O'Malley S. Caring for people with AIDS. *Provider*. November 1994:25–34.

Parsons Y. Healing more than wounds. *Contemp Long-Term Care*. June 1995:57–76.

Squires RW, Gau GT, Miller TD, et al. Cardiovascular rehabilitation: Status. *Mayo Clin Proc*. 1990; 65:731–755.

Walker FJ, Walker M. Experience with a prolonged respiratory care unit—revisited. *Chest*. 1991; 98:616–620.

Wound care: A natural subacute specialty. *Briefings Subacute Care*. 1994; 1(4):1, 9–10.

TABLE 5–1   COMMON SUBACUTE CARE PROGRAMS

- AIDS care
- Cardiac recovery
- Dialysis/renal failure
- Medically complex care: general, oncology/cancer care, pain management, hospice/terminal care
- Orthopedic care
- Pediatric care
- Postoperative care
- Psychiatric care
- Pulmonary care
- Rehabilitation services: general, brain and spinal cord injury, burns, stroke, trauma
- Wound care

TABLE 5–2   CATEGORIES AND DESCRIPTIONS OF COMMON TREATMENTS AND PROCEDURES IN SUBACUTE PATIENTS

Category/Item	Description
Medication Administration	
Chemotherapy administration	Administration of chemotherapy (antineoplastic drugs) to treat various types of neoplasms
IV medication administration	The IV administration of medications such as antibiotics
IM/SC medication administration	Administering intramuscular or subcutaneous medications
Administration of Nutrients/Fluids	
Hyperalimentation (total parenteral nutrition)	Administration of nutrients via percutaneous catheter to persons who are unable to eat or absorb food
IV fluid administration	The IV administration of fluids for hydration and delivery of medications
Tube feeding	The use of nasogastric or gastric tubes as the primary methods of feeding
Nonmedication Treatments	
Blood transfusion	Infusions of blood or any blood products (e.g., platelets)
Hemodialysis/peritoneal dialysis	Removal of wastes (short-term or chronic, long-term treatment) from the blood or peritoneal fluid of persons whose kidney function has ceased or is inadequate
Occupational therapy	Occupational therapy services provided for rehabilitation including treatment for daily living skills, perceptual motor skills, and upper extremity range-of-motion strength and coordination, as well as fabrication of adaptive equipment
Physical therapy	Services provided for the purpose of rehabilitation or restoration of physical function and mobility
Respiratory, oxygen, medical gas therapy	Specialized care involving the administration of oxygen or aerosol therapy as part of respiratory care. This does not include patients who administer their own oxygen nebulizers, vaporizers, or atomizers; or one-time STAT emergency administration of oxygen
Specialty beds	Care involving the use of an air-fluidized bed (e.g., Clinitron, Mediscus, KCI Fluidaire) or low-air-loss bed (e.g., KCI Kinair, SSI Flexicare, Mediscus) for treatment of advanced pressure ulcers, flaps, grafts, burns, pain management, and other conditions for patients who are bedridden or whose mobility is either physically or conditionally restricted (does not include egg crates and air- or water-filled mattresses)

TABLE 5–2   CATEGORIES AND DESCRIPTIONS OF COMMON TREATMENTS AND PROCEDURES IN SUBACUTE PATIENTS (CONTINUED)

Category/Item	Description
Speech/language therapy	Speech/language pathology services provided by a licensed speech/language pathologist for the purpose of preventing or modifying speech/language disorders or to assist a person's cognition-language and communication skills, or treating dysphagia, oral or pharyngeal swallowing disorders
Suctioning	Ongoing intermittent removal of secretions from upper and/or lower airway to maintain the airway
Ventilator care	Care involving the use of a mechanical device to assist or to perform the function of respiration
Ventilator weaning process	Process of gradually reducing ventilatory support toward eventual discontinuation of the ventilatory and/or tracheostomy support, including monitoring of patients who are being permitted to breathe on their own for gradually increasing periods of time
Wound/decubitus care (stages III and IV)	Care given to treat a stage III or IV pressure stasis, vascular, surgical, or other ulcer of sufficient size and extent to be through muscles or down to bone, caused by conditions such as wound dehiscence, fistulas, progressive cancers, and stump ulcerations (but not usually due to traumatic injuries such as lacerations or burns)
Insertion of Tubes/Catheters to Enable Treatments	
Insertion of central line	Placement of a central venous catheter to permit administration of total parenteral nutrition, fluids, or other medications
Insertion of peripheral IV line	Placement of a catheter in a peripheral vein to permit administration of fluids, nutrients, or medications
Care of Tubes/Catheters Inserted to Enable Treatments and Care	
Chest tube drainage	Management of a tube inserted into the chest cavity to remove excess fluids, treat pneumothorax, or administer treatments
Drainage tube (other than chest tube or Foley catheter)	A tube, catheter, or surgical drain into a body cavity or tissue compartment for the purpose of draining, decompressing, evacuating, or irrigating excess fluids/and or fluids caused by infection (e.g., Penrose drains, NG tubes connected to Gomco suction)
Percutaneous catheters	Insertion of a catheter through the skin to administer medications, and care given to maintain the patency of the line on days when infusions are not administered
Tracheostomy care	Care directed toward maintaining airway patency and preventing infection of a tracheostomy site, including tracheostomy tube cleansing and/or changes and wound site care
Management of peripheral or central IV lines	Care of IV catheters and associated dressings
Monitoring	
Suicide precautions	Prescribed continuous monitoring of patient to prevent suicide
Blood gas monitoring	Drawing of arterial blood to screen for abnormal blood gas values, usually in persons experiencing respiratory decompensation
Communicable disease care/isolation	Precautions and other care given to a patient who has a disease that is transmitted primarily by blood, blood products, and/or body fluids

TABLE 5–3   FACETS OF AN **AIDS** CARE PROGRAM

Item	Components
Description	• Care for those with recent complications of AIDS or AIDS-related illnesses
Objectives	• Manage medical and psychosocial complications of the illness • Plan for subsequent care
Program components	• Assessment and management of medications • Pain management • Rehabilitation and restorative care as indicated • Medical management of complications, especially infections • IV therapy as needed • Provision of nutrition • Support for coping with illness and its prognosis
Admission criteria	• Need for continuing management of multiple problems complicating recovery, including recurrent or complicated infections • Terminal state requiring frequent care and treatment adjustment • No more than moderately unstable vital signs
Common problems to be treated/managed/monitored	• Infection/contagion • Prolonged disease/disability • Activity intolerance • Self-esteem disturbance • Depression • Ineffective individual coping • Spiritual distress
Anticipated risks/complications of current illness	• Multiple recurrent or new-onset infections • Continued decline despite treatment
Principal care providers	• Physician, nurse, social worker, dietitian, clinical pharmacist, rehabilitation therapists, activities therapists
Physical plant, equipment, and supplies	• Isolation capabilities • Uncommon, expensive anti-infective agents
External resources/referrals	• Infectious disease specialists
Potential problems/risk-management issues	• Exposure of staff and other patients to blood-borne and opportunistic pathogens (TB, hepatitis, HIV virus, uncommon bacterial infections) • Patient's social and lifestyle issues (drug and alcohol use, etc.)
Staff education and training/policies and procedures	• Pathophysiology/complications/prognosis of HIV infection • Universal precautions • Terminal care • Appropriate preparation, storage, and administration of IV medications • Management of manipulative behaviors • Psychosocial influences on response to illness
Discharge parameters	• Resolution of significant infection • Adequate pain relief on oral or cutaneous medications • Afebrile, vital signs stable • Adequate arrangements for follow-up and support of ADL deficits at transfer site
Patient/family education	• Prognosis for illness • Options for ethical decision making, including possible future limitations on aggressive medical care • Coping with consequences of irreversible illness • Recognition of signs/symptoms of recurrent complications

TABLE 5–4   FACETS OF A CARDIAC RECOVERY PROGRAM

Item	Components
Description	• Care for patients with complications of heart disease or needing continuing management after surgery or other treatment for heart disease • Case examples: recent cardiac surgery, postmyocardial infarction (MI), continuing management of endocarditis, heart failure/shock
Objectives	• Monitor and assess during recuperative phase • Prevent complications where possible; identify and manage them in a timely fashion when they occur • Administer medications and treatments • Improve functional capabilities
Program components	• Rehabilitation therapies to optimize mobility and function • Assessment and management of medications • Pain management • Risk factor management (diet, lifestyle, cultural and social factors) • Monitoring of respiratory status, fluid volume status, cardiac stability • Assessment and management of problems of mobility and endurance that may affect cardiovascular function
Admission criteria	• Vital signs no more than moderately unstable • No active angina • Stable cardiac enzymes (post-MI) • Arrhythmias controlled or controllable by oral medication • No more than moderate fluid excess, such as manifest by edema • No more than minimal pulmonary edema • Ability to transfer from bed to chair with assistance
Common problems to be treated/managed/monitored	• Prolonged disease/disability • Fluid volume excess • Instability • Activity intolerance • Ineffective breathing pattern • Impaired gas exchange • Decreased cardiac output • Self-care deficit • Depression • Arrhythmia
Anticipated risks/complications of current illness	• New or recurrent acute cardiac event (MI, myocardial or valvular rupture, failure) • Pulmonary edema • Cardiopulmonary arrest • Pulmonary embolism
Principal care providers	• Nurses, nursing assistants, rehabilitation therapists, dietitians, physicians (attending/cardiologist)
Physical plant, equipment, and supplies	• Emergency cart for cardiac resuscitation • EKG machine and supplies • Adequate space for any monitoring equipment
External resources/referrals	• Cardiologist • Community Emergency Medical Services and coronary care unit
Potential problems/risk-management issues	• Rapidity and scope of intervention for abrupt change in condition • Capacity for rapid transfer to acute care hospital • Clarity of resuscitation and other emergency intervention orders • Patient/family understanding of scope and limits of care at subacute site
Staff education and training/policies and procedures	• Basic principles of cardiac function • Identifying potential complications in cardiac patients • Cardiopulmonary resuscitation procedures

(continued)

TABLE 5–4   FACETS OF A CARDIAC RECOVERY PROGRAM (CONTINUED)

Item	Components
	• Appropriate use of cardiotonic medications • Identifying and managing significant signs/symptoms of condition change
Discharge parameters	• Correction of excess fluid volume • Stable vital signs • Control of arrhythmias on oral medication • Improved activity tolerance to allow function in discharge setting • Tolerable dyspnea at rest and on exertion • Stable blood gases or oxygenation status • Improvement of cardiac output to enable adequate function, with help as needed • Adequate home or facility-based ADL and IADL support consistent with cardiac limitations on self-care
Patient/family education	• Coping with functional limitations • Recognition of prognosis and possible recurrent problems • Proper medication administration • Recognizing significant complications/condition changes • Ability to recognize medication side effects/complications • Options for ethical decision making, including possible future limitations on aggressive medical care

TABLE 5–5   FACETS OF A DIALYSIS/RENAL FAILURE PROGRAM

Item	Components
Description	• Care for those with acute or chronic renal failure, sometimes including dialysis
Objectives	• Manage complications of renal failure • Stabilize or improve condition to allow continued function elsewhere
Program components	• Provision of dialysis as indicated • Careful management of fluid and electrolyte balance • Assessment and regulation of medications, in the light of significant renal impairment • Monitoring of cardiovascular stability • Assessment and management of problems of mobility and endurance caused by chronic illness • Recognition and management of complications arising from those problems • Pain management, as indicated • Rehabilitative/restorative care • Follow-up after hospitalization • Maintenance of adequate nutrition, adjusted for renal dysfunction • Patient and family teaching/training
Admission criteria	• Need for continued management of recent onset acute renal failure or exacerbation of chronic renal failure • Need for dialysis that cannot be given as an outpatient • Causes of renal failure already identified • Vital signs and overall status mostly stable • No more than moderate fluid and electrolyte imbalance • No active peritonitis for peritoneal dialysis patients • Contingency plan established in case of increased instability
Common problems to be treated/managed/monitored	• Infection/contagion • Prolonged disease/disability • Fluid volume deficit

TABLE 5–5   FACETS OF A DIALYSIS/RENAL FAILURE PROGRAM (CONTINUED)

Item	Components
	• Fluid volume excess • Decreased cardiac output • Bleeding/anemia • Altered nutrition • Activity intolerance • Impaired mobility • Self-care deficit • Pain
Anticipated risks/complications of current illness	• Hypotension • Fluid/electrolyte imbalance • Shunt infection • Peritonitis • Bleeding from shunt • Clotting of shunt
Principal care providers	• Physician, nurse, nursing assistant, social services, dietitian, clinical pharmacist • Rehabilitation therapists, activities therapists • Nephrologist
Physical plant, equipment, and supplies	• Equipment and supplies for dialysis • Adequate space for dialysis equipment in room
External resources/referrals	• Outpatient dialysis center • Mobile dialysis teams
Potential problems/risk-management issues	• Consistent knowledge and training of staff to perform dialysis, recognize problems and complications
Staff education and training/policies and procedures	• Proper techniques for dialysis • Pathophysiology of fluid/electrolyte balance • Complications of acute and chronic renal failure • Medication adjustments in renal failure • Dietary issues in renal failure
Discharge parameters	• Resolution of any infection • Stable, corrected fluid volume • Control of any bleeding • Stabilization or progressive improvement of nutritional status • Improvement of strength, endurance, self-care capabilities • Management of pain with oral or cutaneous medications
Patient/family education	• Purpose, administration, and potential complications of medications • Recognizing common complications of dialysis patients • Follow-up care arrangements • Options for ethical decision making, including possible future limitations on aggressive medical care

TABLE 5–6   FACETS OF A MEDICALLY COMPLEX CARE PROGRAM

Item	Components
Description	• Continuing care for patients with multiple medical and functional problems and complications prolonging their recuperative period • Management of terminally ill individuals with complications or need for specialized management **Typical cases:** • Gastrointestinal disorders with recent major bleeding and/or weight loss • General debility from multiple chronic conditions and complications • Renal failure with chronic or acute debilitation • Diabetes with recent major complications • Septicemia with prolonged treatment course in hospital with complications and recurrences • Terminal patient with fluctuating pain medication management
Objectives	• Manage both primary and secondary medical conditions • Stress secondary and tertiary prevention • Improve functional impairments due to prolonged or severe illness **Terminally ill:** • Facilitate a dignified, comfortable death • Help family and patient cope with implications of patient's death • Limit aggressive medical interventions not consistent with plan of care
Program components	• Treatment of medical illnesses and functional problems • Prevention and management of complications arising from those problems • Medication regulation • Rehabilitative/restorative care
Admission criteria	• Need for continued management of prolonged medical problem • Need for continued assessment and monitoring that cannot be given at another site • Major causes of problems already identified • No more than moderate instability
Common problems to be treated/managed/ monitored	• Risk for injury • Infection/contagion • Prolonged disease/disability • Fluid volume deficit • Bleeding • Altered nutrition • Impaired skin integrity • Altered body temperature • Activity intolerance • Impaired mobility • Self-care deficit
Anticipated risks/ complications of current illness	• Further decline in condition despite treatment • Decline due to irreversible underlying conditions • Complications of prolonged immobility • New-onset illnesses related or unrelated to primary problem
Principal care providers	• Physician, nurse, nursing assistant, social services, dietitian • Clinical pharmacist, rehabilitation therapists, activities therapist
Physical plant, equipment, and supplies	• Adequate space for rehabilitative therapies
External resources/referrals	• Lab/radiology for follow-up testing
Potential problems/ risk-management issues	• Need for clear, mutually accepted plan if condition declines or does not improve • Failure to identify treatable versus irreversible conditions causing symptoms or condition changes • Understanding by patient and family of prognosis and possible complications

TABLE 5–6	FACETS OF A MEDICALLY COMPLEX CARE PROGRAM (CONTINUED)

Item	Components
Staff education and training/ policies and procedures	• Management of complex illness and associated problems • Management of individuals with multiple chronic impairments • Ethical decision-making procedures
Discharge parameters	• Stable vital signs/afebrile • Resolution of any major infections • Correction of significant fluid volume deficit • Control of any significant bleeding • Established adequate oral intake or alternate nutrition • Sufficient correction of impaired mobility and self-care deficit to enable function with support as needed in discharge setting
Patient/family education	• Purpose, administration, and potential complications of medications • Recognizing common complications of conditions, problems • Continuing improvement in mobility and function • Likely continued course of illness, chance for recurrence • Options for possible future limitations on aggressive medical care

TABLE 5–7	FACETS OF AN ONCOLOGY/CANCER CARE PROGRAM

Item	Components
Description	• Continuing care for patients who have undergone surgery, chemotherapy, radiation, immunotherapy or hormone therapy as a result of cancer **Typical cases:** • Malignancies of the respiratory, digestive, hepatobiliary, nervous, or reproductive systems • Postacute leukemia/lymphoma • Treatment and support needed after chemotherapy, immunotherapy, hormone therapy, or radiation therapy • Recent treatment or surgery requiring ongoing clinical monitoring not feasible at alternative site
Objectives	• Minimize and manage pain and discomfort • Maximize functional capacity and endurance • Educate and prepare patient and family for subsequent course of illness • Administer treatments where needed • Identify, monitor, and address complications of illness and treatments
Program components	• Administration of chemotherapy • Management of complications secondary to cancer or to treatment • Pain management • Care specific to functional problems of body systems affected by cancer (respiratory, digestive, nervous, hepatobiliary, reproductive, etc.) • Intravenous therapy as needed through peripheral or central lines • Parenteral nutrition as indicated
Admission criteria	• Afebrile, no more than moderate instability • Treatment regimen completed or well established • Clear plan for follow-up testing and treatment • Adequate hematologic parameters (WBC, hematocrit, platelet count) • Complications stabilized or resolved, at least for present

(continued)

TABLE 5–7   FACETS OF AN ONCOLOGY/CANCER CARE PROGRAM (CONTINUED)

Item	Components
Common problems to be treated/managed/monitored	• Infection/contagion • Prolonged disease/disability • Bleeding • Altered oral mucous membranes • Altered body temperature • Activity intolerance • Self-esteem disturbance • Depression • Dysfunctional grieving • Ineffective individual coping • Spiritual distress
Anticipated risks/ complications of current illness	• Nutritional deficits • Impairment of vital organ function/skin breakdown due to treatments • Organ systems dysfunctions due to tumor effects • Increased potential for infection • Bleeding and clotting disturbances
Principal care providers	• Physician, nurse, nursing assistant, social services, dietitian, clinical pharmacist, rehabilitation therapists, activities therapists • Oncologist
Physical plant, equipment, and supplies	• IV and central line infusion supplies and fluids • Chemotherapeutic agents
External resources/referrals	• Oncologist • Radiation therapist • Nuclear medicine
Potential problems/ risk-management issues	• Realistic patient and family understanding and acknowledgement of illness and its complications • Complications related to administering chemotherapy IV
Staff education and training/ policies and procedures	• Types of cancers and their course and complications • Proper administration of medications and treatments • Anticipation and identification of complications of treatments and conditions • Ethical decision-making processes • Principles of pain management
Discharge parameters	• Resolution of complicating infections • Sufficient recovery from prolonged disease/disability to function in discharge setting with support as needed • Availability of sufficient support in discharge setting • Control of any internal or external bleeding • Tolerable chemotherapy side effects/complications • Identification and initial management of depression, disturbed self-concept, other emotional responses to illness • Adequate pain relief through oral or cutaneous medications or mechanical devices
Patient/family education	• Likely course of illness • Complications of chemotherapies • Recognition of subsequent complications of illness • Use and monitoring of routine medications • Medication titration for pain relief • Options for ethical decision making, including possible future limitations on aggressive medical care

TABLE 5–8   FACETS OF A PAIN MANAGEMENT PROGRAM

Item	Components
Description	• Care for individuals with severe, frequent pain requiring titration of medications and possible use of other pain relief modalities
Objectives	• Relief of pain • Address medical and psychosocial issues that may be influencing or causing pain • Improvement or restoration of function
Program components	• Assessment of causes of pain • Titration of pain medications • Treatment of associated medical illnesses and functional problems • Use of physical pain relief modalities, where possible • Rehabilitative/restorative care to reduce pain, improve function
Admission criteria	• Relatively stable vital signs • Substantial, persistent, or recurrent pain requiring frequent dosage adjustment, continuing treatment of underlying causes, or frequent administration of parenteral medications
Common problems to be treated/managed/monitored	• Prolonged disease/disability • Constipation • Activity intolerance • Self-care deficit • Depression • Social isolation • Ineffective individual coping
Anticipated risks/complications of current illness	• Worsening of condition causing pain • Side effects of narcotics: tolerance, confusion, constipation
Principal care providers	• Physician, nurse, nursing assistant, social services, clinical pharmacist, rehabilitation therapists, activities therapists
Physical plant, equipment, and supplies	• Infusion pumps and other equipment • External pain devices such as TENS units
External resources/referrals	• Pain management centers
Potential problems/risk-management issues	• Psychosocial instability exacerbating or caused by pain state • Serious complications due to high or excessive dosing of narcotics
Staff education and training/policies and procedures	• Medical and psychosocial factors influencing pain • Strategies for handling the chronic pain patient • Sequential approach to selecting analgesics
Discharge parameters	• Tolerable level of pain on oral or cutaneous medications or other treatments • Control of medication side effects such as constipation • Improvement in self-care to allow function in discharge setting with available support • At least some progress in addressing psychological complications such as depression • Some support established for improving individual coping with pain and its causes
Patient/family education	• Strategies for coping with chronic pain/living with a chronic pain patient • Proper use of standing and PRN pain medications • Recognition of interactions of analgesics with other medications • Proper use of any mechanical pain relief devices

TABLE 5–9   FACETS OF A HOSPICE/TERMINAL CARE PROGRAM

Item	Components
Description	• Management of terminally ill individuals with complications or need for specialized management • Support for family of terminally ill individuals **Typical cases:** • Terminal patient with fluctuating pain medication management • AIDS patient with short-term prognosis • Individual dying from Alzheimer's disease, multisystems failure, major stroke, or injuries needing multidimensional care
Objectives	• Facilitate a dignified, comfortable death • Relieve pain and provide comfort measures • Help family and patient cope with implications of patient's death • Limit aggressive medical interventions not consistent with plan of care
Program components	• Medication and nonmedication treatment of pain and discomfort • Supportive care • Development and implementation of limited treatment plans
Admission criteria	• Terminal condition with prognosis of imminent death • Need for complex adjustment of pain medications or treatments • Complications of previous treatment requiring continuing management until death
Common problems to be treated/managed/monitored	• Risk for injury • Impaired skin integrity • Altered body temperature • Impaired mobility • Self-care deficit • Self-esteem disturbance • Depression • Dysfunctional grieving • Altered family processes • Ineffective individual coping • Spiritual distress • Family coping: potential for growth
Anticipated risks/ complications of current illness	• Complications of prolonged immobility • Complications of medications and treatments • Conflicts among patient, family members regarding limitations on treatment or aggressiveness of interventions • Strain or breakdown of normal family relationships, roles
Principal care providers	• Physician, nurse, nursing assistant, social services, dietitian, clergy • Clinical pharmacist, rehabilitation therapists, activities therapist, ethicist
Physical plant, equipment, and supplies	• Adequate space for families to remain overnight, for family conferences and patient/family privacy • Mechanical pain relief modalities
External resources/referrals	• Pain management consultant • External hospice program
Potential problems/ risk-management issues	• Inadequate clarification of conditions not to be treated and aggressiveness of any medical testing and interventions • Unclear advance directives or patient wishes • Unclear understanding of identity and roles of any substitute decision makers • Resolution of conflicts among patient, family members regarding limitations on treatment or aggressiveness of interventions • Insufficient pain relief • Unexpectedly severe side effects of medications • Understanding by patient and family of prognosis and possible complications of using large doses of potent analgesics

TABLE 5–9   FACETS OF A HOSPICE/TERMINAL CARE PROGRAM (CONTINUED)

Item	Components
Staff education and training/ policies and procedures	• Management of complex illness and associated problems • Management of individuals with multiple chronic impairments • Ethical decision-making principles and procedures • Helping family/patient adjust roles, dynamics • Helping family manage loss and grief
Discharge parameters	• Death • Unexpected rally or recovery that makes death less imminent
Patient/family education	• Options for effective pain management • Likely course of the patient's illness • Adjustment of family/patient roles, dynamics • Managing loss and grief • Recognizing signs of impending death • Making additional or revised choices about limitations on aggressive medical care

TABLE 5–10   FACETS OF AN ORTHOPEDIC PROGRAM

Item	Components
Description	• Care for patients with musculoskeletal disorders, injuries, or treatments
Objectives	• Restore optimal function after surgery, injury, hospitalization • Prevent complications
Program components	• Pain management • Anticoagulant therapy • Maintain vascular integrity of affected limbs • Manage traction, casts, braces • Address deficits of activities of daily living and mobility • Provide comprehensive physical and occupational therapy
Admission criteria	• Proper reduction, splinting, casting, or replacement of fractures • No evidence of prosthetic dislocation or infection • Cognitive ability and general potential for participation in rehabilitation • Substantial healing of any amputation sites • No active bleeding • Stable vital signs • Clear game plan from orthopedist or other surgeon
Common problems to be treated/managed/ monitored	• Risk for injury • Bleeding • Activity intolerance • Impaired mobility • Self-care deficit • Potential for infection at operative site
Anticipated risks/ complications of current illness	• Venous thrombosis/pulmonary embolism • Infection of wound site or prosthesis
Principal care providers	• Physician, nurse, nursing assistant, social services, dietitian, rehabilitation therapists, activities therapists • Consultants: orthopedist, general surgeon
Physical plant, equipment, and supplies	• Equipment and supplies for traction, cast care, joint alignment • Proper beds and bed equipment for joint immobilization/traction

(continued)

TABLE 5–10   FACETS OF AN ORTHOPEDIC PROGRAM (CONTINUED)

Item	Components
External resources/referrals	• Orthopedist
Potential problems/ risk-management issues	• Improper handling of cast, traction, splints, or other equipment that could lead to further injury or misalignment • Skin breakdown under appliances, casts, splints • Incomplete or incorrect orders regarding weight-bearing status, precautions
Staff education and training/policies and procedures	• Proper techniques for handling joint replacement patients • Proper handling of splints, traction equipment • Techniques for patient transfer and assistance with bed mobility
Discharge parameters	• Progressive improvement in function • Good wound site healing • Improved activity tolerance and mobility • Adequate function with supportive equipment such as cane, walker
Patient/family education	• Proper use of any orthopedic devices • Precautions such as limited weight bearing • How to monitor for complications of condition

TABLE 5–11   FACETS OF A PEDIATRIC CARE PROGRAM

Item	Components
Description	• Care for children with significant medical, functional, and developmental problems requiring complex short-stay or continuing care **Typical cases:** • Tracheostomy or ventilator dependent, or need for supplemental oxygen, due to acute illness, injury, reactive airway disease, or pulmonary/respiratory tract developmental problem • Traumatic brain and spinal cord injury • Complications of cystic fibrosis • Childhood malignancies
Objectives	• Manage both primary and secondary medical conditions • Accommodate child's developmental, educational, and psychological needs • Provide appropriate recreation, therapies • Address child's and family's psychosocial and educational needs • Stress secondary and tertiary prevention • Improve functional impairments due to prolonged or severe illness
Program components	• Treatment of medical illnesses and functional problems • Prevention and management of complications arising from those problems • Medication regulation • Rehabilitative/restorative care • Support for psychosocial problems and development
Admission criteria	• Childhood illness, injury, or developmental disorder causing need for continued assessment, monitoring, and management that cannot be given at another site • Major causes of problems already identified • No more than moderate instability
Common problems to be treated/managed/monitored	• Potential for injury • Infection • Prolonged disease/disability • Ineffective breathing pattern

TABLE 5–11	FACETS OF A PEDIATRIC CARE PROGRAM (CONTINUED)

Item	Components
Anticipated risks/ complications of current illness	• Altered nutrition • Impaired mobility • Further decline in condition despite treatment • Injury due to behavior, wandering, inattention • Decline due to irreversible underlying conditions
Principal care providers	• Pediatrician, nurse, nursing assistant, social services, dietitian • Clinical pharmacist, rehabilitation therapists, activities therapist • Developmentalist or child life specialist
Physical plant, equipment, and supplies	• Equipment, supplies, furniture, and environment compatible with needs and risks of this younger age group
External resources/referrals	• Pediatric surgeons/specialists
Potential problems/ risk-management issues	• Need for clear, mutually accepted plan if condition declines or does not improve • Failure to identify treatable versus irreversible conditions causing symptoms or condition changes • Understanding by family of prognosis and possible complications
Staff education and training/ policies and procedures	• Management of complex illness and associated problems in children • Educational, developmental, recreational, psychological needs and problems of children • Ethical decision-making procedures
Discharge parameters	• Stable vital signs/afebrile • Resolution of any major infections • Consolidation of problems so that they can be managed effectively in another setting • Established adequate oral intake, formula, tube feeding, or alternate nutrition
Patient/family education	• Purpose, administration, and potential complications of medications • Recognizing common complications of conditions, problems • Expected improvements in function and self-care • Likely continued course of illness, chance for recurrence • Options for possible future limitations on aggressive medical care

TABLE 5–12	FACETS OF A POSTOPERATIVE CARE PROGRAM

Item	Components
Description	• Continuing management after surgery, needed because of complications, prolonged recovery, or problems with the surgical wound site(s)
Objectives	• Provide support for complex needs after surgery • Help achieve maximum possible functional recovery • Manage medical complications of surgical problems
Program components	• Management of tubes, drains, catheters • Care of operative wound site(s) • Close management of nutrition, hydration, and electrolyte balance • Assessment and regulation of medications • Monitoring of cardiovascular stability • Provision of therapies as indicated to improve mobility and endurance • Recognition, management, and attempted prevention of complications of surgery or medical conditions • Pain management, as indicated

(continued)

TABLE 5–12   FACETS OF A POSTOPERATIVE CARE PROGRAM (CONTINUED)

Item	Components
Admission criteria	• Recent complicated surgery requiring frequent continuing postoperative management • Prolonged postoperative course complicated by multiple medical and functional problems • General debilitation due to surgery, convalescence, and possibly other coexisting conditions • Management of nosocomial or iatrogenic conditions such as skin breakdown or urinary incontinence resulting during postoperative period
Common problems to be treated/managed/monitored	• Risk for injury • Infection/contagion • Prolonged disease/disability • Instability • Fluid volume deficit • Bleeding • Altered nutrition • Impaired skin integrity • Altered body temperature • Urinary incontinence • Activity intolerance • Ineffective airway clearance • Impaired mobility • Self-care deficit
Anticipated risks/complications of current illness	• Internal or operative site infection • Internal bleeding • Progressive decline • Recurrence of condition for which surgery performed • Venous thrombosis/pulmonary embolism • Postoperative or postanesthesia confusion, altered mental status
Principal care providers	• Physician, nurse, nursing assistant, social services, clinical pharmacist, rehabilitation therapists, activities therapists • Surgeon
Physical plant, equipment, and supplies	• Dressings and instruments for suture removal, wound care, etc.
External resources/referrals	• Surgical consultant • Hospital-based or ambulatory surgery center or special procedure site
Potential problems/risk-management issues	• Failure to recognize or respond to surgical complications in a timely fashion • Insufficient coordination between surgical and medical physicians
Staff education and training/policies and procedures	• Understanding of common surgical procedures • Management of postoperative conditions • Anticipation and recognition of common postoperative complications, including nosocomial and iatrogenic problems • Principles of postoperative pain management
Discharge parameters	• Healing of wound site • Absence of local or systemic infection • Minimal pain, controllable by oral medications • Ability to function adequately with available support • Substantial resolution of reversible complications, problems
Patient/family education	• Understanding prognosis, time frame for recovery • Recognition and reporting of complications • Appropriate use of medications, devices • Plans for follow-up care

TABLE 5–13   FACETS OF A PSYCHIATRIC CARE PROGRAM

Item	Components
Description	• Comprehensive medical, nursing, and rehabilitative care to individuals with unstable behavioral, cognitive, emotional, and mood disturbances **Typical cases:** • Alzheimer's disease patient with recent-onset psychotic features • Major depression • Recent increase in physically aggressive behaviors
Objectives	• Systematically provide appropriate psychiatric, medical, nursing, and rehabilitative and restorative care to stabilize and improve condition and enable return to previous or less restrictive setting • Enable relearning activities of daily living functions such as basic bathing, grooming, and dressing • Maximize level of independent functioning
Program components	• Psychiatric management • Physical and occupational therapy • Management of medical causes and conditions • Psychological testing and counseling • Therapeutic recreation
Admission criteria	• No more than minor medical instability • Moderately unstable cognition, mood, behavior • Potential response to multidimensional support and interventions
Common problems to be treated/managed/monitored	• Prolonged disease/disability • Risk for injury • Altered health maintenance • Self-care deficit • Altered cognitive function • Self-esteem disturbance • Depression • Altered family processes • Social isolation • Impaired verbal communication • Ineffective individual coping
Anticipated risks/complications of current illness	• Progression of symptoms to greater instability • Recurrence or exacerbation of medical conditions
Principal care providers	• Psychiatrist, nurse, nursing assistant, activities therapist, social services, dietitian, attending physician
Physical plant, equipment, and supplies	• Restricted area for wandering • Security of windows, doors, stairways • Limited access to objects with high potential to harm self or others
External resources/referrals	• Psychologist • High-acuity or secured psychiatric facility
Potential problems/risk-management issues	• Injury inflicted to self or others by wandering, physical aggression • Side effects or complications of medications • Suicide attempt
Staff education and training/policies and procedures	• Principles of care of unstable mood, behavior • Recognition and management of dangerous escalations of aggressive behavior • Recognition of escalating risk of suicide • Proper delivery of treatments and therapies • Appropriate management of dementia
Discharge parameters	• Achievement of sufficient psychiatric stability to enable treatment and monitoring to continue in a less intensive or restrictive setting

(continued)

TABLE 5–13   FACETS OF A PSYCHIATRIC CARE PROGRAM (CONTINUED)

Item	Components
Patient/family education	• Sufficient improvements in activity tolerance, self-care, and mobility to allow adequate function in discharge setting • Coping with functional and behavioral limitations likely to remain after treatment is concluded • Plan for follow-up care, supervision, and management

TABLE 5–14   FACETS OF A PULMONARY CARE PROGRAM

Item	Components
Description	• Care for individuals whose pulmonary function is compromised by acute or chronic illness, or both, requiring closer monitoring and treatment • Chronic ventilator care: Care of individuals needing mechanical ventilatory support for at least 6 hours of each 24-hour period and who have been receiving mechanical ventilation for 30 days or more (American Association of Respiratory Care) **Typical cases:** • Serious respiratory infections (pneumonia/bronchitis) compromising respiratory status • Continued care after surgical chest procedures • Postacute respiratory failure secondary to pulmonary edema, chronic lung disease, or neurological disease
Objectives	• Maintain adequate oxygenation and CO_2 elimination • Control factors increasing ventilatory dependency • Minimize ventilator dependency or wean from ventilator, where possible • Try to prevent complications of respiratory impairment • Manage pulmonary infections • Prevent deterioration • Provide pulmonary rehabilitation
Program components	• Monitoring vital signs, oxygen saturation, end-tidal CO_2 level, respiratory rate, patterns of breathing, respiratory mechanics, lung volumes, and peak flow • Medication administration • Respiratory and inhalation therapies • Mechanical ventilatory support as needed • Chest physiotherapy • Tracheostomy care • Tracheostomy and ventilator weaning and management
Admission criteria	• Requires respiratory therapies/treatments • Causes of current problems well defined • No more than moderate medical instability • Significant uncompensated alterations in oxygenation, CO_2 elimination • Respiratory status stable on facility ventilator • Stable tracheostomy • Placement also based on coexisting problems, arterial blood gases, FiO_2, and current ventilator settings if ventilator dependent
Common problems to be treated/managed/monitored	• Infection/contagion • Prolonged disease/disability • Instability • Excess fluid volume • Altered nutrition • Altered body temperature • Activity intolerance • Ineffective airway clearance

TABLE 5–14	FACETS OF A PULMONARY CARE PROGRAM (CONTINUED)

Item	Components
	• Ineffective breathing pattern • Impaired gas exchange • Impaired mobility • Self-care deficit • Social isolation • Altered family processes
Anticipated risks/ complications of current illness	• Recurrent pneumonia/tracheobronchitis • Airway obstruction • Heart failure • Complications of immobilization • Progressive ventilatory failure
Principal care providers	• Physician (primary attending and pulmonologist), nurses, nursing assistant, respiratory therapists, dietitians, social services, physical therapists, occupational therapists
Physical plant, equipment, and supplies	• Oxygen and other medical gases • Ventilators suitable to a subacute program • Tracheostomy tubes of various sizes • Tubing, canisters, and masks for medical gas administration • Inhalation therapy equipment • Pulse oximeter • Ventilator and patient monitors • Alarms with remote signaling units for the nurse's station • Oxygen concentrator • Manual resuscitator • Suction machine or wall suction units • Effective control of room temperature and ventilation • Rooms of sufficient size to accommodate two ventilators, suctioning and other equipment, supplies, and staff • Electrical system must handle ventilators and other equipment • Backup power in case of electrical outage
External resources/referrals	• Blood gas analysis • Laboratory • Radiology • Respiratory therapy
Potential problems/ risk-management issues	• A minimum number of beds (typically 4 to 10) is needed for the unit to be financially viable • Equipment needs can vary dramatically depending on the acuity of the patients accepted for admission to the unit • Costs of modifying physical plant can be substantial unless patients selected for admission are limited to those persons whose medical needs can be treated with equipment designed for home use • For patients with more complex ventilator needs, space and power requirements increase significantly • Ventilators designed for hospital use can be quite bulky and have a greater power requirement; they may not be suitable for subacute care • Bulk oxygen systems are cheaper to use than tanks • In-room tanks and oxygen concentrators can serve many patients adequately • Patients requiring PEEP are usually more unstable and require more complex equipment and technology • Risk areas: related to equipment malfunctions/failures
Staff education and training/ policies and procedures	• Proper operation of equipment and use of supplies • Recognizing and managing problems with equipment • How to get help with mechanical problems • Managing complications of ventilatory failure • Tactics for effectively weaning patients from ventilators • Proper techniques (suctioning, chest physiotherapy, etc.)

(continued)

TABLE 5–14   FACETS OF A PULMONARY CARE PROGRAM (CONTINUED)

Item	Components
	• Cardiopulmonary resuscitation • Obtaining and analyzing blood samples • Pulmonary function testing • Therapeutic chest percussion • Bronchopulmonary drainage • Coughing and breathing exercises • Mechanical ventilatory and oxygenation support • Aerosol, humidification, and therapeutic gas administration • Assembly and sequential operation of equipment and accessories to implement therapeutic regimens • Procurement, handling, storage, and dispensing of therapeutic gases
Discharge parameters	• No more than moderate instability • Stable or improving oxygenation/CO_2 elimination • Ability to clear secretions (either spontaneously or by tracheal suctioning) • Absence of significant aspiration • Optimal or improving nutrition and hydration status • Stable acid-base status • Evidence of gag/cough reflex or protected airway • Relatively stable FiO_2 anticipated for ventilator patient
Patient/family education	• Tactics for patient energy conservation and stress management • Ensuring proper training in operating equipment and recognizing problems • Breathing retraining • Pulmonary hygiene • Possible subsequent limits on aggressive medical interventions • Proper nutrition and hydration

TABLE 5–15   FACETS OF A REHABILITATION PROGRAM

Item	Components
Description	• Comprehensive rehabilitative care for individuals with medical and functional problems that may be helped by such treatments • May be given as part of an overall medical program or as the primary service objective **Typical cases:** • Traumatic brain or spinal cord injury • Post-hip fracture • Post-joint replacement • General deconditioning • Patients recovering from a cerebrovascular event as a result of infarction or hemorrhage
Objectives	• Systematically provide appropriate rehabilitative and restorative care that maintains or improves function, assists recovery from illness and injury, and supports the provision of other medical and nursing services • Help individuals adapt to significant irreversible changes in physical and functional status • Enable relearning activities of daily living functions such as basic bathing, grooming, and dressing • Maximize level of independent functioning • Prevent and manage complications

TABLE 5–15	FACETS OF A REHABILITATION PROGRAM (CONTINUED)

Item	Components
Program components	• Facilitate reentry into the community • Optimize psychosocial adaptation • Physical therapy • Occupational therapy • Speech therapy • Psychological testing and counseling • Therapeutic recreation • Vocational rehabilitation • Orthotics/prosthetics • Traumatic brain injury (TBI): coma stimulation
Admission criteria	• No more than moderate medical instability • Adequate level of alertness and cognitive functioning to allow participation in therapies (except for head injury patient) • Presence of functional deficits likely to respond to therapies • Need for specialized assistive devices
Common problems to be treated/managed/ monitored	• Risk for injury • Prolonged disease/disability • Activity intolerance • Impaired mobility • Self-care deficit • Altered cognitive function • Altered family processes • Social isolation • Impaired verbal communication • Ineffective individual coping • Spiritual distress • Family coping: potential for growth
Anticipated risks/complications of current illness	• Recurrence or exacerbation of medical conditions
Principal care providers	• Primary: physical therapy, occupational therapy • Other specialized services: psychologist, activities, vocational rehabilitation, orthotics, prosthetics, speech therapist • Physician, social services, nursing, nursing aide, dietitian
Physical plant, equipment, and supplies	• Appropriate centralized area for delivering rehabilitation services • Availability of assistive devices • Room size sufficient to allow movement and transfer using assistive devices, wheelchairs, bathroom support
External resources/referrals	• Prosthetics/orthotics • Electromyography (EMG) testing • Physiatrist
Potential problems/ risk-management issues	• Injury during treatment or due to faulty devices or equipment
Staff education and training/ policies and procedures	• Principles of rehabilitative care • Proper delivery of treatments and therapies • Supportive roles of nonrehab personnel
Discharge parameters	• Achievement of functional and overall improvement relative to specific objective goals determined at outset • Sufficient improvements in activity tolerance, self-care, and mobility to allow adequate function in discharge setting
Patient/family education	• Understanding of goals and prognosis • Coping with functional limitations likely to remain after treatment is concluded • Recognition of potential complications of illnesses, conditions • Plan for follow-up care and treatment • In-home adjustments, equipment, supplies to enable adequate function

TABLE 5–16   FACETS OF A WOUND CARE PROGRAM

Item	Components
Description	• Treatment of complicated or extensive acute or chronic wounds and management of the predisposing factors and complications (acute: postoperative, recent skin breakdown; chronic: little or no progress toward healing a week or more after onset) **Typical cases:** • Multiple pressure sores (primarily stages III and IV) • Recent skin grafts • Recent debridement procedures • Infectious complications such as cellulitis, osteomyelitis • Skin ulcerations due to amputation, malignancy • Surgical wounds
Objectives	• Intensive wound treatment to enable improvement or healing • Management of complications • Control of risk factors
Program components	• Identify acuity or chronicity of wound • Identify course of wound development (causative factor, onset, duration, recurrence) • Identify and address causes (surgical wound dehiscence, pressure, vascular insufficiency, edema, skin destruction from gangrene, malignancy, etc.) • Accurately characterize the wounds (type, location, size, drainage [color, amount, texture, odor], tissue integrity [intact, partial thickness, full thickness, undermining, tunneling, necrosis], tissue viability [phase of healing], and vascular status [erythema, hematoma, edema, ischemia]) • Identify and manage predisposing factors • Improve tissue integrity and viability • Aggressive management of nutrition, hydration • Assessment and management of infection • Identify and manage complications such as infection, hidden extension such as fistulas and tunneling • Promote wound healing through surgical and chemical debridement • Rehabilitative and restorative care to improve mobility, where feasible • Pain management • Manage devices inserted to facilitate wound drainage • Prepare patient for subsequent surgery (debridement, flaps, grafts) • Manage postoperatively skin grafts, flaps, or other repairs
Admission criteria	• Patient requires aggressive, frequent management of wounds or ulcers, with anticipated progress toward healing • No more than moderate instability of vital signs • Afebrile or have treatment plan prior to transfer for elevated temperatures • If infection apparent, appropriate treatment protocols should be initiated
Common problems to be treated/managed/monitored	• Risk for injury • Infection/contagion • Prolonged disease/disability • Fluid volume deficit • Altered nutrition • Impaired skin integrity • Altered body temperature • Urinary incontinence • Bowel incontinence • Activity intolerance • Impaired mobility • Self-care deficit • Depression

TABLE 5–16	FACETS OF A WOUND CARE PROGRAM (CONTINUED)

Item	Components
Anticipated risks/ complications of current illness	• Impaired verbal communication • Further necrosis/breakdown • Infections at site, progressing to septic complications • Recurrent surgical wound dehiscence • Development of new wound infections • Potential for problems increased by multiple wound sites, chronicity of wounds, poor nutrition/dehydration, diabetes mellitus, neurologic/vascular impairments, medical instability, paralysis, immobility, edema, advanced age, impaired cognition
Principal care providers	• Dietitian, nursing assistant, nurses, physician • Plastic surgeon/physical therapist/occupational therapist/wound care nurse specialist
Physical plant, equipment, and supplies	• Whirlpool and treatment areas • Variety of dressings • Topical debriding and anti-infective agents • Surgical debridement and suture removal kits • Swabs and other material to collect specimens • Irrigation solutions and syringes • Sterile adherent and nonadherent gauze pads of various sizes • Transparent colloidal wound dressings • Materials to manage infectious waste
External resources/referrals	• General surgeon • Plastic surgeon • Infectious waste disposal site
Potential problems/ risk-management issues	• Failure of healing • Development of new pressure ulcers • Infectious waste exposure and disposal
Staff education and training/ policies and procedures	• Appropriate assessment and documentation of characteristics and changes in wounds (size, drainage, tissue integrity, viability, etc.) • Various causes and underlying pathophysiology of skin breakdown • Principles of maintaining skin integrity • Principles of reducing skin pressure and preventing skin breakdown • Recognition of complications such as infection and undermining • Care of surgical repairs such as flaps and grafts • Proper operation of special beds
Discharge parameters	• Progress in minimizing negative impact of prolonged disease/disability • Correction of any hydration deficits • Progress in improving nutritional deficits • Afebrile • Adequate control or management of urinary and bowel incontinence to minimize wound contamination • Institution of measures to enhance mobility and self-care • Minimal or no infection of wound sites • Wound healing or close to healing • Treatable risk factors for additional skin breakdown addressed
Patient/family education	• Dressing changes and other wound site care • Recognition of infection • Turning and positioning

TABLE 5–17 CORE FUNCTIONS OF THE VARIOUS PRACTITIONERS AND PROVIDERS IN A SUBACUTE PROGRAM

Discipline	AIDS	CARD	DIAL	MED	ONCO	PAIN	TERM	ORTH	PEDS	POSTOP	PSYCH	PULM	REHAB	WOUND
Activities														
Provide appropriate therapeutic and recreational activities.	✓	✓	✓	✓	✓	✓	✓	✓	✓	✓	✓	✓	✓	✓
Observe and document behaviors, function, and cognition during activities.	✓	✓	✓	✓	✓	✓	✓	✓	✓	✓	✓	✓	✓	✓
Clinical Pharmacist														
Evaluate medications, and advise physician on doses and options.	✓	✓	✓	✓	✓	✓	✓	✓	✓	✓	✓	✓	✓	✓
Help monitor for medication side effects and suggest alternatives where pertinent.	✓	✓	✓	✓	✓	✓	✓	✓	✓	✓	✓	✓	✓	✓
Educate staff, patients, family on purpose, complications, and appropriate compliance with medications.	✓	✓	✓	✓	✓	✓	✓	✓	✓	✓	✓	✓	✓	✓
Assist adjustment of routine medications that may be necessitated by condition or other treatments.	✓	✓	✓	✓	✓	✓	✓	✓	✓	✓	✓	✓	✓	✓
Recommend appropriate topical debriding agents, anti-infectives.	✓	✓	✓	✓	✓	✓	✓	✓						✓
Dietitian														
Ensure appropriate, realistic diet.	✓	✓	✓	✓	✓	✓	✓	✓	✓	✓	✓	✓	✓	✓
Educate patient and family on dietary issues.	✓	✓	✓	✓	✓	✓	✓	✓	✓	✓	✓	✓	✓	✓
Assess special dietary restrictions/supplementation/ special needs.	✓	✓	✓	✓	✓	✓	✓	✓	✓	✓	✓	✓	✓	✓
Help patient adjust eating patterns if appetite is affected by illness or treatments.	✓	✓	✓	✓	✓	✓	✓	✓	✓	✓	✓	✓	✓	✓
Advise about diets that may be too loose (e.g., more sodium restriction needed) or too stringent (e.g., tight fluid restriction contributing to dehydration).	✓	✓	✓	✓	✓	✓	✓	✓	✓	✓	✓	✓	✓	✓

	C1	C2	C3	C4	C5	C6	C7	C8	C9	C10	C11	C12	C13
• Advise physicians and nurses on change in meal frequency or size, or on IV or parenteral feeding as indicated.	✓	✓	✓	✓	✓	✓	✓	✓	✓	✓	✓	✓	✓
• Nutritional teaching to try to maintain or restore lost body weight.	✓	✓	✓	✓	✓	✓		✓	✓	✓	✓	✓	✓
• Recommend diet to ensure adequate nutrition in face of increased metabolic demand due to wounds, recent postoperative state, etc.	✓	✓	✓	✓	✓	✓		✓	✓	✓		✓	✓

Nurse

	C1	C2	C3	C4	C5	C6	C7	C8	C9	C10	C11	C12	C13
• Administer medications and treatments.	✓	✓	✓	✓	✓	✓	✓	✓	✓	✓	✓	✓	✓
• Assess functional and physical status.	✓	✓	✓	✓	✓	✓	✓	✓	✓	✓	✓	✓	✓
• Identify and report potentially or actually serious complications or new-onset conditions.	✓	✓	✓	✓	✓	✓	✓	✓	✓	✓	✓	✓	✓
• Help patient and family cope with feelings about possible activity and role changes.	✓	✓	✓	✓	✓	✓	✓	✓	✓	✓	✓	✓	✓
• Assess patient's risks.	✓✓✓	✓✓✓	✓✓✓	✓✓✓	✓✓✓	✓✓✓	✓✓✓	✓✓✓	✓✓✓	✓✓✓	✓✓✓	✓✓✓	✓✓✓
• Monitor posttreatment status.	✓	✓	✓	✓	✓	✓	✓	✓	✓	✓	✓	✓	✓
• Educate and train patient/family in aspects of rehabilitation and self-care.	✓	✓	✓	✓	✓	✓	✓	✓	✓	✓	✓	✓	✓
• Provide some aspects of rehabilitative/restorative care.	✓	✓	✓	✓	✓	✓	✓	✓	✓	✓	✓	✓	✓
• Assess and document response to treatment and overall progress.	✓	✓	✓	✓	✓	✓	✓	✓	✓	✓	✓	✓	✓
• Help assess nutrition and hydration status.	✓	✓	✓	✓	✓	✓	✓	✓	✓	✓	✓	✓	✓
• Help identify medications that may be causing or contributing to signs, symptoms, or complications.	✓	✓	✓	✓	✓	✓				✓	✓	✓	✓
• Manage fluctuations in behavior and socially inappropriate or risky behaviors.	✓					✓		✓	✓			✓	
• Review with patient and family measures to deal with limited pulmonary reserve, such as energy conservation and good nutrition and hydration.	✓							✓	✓	✓		✓	

(continued)

TABLE 5–17   Core Functions of the Various Practitioners and Providers in a Subacute Program (Continued)

Discipline	AIDS	CARD	DIAL	MED	ONCO	PAIN	TERM	ORTH	PEDS	POSTOP	PSYCH	PULM	REHAB	WOUND
• Teach patient techniques to relieve pain, including use of mechanical devices.	✓	✓	✓	✓	✓	✓	✓	✓	✓	✓	✓	✓	✓	✓
• Manage pressure-relieving devices such as air-fluidized beds or airflow mattresses.	✓			✓	✓	✓	✓	✓	✓	✓		✓	✓	✓
• Help improve immobility or prevent its complications.	✓	✓	✓	✓	✓	✓		✓	✓	✓	✓	✓	✓	✓
• Help patient and family cope with defined terminal condition.	✓	✓	✓	✓	✓	✓	✓	✓	✓	✓	✓	✓	✓	✓
• Help clarify expectations for, and limitations on, medical testing and treatment.	✓	✓	✓	✓	✓	✓	✓	✓	✓	✓	✓	✓	✓	✓
• Educate and train family in aspects of illness and role in care of child.		✓						✓	✓	✓	✓	✓	✓	✓
• Monitor for, and manage, complications of surgery.								✓	✓	✓		✓	✓	✓
• Assist in weaning from tracheostomy/ventilator.									✓			✓		
Nursing Assistant														
• Help provide personal and rehabilitative/restorative care.	✓	✓	✓	✓	✓	✓	✓	✓	✓	✓	✓	✓	✓	✓
• Help manage fluctuations in behavior and socially inappropriate or risky behaviors.	✓								✓		✓			
• Help monitor for and report changes in signs and symptoms (e.g., dyspnea, pain, decreased endurance) or possible complications observed during care.	✓	✓	✓	✓	✓	✓	✓	✓	✓	✓	✓	✓	✓	✓
• Help improve mobility or prevent complications of immobility.	✓	✓	✓	✓	✓	✓	✓	✓	✓	✓	✓	✓	✓	✓
Physical/Occupational Therapist														
• Recommend and provide appropriate therapeutic program.	✓	✓	✓	✓	✓	✓	✓	✓	✓	✓	✓	✓	✓	✓

- Educate and train patient/family in aspects of rehabilitation and self-care.
- Provide prescribed program for improving endurance, strength, exercise tolerance, ADL and IADL performance.
- Apply prescribed exercise programs designed to facilitate joint range of motion, muscle strengthening, improved mobility and transfers, and prosthesis training.
- Teach patient to monitor heart rate and rhythm before and after exercise.
- Train patient to use specialized equipment such as braces, crutches, walkers, and wheelchairs.
- Assess home situation for potential obstacles to adequate function (steps, distances, etc.).
- Teach patient techniques to relieve pain, including use of mechanical devices.
- Monitor and document progress toward achieving functional objectives.
- Give whirlpool treatments to clean wounds and promote healing.
- Change dressings following the treatment (as arranged with nursing).
- Instruct patient and family in tactics to improve mobility or prevent complications of immobility.

Physician
- Make staff aware of significant risks and possible complications.

(continued)

Discipline	AIDS	CARD	DIAL	MED	ONCO	PAIN	TERM	ORTH	PEDS	POSTOP	PSYCH	PULM	REHAB	WOUND
• Coordinate management of primary and secondary problems and significant risk factors.	✓	✓	✓	✓	✓	✓	✓	✓	✓	✓	✓	✓	✓	✓
• Order medications, treatments, and preventive measures/precautions.	✓	✓	✓	✓	✓	✓	✓	✓	✓	✓	✓	✓	✓	✓
• Identify and manage complications.	✓	✓	✓	✓	✓	✓	✓	✓	✓	✓	✓	✓	✓	✓
• Assess for wound site healing and absence of infection.	✓	✓	✓	✓	✓			✓	✓	✓				✓
• Supervise weaning from tracheostomy/ventilator.			✓						✓	✓		✓		✓
• Explain condition and its implications to patient and family.	✓	✓	✓	✓	✓	✓	✓	✓	✓	✓	✓	✓	✓	✓
• Help explain realistic prognosis.	✓	✓	✓	✓	✓	✓	✓	✓	✓	✓	✓	✓	✓	✓
• Discuss game plan in case of worsening condition.	✓	✓	✓	✓	✓	✓	✓	✓	✓	✓	✓	✓	✓	✓
• Review code status with patient and family.	✓	✓	✓	✓	✓	✓	✓	✓	✓	✓	✓	✓	✓	✓
• Clarify expectations for, and limitations on, medical testing and treatment.	✓	✓	✓	✓	✓	✓	✓	✓	✓	✓	✓	✓	✓	✓
• Limit medical treatment when consistent with patient condition and wishes.	✓	✓	✓	✓	✓	✓	✓	✓	✓	✓	✓	✓	✓	✓
• Interpret test results (lab, EKG, X-ray, etc.).	✓	✓	✓	✓	✓	✓	✓	✓	✓	✓	✓	✓	✓	✓
• Titrate medications as indicated.	✓	✓	✓	✓	✓	✓	✓	✓	✓	✓	✓	✓	✓	✓
• Oversee selection of rehabilitation therapies.	✓	✓	✓	✓	✓	✓	✓	✓	✓	✓	✓	✓	✓	✓
• Anticipate and prevent iatrogenic problems.	✓	✓	✓	✓	✓	✓	✓	✓	✓	✓	✓	✓	✓	✓
• Perform appropriate procedures.	✓	✓	✓	✓	✓	✓	✓	✓	✓	✓	✓	✓	✓	✓

Respiratory Therapist

- Administer respiratory therapies.
- Assess response to ventilator support.
- Monitor operation of ventilator and other respiratory equipment.
- Help wean appropriate patients from ventilator/tracheostomy.

Social Worker

- Help arrange for any needed home-based or other supplemental services after discharge.
- Help assess alternative placement if return home is not feasible.
- Help patient/family express and cope with implications of future functional limitations or anticipated decline.
- Assess psychosocial functioning of patient and family.
- Evaluate available resources for postdischarge care at home.

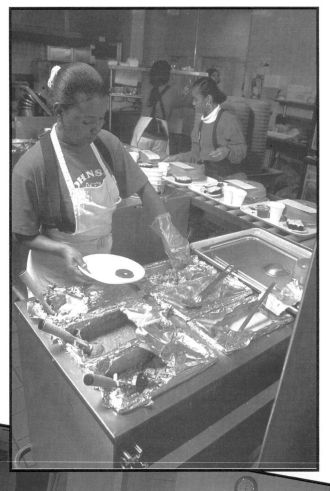

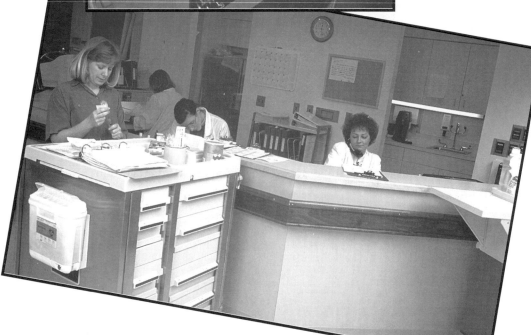

Roles and Responsibilities of the Players

*H*ealth care provision is changing from territoriality and excessive competitiveness and individualism to a more collaborative interdisciplinary and community-wide approach. These changes are important because they are much more compatible with essential natural principles that seek to find and maintain appropriate balance. This balance is important at all levels: in the care of individuals, in the systems that provide the care, in the relationships among various parts of the health care system, and in the relationship of the health care system to other social systems.

Many disciplines and individuals are involved in the care of subacute patients and in the support systems for practitioners providing the care. All players—from owners to nursing assistants—have a vital direct or indirect role in the care. Finding their appropriate roles is vital to trying to ensure these balances. The team approach works best only with the proper conceptual foundation and culture.

The objectives of this chapter are to define the various participants in subacute care provision, to explain those important balances involving these participants, to consider how they can help achieve those balances, to define an effective team approach, and to examine the functions and essential knowledge and skills of the participants.

Everything in nature tries to maintain an essential balance within certain boundaries. Homeostasis ("remaining constant") is one of the most fundamental natural principles. Despite considerable flexibility, natural systems suffer when conditions become too extreme or fluctuate too widely or too frequently. The subsequent attempt to restore at least some balance may cause catastrophic responses. For instance, climatic extremes such as prolonged heat buildup or a clash of markedly different weather systems may result in violent weather such as hurricanes or tornadoes. Pent-up pressures inside the earth may lead to volcanic eruptions or earthquakes. These natural "disasters" serve an important purpose to restore balance to systems that have gone too far astray.

Living organisms have complex systems to help maintain a delicate balance despite internal and external variances. For example, in humans the kidneys, lungs, liver, and various hormones and neurochemical mechanisms help maintain an acceptable internal fluid and chemical balance. Another common example is body temperature. Various individuals have different normal temperature ranges. A low-grade fever for one person may be a normal temperature for another. But when a person's temperature varies too widely from its norm, the body initiates compensatory mechanisms such as shivering or sweating. However, too much imbalance overwhelms internal regulatory mechanisms. No one can survive with an internal temperature too low (below 90°F) or too high (above 106°F) for long. Drastic intervention may be needed to prevent death.

As discussed in earlier chapters, many illnesses can disrupt an individual's internal balance. Patients who need complex health care often have profound imbalances (such as heart failure or major nutritional deficits) that can be restored only through extensive effort. Or their previous balance center may have been permanently reset—for example, by cancer or a stroke—requiring extensive efforts to help them adjust and function adequately. Thus, although acute care focuses on correcting extreme imbalance incompatible with survival, subacute care is largely about restoring a lasting internal balance or finding a new one.

The same principles that apply to patient management are also relevant to the systems and processes providing the care. Successful human systems must recognize and respect the natural laws, such as homeostasis, that govern human physiology and psychology. Health care organizations and systems represent a collection of individuals and groups with many different psychological and biological starting points. All individuals and groups have certain needs and perspectives that form their own boundaries. Although they may function well within those boundaries, they may or may not be flexible enough to function successfully in conjunction with others who have different needs, perspectives, and roles.

Effective social systems therefore require some balance between common objectives and limited self-interest. But so many competing needs and interests make it hard to determine and maintain the proper balance, to define the appropriate boundaries, and to either select or train those who are comfortable within them. Systems may become unbalanced when the individuals within them cannot reconcile their different needs or perspectives sufficiently to achieve desirable objectives. Moderate imbalances lead to dysfunction, and serious imbalances can become very destructive.

Because no one is immune to the laws of nature or of human nature, it is better to respect than to try to defy them. Any complex system of health care delivery must therefore consider the many overlapping and contrasting centers of interest of both the providers and the recipients of care. Both as patients and as practitioners, individuals tend to relate in terms of their own needs and attitudes. Yet the system must preserve a broad enough balance to function effectively. As a complex system dealing with complex problems, successful subacute care must also deal with these issues effectively.

After many decades of excessive emphasis on competition and control, health care provision is necessarily moving away from territoriality and excessive competitiveness toward broader collaboration; from sharp divisions of individual roles and responsibilities toward shared functions and mutual support; and from sharp divisions between clinical and administrative functions in health care organizations toward recognizing their close interdependence.

Subacute Care as an Interdisciplinary Undertaking

For most people, personal satisfaction is enhanced by optimal physical and psychological well-being and minimal distress. Therefore, the primary focus of all health care programs and practitioners should be to help individuals achieve such objectives. Many factors, including illness and injury, can make the result only partially successful. Sometimes the objective can be accomplished by individual practitioners (nurses, therapists, physicians, and so on), or by only a few individuals acting together. At other times, the effective interactions of a broad assortment of individuals are needed.

Transitional and long-term care require this latter approach. As discussed in earlier chapters, individuals with complex conditions often require complex care—repeatedly rather than occasionally—until their complex condition has stabilized, improved, or become otherwise manageable. Subacute care is thus much more than just a business, or the delivery of specific services or treatments. It is a package of services delivered systematically and repeatedly, within a limited time frame, by various individuals performing specific roles to help those who need the services to achieve a desired level of stability or improvement. It requires the effective coordination of a series of complex processes. In addition to the care processes, it requires many support and management processes that directly or indirectly affect practitioner performance or some aspect of care provision.

Influence of Changes in the Health Care System.   Traditionally, health care practitioners have not ordinarily considered cost or efficiency in their decision making ("cost is no object to achieve quality"), often equating both with interference with their professional judgment. Increasingly, decisions about care and services are influenced by those paying for care as much as or more than those providing it. However, although practitioners must also consider the economics of the care, payers must recognize that excessive cost cutting that fails to manage real problems will likely result in persistent or recurrent problems that eventually cost even more to manage. Physicians and payers alike must seek a proper balance between financial and care considerations in their decision making and in care systems.

In summary, the principle and challenge of achieving homeostasis applies at several levels in subacute care: in the objectives of care in individual cases, in the relationships among the various players, in the systems that support the care provision, between the care providers and those paying for the care, and in the relationship of subacute programs with other parts of the health care continuum.

Roles and Relationships Among Individuals

Health care delivery has sometimes been plagued by the lack of skilled individuals, but it is probably most often plagued by the use of the wrong conceptual models to try to optimize those individuals' performance. One common mistaken notion is that skilled individuals who are assembled and allowed to do their thing without interference will do the right thing. This outmoded interpretation overlooks several realities: (1) there are many different interpretations of the right thing, depending on the knowledge, skills, background, experience, motives, perceptions, and personalities of involved individuals; (2) knowledge of what is right does not assure that the right thing will occur; and (3) there is a substantial difference between treating illnesses and fixing problems.

Some physicians have contributed to these problems by promoting—and often forcing—the model of rugged individualism, that is, physicians should be left to function as independent practitioners who know what is best for each patient. Outsiders have been seen as interfering with this relationship and inhibiting the physician from exercising the best possible judgment.

However, changing times require modifying attitudes. The total quality management (TQM) philosophy—more compatible with the principle of homeostasis—suggests that any enterprise's products or services are the result of the combined efforts of those who are directly or indirectly involved in, or who influence, a system. It appreciates both the skill and contributions of individuals and the system's need to properly balance their roles and functions. It acknowledges the need to recognize and optimize different perspectives, backgrounds, attitudes, and motivations, and to define reality and responsibility through a common approach derived from multiple perspectives, not by trying to pick from among multiple separately developed, incompatible approaches. Thus, health care is best viewed as an interdisciplinary effort involving all parties, not just those—such as nurses and physicians—who directly give the care. No one should claim "ownership" of the patient, and each must practice his or her discipline and specialty in the proper context.

Successful transitional and long-term care require a balanced approach. Achieving common objectives requires the cooperative participation of all individuals who influence or have a stake in the outcome. Different systems and individuals may function at various times and by diverse means, but they need common goals and objectives and coordination of methods. Although some individuals may compensate for the weaknesses of others, too much need for compensation may overload the system and cause significant performance failures.

The Team Approach

Effective subacute care requires a team approach. Yet what does that mean? Even those who advocate for this approach in subacute care may not understand or clarify what kind of team approach is needed. Table 6–1, p. 145, describes several different team models. Choosing the wrong team approach can be as problematic as not choosing any type.

For instance, in providing home care, multiple individuals provide various services at different times, but rarely interact simultaneously. Any case manager or care coordinator is expected to coordinate the care but rarely to synchronize individual performances. Similarly, the traditional approach to acute care has been more akin to the bowling team or home care model, with the physician as a central figure and others playing a subordinate role.

In contrast, subacute care has features of several other models, because:

- Team members have unique varied skills, which must be integrated toward a common goal (symphony orchestra model).
- Team members must cross-coordinate closely (symphony orchestra model).
- Different team members perform functions at various times, with the timing of their participation often being essential (football team model).
- Many actions or jobs of most team members require participation or support from other team members for their successful completion (football team model).

A team has been defined as "a small number of people with complementary skills who are committed to a common purpose, performance goals, and approach for which they hold themselves mutually accountable" (Katzenbach & Smith, 1993). In an orchestra, or on a football team, everyone has a common objective (perform the music; win the game). All positions are important to achieving that objective, despite differences in the frequency and scope of the performance of various individuals. In playing a musical composition, the strings may have the biggest part and the first violins may play the melody most often, but the timpanist and the bassoonist have equally important roles, even though they only participate intermittently and rarely play the melodies. On a football team, even a highly skilled quarterback cannot achieve the objectives (score points and win the game) without the effective participation of those at all other positions, including the defense and special teams. Both in an orchestra or on any sports team, some players may be able to compensate for the weaknesses of others, but eventually too many weaknesses affect the outcome and can undermine even the best individual performances.

Furthermore, individual roles may change, depending on the context in which performance occurs. For instance, musicians playing chamber music or solo recitals have different roles than when they play the same instruments with an orchestra. Similarly, practitioners must appreciate that their roles and functions in subacute care may differ in important ways from those in other settings, even though they are practicing the same professions, treating the same patients, and managing the same diseases.

For instance, physicians manage many of the same medical conditions in subacute programs as they do in hospitals, in their offices, or even in the home. But they play a different role because the patient is in a different phase of illness, and the care must manage problems—including the consequences of the conditions—and not just causes. The effects of medical treatment may range from cure to making things worse. Other care providers including nurses, nursing assistants, dietitians, and physical and occupational therapists render much of the care.

Practitioner Concerns.   Some individuals and disciplines, especially physicians, are concerned and skeptical about the idea of value for all players, and the possible intrusion of others on the care of "their" patients. This concern may be valid when it comes to the specialized skills involved in medical practice (making diagnoses, choosing relevant treatments, and performing specific procedures such as surgery). For example, it takes many years and specialized training to learn the intricacies of managing complicated heart disease or to perform neurosurgery. But other matters, such as the desirable extent and limits of care or the best way to manage functional impairment, are not strictly medical issues.

Practitioners and managers alike must also recognize that the responsibility or authority to make certain decisions is not the same as the right to control the environment or restrict the input of others into those decisions. In any health care environment, practitioners must consider the perspectives of those who are affected by their performance—just as woodwind players may not be in a position to tell violinists how to play the violin, but may have relevant suggestions about the impact of the violin playing on the orchestra's overall performance.

Processes and Functions.   The factors essential to a successful team approach to subacute care will be considered throughout the remainder of this book. Chapter 7 discusses the many processes of care for subacute patients, including assessment, monitoring, treatment, and follow-up. Table 6–2, p. 145, lists various disciplines involved in these processes. Chapters 8 and 9 consider other processes indirectly related to the care such as planning, policy setting, and various support functions and basic "generic" functions such as information gathering, reasoning, communications, and problem solving.

Therefore, all players have a direct or indirect relationship to the care (Figure 6–1). Their roles must be viewed both in relation to patients and to the greater system within which the care is provided, including other disciplines and individuals. Everyone's actions are in turn influenced by many internal and external forces, including the changing nature of health care delivery and the expectation for increasing cost-effectiveness. These external forces may stress or weaken the system severely. Appropriate attitudes and processes (Table 6–3, p. 146) constitute the cement that reinforces this system and enables the players to keep it together effectively.

In subacute care, the participants—the care providers and recipients—primarily determine the game plan. Once that game plan is determined, the players must contribute appropriately and must synchronize their contributions. Usually, they can find common ground among themselves, but they may need appropriate coaching, directing, or refereeing under several circumstances: when they disagree about their individual roles and responsibilities in the processes of care; when they disagree about the game plan or about its execution; when players do not perform their functions appropriately or in a timely fashion; or when the game plan needs to be reconsidered because of new information, undesirable results, or changes in patient wishes or needs.

The Subacute Culture

Culture has been defined as "the prevailing pattern of values, myths, beliefs, assumptions, and norms and their embodiment in language, symbols, and artifacts . . . in management goals and practices, and in participant sentiments, attitudes, activities, and interactions." Like much of the health care system, organizations and subacute care programs have their own identifiable cultures (Singleton, 1995).

FIGURE 6–1   THE DIRECT OR INDIRECT RELATIONSHIP OF ALL PLAYERS TO PATIENT CARE

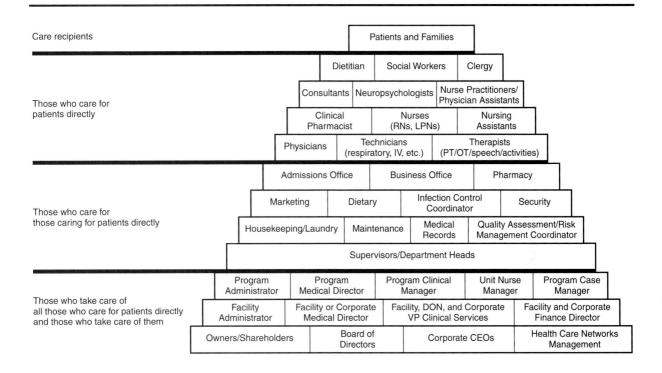

Subacute care combines aspects of acute medical, long-term nursing, and rehabilitative care (Table 6–4, p. 146). An effective subacute culture must accommodate relevant aspects of each of these. A common mistake, with often unfortunate consequences, is to simply mix together individuals and hope for the best. This approach often results in an uneasy coexistence of individuals who fear and mistrust one another. Given the difficulty of finding staff with the appropriate knowledge, skills, experience, and attitudes, management must help individuals adapt appropriately in an often unfamiliar environment. The strengths of various individuals must be emphasized and the weaknesses identified. Roles and responsibilities must be clarified through mutual discussion, not imposed by one group upon another.

The Various Players

Subacute care's many players may be classified as providers and recipients. Providers may be categorized as owners and owner representatives (governing bodies or boards), management (chief executive officers [CEOs], administrators, and program directors), clinical leadership, practitioners, and support staff. Recipients include patients, families, and others who directly or indirectly support or influence either (for example, payers).

Core practitioners and care providers in subacute care include activities or recreational therapists, clinical pharmacists, dietitians and nutritionists, generalist and specialist physicians, nurses, nursing assistants, social workers, and physical and occupational therapists. Other participants and practitioners may include clergy, dentists, ethicists, neuropsychologists, and respiratory and speech therapists. Health care support players include owners, boards of directors, chief executives and administrators, department heads, internal case managers, and support staff such as housekeeping, maintenance, and dietary departments. The remainder of this chapter considers their various roles and responsibilities in helping achieve the overall care goals and objectives.

VITAL SUPPORTING ROLES

Owners and Boards

Subacute care is typically provided within facilities owned and operated by proprietary (for-profit), governmental, or nonprofit health care organizations. Most nonprofit facilities are owned by community-based, usually tax-exempt organizations. Governmental facilities are owned and managed by government entities or agencies, and for-profit (proprietary) facilities are owned by private or public shareholders.

In each case, the management answers to an owner or owner representative, whether an individual or a group such as a board of directors. In nonprofit organizations, boards typically consist of local community individuals with an interest in the organization and its programs. In governmental facilities, the governing body is usually a mix of business people and political appointees. For-profit boards consist of individuals from the corporate and health care worlds who have a legal responsibility to make decisions that benefit the company's value to shareholders. Despite these structural and organizational differences, all health care programs must deal with the same care and management issues. Like all players, owners and governing bodies substantially influence the care.

Roles.   Whether an individual or part of a group, corporation, or government agency, the governing body has ultimate responsibility and authority for the operation of the organization and all of its programs, including subacute care. It is also responsible for establishing an organization's mission and major goals and objectives, and for ensuring that they are carried out appropriately. Owners and boards must approve program plans and budgets, oversee the proper evaluation of the program's results, and ensure that the program's successes and weaknesses are evaluated and addressed appropriately. Their important functions may be categorized as follows.

Establish and Reinforce the Appropriate Organizational Culture.   Owners and boards have a tremendously important role in setting a tone for the whole organization by establishing and reinforcing an appropriate organizational culture. Because they rarely have substantial knowledge or experience in providing the care they are overseeing, they tend to focus on the business side of care and on making major policy decisions. Also they are several times removed from direct care provision (Figure 6–1). However, an imbalance at the top between running the business and helping support the care is unworkable and short-sighted. Therefore, they must fulfill their responsibilities to patients via their responsibility to—and their influence upon the performance of—the management and the direct care providers.

Because most health care organizations offer more than one program and level of care, the roles and functions of governing bodies and owners are not likely to be specific to a subacute program. However, many principles of appropriate governance and management are generic, and the organization's goals and activities must be compatible with all of its programs and services. Any organization that offers subacute care must enable it to succeed by having the essential attitudes, systems, and processes as discussed throughout this book.

To do this, governing bodies and owners must choose their own leadership carefully and recognize the potentially damaging effects of personality-based politics at any level of the organization, including their own. They must hire and guide appropriate management such as CEOs and administrators to ensure that these individuals support and display the appropriate values and behaviors. They cannot just assume that the management and care providers are doing what they should. Instead, they must ensure that a system exists to reinforce effective performance and to improve on suboptimal performance.

Establish Bylaws and Organizational Policies. Owners and boards should adopt or modify bylaws or comparable policies that describe the organizational structure and establish appropriate authority and responsibility. Boards should establish appropriate criteria for appointment and continued board membership. These should go beyond such traditional criteria as attendance requirements, political influence, and donations history. They must emphasize appropriate leadership potential to influence the attitudes and performance of the management and staff as well as some understanding of how to create effective systems and monitor that performance.

Approve Organizational Policies. The board should approve the organization's general operating policies. It should ensure that they are compatible with relevant principles of clinical practice and professional standards, and that they support appropriate, efficient performance at all levels.

Select and Guide Appropriate Management. The owner or governing body must appoint a principal facility manager (CEO or administrator) as official representative, and must specify how this individual will be held accountable. It should formalize the CEO/administrator's responsibilities and authority both from its own perspective and from the vantage point of management staff and care providers who need this person's support and guidance. It should create a mechanism for the CEO/administrator to periodically provide it with relevant information regarding various aspects of the organization and its programs. It should ensure that the appropriate criteria are used to select the leadership and managers throughout the organization.

Establish Guidelines for Physician Participation. Although boards have ultimate legal authority for physician privileges in hospitals, subacute programs may exist in facilities without governing bodies or formal medical staffs. Nevertheless, the owner/owner representative/board is ultimately responsible for the care delivered by the organization's programs. The owner/board should define some system for ensuring effective physician participation in the subacute program. Some form of physician privileges relevant to this level of care is desirable. The CEO/administrator may serve as the governing body representative to approve such privileges and to appoint a medical director. The physicians should have appropriate access to the governing body.

Ensure Appropriate Balance Between Resources and Care Demands.

Every health care organization must deal with the issue of limited funds and resources. Providing consistently effective and efficient care requires finding the proper balance between the demands of the care and resources to provide it. Traditionally, the "more is better" approach has often been wasteful, and the "lean and mean" approach of cutting corners can severely overtax staff performance and impair the patient care.

Although resources (for example, physical plant and equipment) and staff are costly, many of the means for their efficient use are not. Boards must ensure both adequate resources and an appropriate environment (attitudes, systems, and processes) for their efficient use. To do this properly, they must understand the care so that they can authorize funds to develop the essential systems and processes, and find and retain staff with appropriate attitudes. They must support the CEO/administrator, who in turn must support the staff. They should ensure that care providers have adequate input into decisions affecting their functioning, and that requests for resources are considered principally based on their relationship to providing the care.

On a systems level, boards must recognize that their planning and program decisions can no longer be made in isolation from the broader health care system. They should consider the needs of the community and state and the roles of other agencies and services. On the other hand, they must temper their organization's enthusiasm to restructure and downsize by recognizing the potential harm of indiscriminate cutting and the failure to adequately involve staff affected by the decisions (Lumsdon, 1995).

Provide Effective Quality of Care Oversight.

Although owners and boards may receive substantial amounts of information about care quality in the program, they usually depend heavily on the management and staff to interpret those results for them. As a result, they may not receive all the information that they should have, or may not recognize the implications of the information they receive. They must be able to distinguish symptoms of operational problems from the causes. If their conclusions and subsequent decisions only address symptoms (for example, reacting to problems by simply demanding replacement of staff), they may worsen the problems or inhibit effective solutions.

Therefore, although owners and boards do not have to know how to deliver care or the details of operating a complex health care system, they need some rational basis for interpreting and responding to the information they receive from the management and staff. They should at least understand the nature of the care, the criteria for determining care quality and efficiency, and basic relevant standards and guidelines. For example, they may not know how to prevent or manage iatrogenic or nosocomial illness, but they should know that it is a major enduring problem in health care, that it should be addressed by the program, and that the program should be able to explain the incidence among its patients and discuss measures to reduce the occurrence. They should refer to available industry standards and benchmarks and be able to relate the program's performance to that of other comparable sites and to specific quality indicators. They should also understand the extent and limits of these various indicators, as well as the virtues and limitations of various program accreditation surveys such as those of the Joint Commission on Accreditation of Healthcare Organizations (JCAHO) or Commission on Accreditation of Rehabilitation Facilities (CARF).

EXAMPLE
Management reports to the board that there have been "only minor quality problems in the subacute program in the past quarter." Board members should request information such as outcome data, patient disposition (including planned versus unplanned transfers), patient/family satisfaction, and staff evaluations of care quality. The board should refer to written indicators and benchmarks to help place the results in the proper context.

To be able to respond appropriately and to ensure that they do not actually make problems worse, owners and boards should recognize basic principles of improving human performance, quality management, and effective problem solving. They should be aware of the general knowledge and skills needed by various practitioners and staff so they can ensure that adequate mechanisms exist to hire, train, and monitor appropriate individuals. Although owners and boards should not interfere in day-to-day management, they must at least spearhead a rational process to improve care and to solve and prevent problems. They also have a major responsibility to ensure effective risk management and safety programs.

Boards and owners must ensure adequate feedback mechanisms and should both give and receive feedback. They must ensure that everyone—including themselves and top management—is considered fairly in efforts to attribute responsibility for causing, solving, and preventing problems; that no one is allowed to evade responsibility or is exempt from receiving and considering feedback about their performance; and that a proper climate enables everyone to feel comfortable in discussing problems and acknowledging responsibility.

Potential Obstacles.   Owners and boards may offer various reasons why they cannot or should not perform the functions just outlined. These include (1) volunteer status (that is, board members in nonprofit organizations are unpaid volunteers); (2) time constraints; (3) skepticism (the belief that these efforts will not make any significant difference); (4) complexity (the issues are too complicated for laymen to grasp sufficiently); and (5) excessive expectations (this is too much to expect of laymen).

Although any of these factors may make it harder to provide effective leadership, none of them justifies failing to do so (Turner, 1995). The tactics discussed later in this chapter for achieving desired performance are all relevant to owners and governing body members. The following additional mechanisms are suggested.

Documentation and Discussion.   Owners and governing bodies should adopt formal written statements of their roles and responsibilities, which they should periodically review and update as needed, in conjunction with those management and staff members whose efforts are affected by their decisions. All new board members should receive an appropriate orientation and should be required to demonstrate that they understand the essential principles.

A Broad Vision.   In the health care of the future, various programs and services will not so much be profit centers as cost centers. Communities and organizations must help find alternatives for providing care and lowering costs. Under managed care, organizations assume much more risk for having excess services and beds. Also, the trend toward networks and alliances of providers requires participants to combine strengths rather than to compete, thereby duplicating services.

Therefore, the desire to view subacute care as a business opportunity, and to capture a market share, should be balanced by the realization of the risk of excess capacity and overstimulated demand. Owners and boards should recognize that their self-interest lies in part in ensuring that a subacute care program fits in with the organization's overall mission, which is in turn related to the community's and state's needs. A mission statement for the subacute program and organization should reflect these principles.

Balance Expectations Appropriately.   Owners and boards have traditionally hired CEOs/administrators to manage the organization's needs and support those who provide the care. Often, however, these individuals wind up directing much of their time and energy to accommodating the expectations and desires of the owners and board members. Despite their nominally dual role, many CEOs are planners and builders, not managers or practitioners, who are often also given the job of primary managers. Good planner/builders may lack the interest or skill for effective management, and their temperaments and tactics may be detrimental to the effective operation of the program. In the changing health care environment of the future, it may be necessary to rethink and reverse the traditional approach of having operations management report to planners/builders.

Overall, owners and boards have vital leadership and preventive roles in their own organizations. Such leadership is needed because health care of the future requires a different framework for doing business and managing those providing the care. The traditional competitive, individualistic, hierarchical, authority-based approach to operating health care organizations is largely incompatible with important goals and objectives (Adams, 1995). Although people can be forced to do anything, they can never be compelled to do it well. Systems must support individual and collective performance so that individuals will make the extra effort that can achieve both effectiveness and efficiency. Neither of these can be achieved consistently in a system where self-serving politics predominates.

Administrators and Program Managers

The administrator not only operates and oversees the business, but also must ensure that the business and care are appropriately matched and mutually supportive; that is, that the business enables the care to be efficient and of good quality, and that good-quality, efficient care enables the business to prosper.

Like a symphony orchestra conductor or the head coach of a football team, administrators are also the key coordinators of all the different aspects of care and the parties who directly or indirectly deliver it. As discussed above, the administrator also must referee the different perspectives of individuals and departments.

EXAMPLE

The physicians complain that they are not getting enough support from the nursing staff. The nursing staff complains that it is hard to get an adequate physician response to their questions. The administrator must help both disciplines look beyond the symptoms (the chief complaints), define the problem (what is meant by "not enough support" and why these things are happening), make sure the medical and nursing directors seek and address the causes of inconsistent performance, and ensure that there is follow-up to keep the problem from recurring. This intervention may be minimal (just being aware that the problem is being addressed) if both disciplines are able to work it out jointly, or it may be extensive if they cannot agree on the facts or on their interpretation.

In larger organizations, there may be several levels of general management between the governing body and those who oversee and provide the care. Many organizations have chief executive officers (CEOs) as the primary liaison between the board or ownership and the management. A chief operating officer (COO) or equivalent may be the one with primary responsibility for day-to-day operations, with the CEO more involved with planning and policy issues. Chains may also have regional and other non-facility-based managers. Any structure can work, provided certain crucial functions occur within clear lines of accountability.

Facility and Program Management.   For organizations with subacute programs, most major management functions at the facility level are vested in an administrator; a program manager may be appointed to oversee a specific program, such as a subacute unit. The various individuals (medical director, nursing manager, and so on) responsible for overseeing the aspects of care in the program should work closely with this individual, even if they report to someone else in the organizational structure.

The program manager should be accountable for the quality of care and overall success of the program, and should ensure appropriate coordination with the rest of the facility and its other programs. For example, a subacute program in a nursing facility (NF) requires additional staffing and resources beyond those customarily available for the facility's long-term care patients. But it is important not to divert too much staff or too many resources from the long-term care section to the point of compromising the care. Therefore, a subacute program manager should help influence and coordinate the acquisition and distribution of staff and resources so that each program is served adequately and none is shortchanged.

The program manager should help develop and implement various aspects of other major facility-wide functions: ensure adequate oversight of care; help establish a system to anticipate and prevent problems; ensure existence of appropriate policies concerning patients' health care, safety, and protection of personal and property rights; ensure the appropriate selection, training, and oversight of personnel; establish appropriate education and information systems; and create systems that support those giving the care. Any facility-wide policies and systems that are used should be tailored as needed to the subacute program.

The administrator must also try to ensure that the time and efforts of direct care staff are maximized, that other staff support them appropriately, and that reasonable efforts are made to reduce obstacles and non-care-related tasks. For example, the activities of nursing personnel should be directed to interaction with patients rather than nonnursing activities such as administrative management, laundry, housekeeping, and dietary duties (JCAHO, 1995, p. 122).

Administrator training and certification programs should explain and promote the idea of the administrator's role as head coach and referee. Such skills are as important as business training and factual knowledge of reimbursement and regulations. Practitioners must learn to recognize this role, and should not contribute to problems by trying to restrict the administrator's understanding of patient care issues.

Clinical Leadership

The clinical leadership consists of those individuals of various disciplines who are responsible for supporting, coaching, assessing, and improving the performance of practitioners and other care providers of various disciplines and departments. In many cases, the subacute leadership will consist of the same individuals who head organization-wide programs and departments. Sometimes, these managers may assign others to fill certain roles in the subacute program. Again, many structures can work as long as the functions are performed effectively. The following sections discuss several key clinical leadership functions: the clinical program manager, medical director, and director of nursing (DON).

Clinical Program Manager.   Some programs assign a nurse or other individual as a clinical coordinator of the subacute program. Typical functions include overseeing individual cases, solving problems, and ensuring that patient and family concerns are addressed and that essential information flows effectively among various practitioners and between practitioners and patients. This individual's roles may overlap or replace those of the case manager, program nursing manager, or program manager. The responsibilities of someone appointed to this role should be closely coordinated with other management in the program. It is important to distinguish the leadership functions of this individual from his or her clinical roles. The program manager has many of the functions of a facility administrator but on a smaller scale. Knowledge of patient care is important, but cannot substitute for the skills of overseeing and helping improve performance and of reconciling the perspectives and differences of various individuals and departments.

Medical Director.   For various reasons, physicians need greater support and leadership at a wider spectrum of sites than ever before. Subacute medical directors, like their long-term care counterparts, have more roles and greater responsibilities than in the past (Levenson, 1993). They also face greater liability and put facilities at much greater risk if they repeatedly fail to prevent and solve significant problems. Their roles should be validated by appropriate support and respect from management, other leadership, and the attending physicians.

Subacute programs need some medical direction, which could be supplied by the facility medical director or by another physician. Program medical direction involves many generic and some program-specific functions. When the subacute program is one of several in an organization, its medical director should be accountable to the organizational or corporate medical director. These latter individuals should at least familiarize themselves with the features and objectives of subacute care so they can support the program medical director and understand the implications of the information they receive about the program and about the physician performance. For example, physician performance in subacute care must be evaluated somewhat differently from that in the acute hospital because of the important differences in physician roles.

EXAMPLE

A nursing facility establishes a subacute program. The facility medical director is a physician with no major background in subacute care. The facility appoints another physician as the subacute program medical director. That physician should be accountable to the facility medical director, who in turn is ultimately responsible for the care in the program. Alternatively, if the subacute medical director is made accountable to another physician (for example, a corporate medical director), then there must be effective accountability and coordination among all these physicians.

Principle: Lines of authority and accountability must enable appropriate oversight and coordination, and be compatible with other programs and services at the same site.

Table 6–5, p. 147, lists basic medical direction functions in a subacute program. In turn, each of those functions involves certain tasks, as follows.

Overall Coordination of Medical Care.   The medical director should review physicians' credentials and recommend privileges to the administration and board to ensure the provision of safe, effective patient care. The medical director should also help ensure the availability of appropriate attending physicians, specialists, and medical consultants for the program.

Physician Performance.   The medical director should develop and implement policies and procedures that define the responsibilities of the medical staff and should oversee physician compliance. The medical director must ensure that physicians participate appropriately in the interdisciplinary team process and should help resolve differences among physicians, staff, patients, families, and others. The medical director should also review physician performance periodically and make recommendations regarding privilege renewals.

Provision of Care.   The medical director should help identify key aspects of care for the overall program or specific services; advise internal and external case managers regarding utilization decisions; help develop appropriate admission and discharge criteria and participate in selected admission and discharge decisions as needed; and help create an effective continuum of care that links various care sites.

Systems and Processes.   The medical director should help create and implement appropriate patient care policies and procedures, help ensure effective coordination between various programs and services, represent the physicians to the administration and board regarding the subacute care program, meet regularly with appropriate clinical and administrative leadership of the subacute care program, help define adequate staffing and resources to provide care safely and effectively, and help create effective communication and information channels and linkages for physicians. Within this area, the medical director should be involved in implementing critical pathways and practice protocols and guidelines based on available standards and relevant medical literature.

Oversight and Improvement of Care.   The medical director should help ensure adequate quality oversight and improvement mechanisms, identify and implement quality indicators for various aspects of subacute care services, review and evaluate the results of quality assessments, and take action to correct and prevent problems. This individual should also consult in specific cases where there are questions about the care, the treatment selections, physician responsiveness, and other related issues.

Education and Training.   The medical director should help explain the subacute care program's goals, objectives, and services to the community as well as the program's physicians, staff, management, patients, and families. This may overlap with a marketing role, as discussed in Chapter 4.

Qualifications for the Medical Director of a Subacute Care Program. Many subacute programs appoint medical directors based on their clinical expertise and experience. But physicians need more than clinical expertise to function effectively in this role. The program medical director does not need expertise in all relevant areas, but should be a clinically competent physician who can also lead, inspire, and help improve physician performance and effectively harmonize the medical care with the rest of the program. This requires certain knowledge and skills in addition to those related to the diagnosis and management of medical conditions. A general internist is often found to serve well as a subacute medical director, but those of other specialties may also be effective. The individual's specialty is less important than managerial and leadership abilities or potential. The medical director should at least be knowledgeable about indicators of quality for all the subacute services.

Table 6–6, p. 147, lists areas of knowledge and skill essential for effective medical direction of subacute care programs. Because relatively few physicians currently understand subacute care or have broad expertise in its various component services, subacute programs may have limited options. However, this should not prevent programs from trying to find individuals who are flexible and willing to learn. The hospital, subacute, and long-term care industries, along with physician organizations and medical training programs, must help improve physician knowledge and skills in these important leadership areas, and should develop more appropriate role models to train such individuals.

Director of Nursing

The nursing care in a subacute program should be directed by a registered nurse. As with the medical director, the organization's DON may also be in charge of the nursing aspects of the subacute program, or may appoint another nurse for this purpose. However, the director of nursing should ordinarily not be the charge nurse, who is responsible for coordinating various daily activities on the unit.

Some programs appoint a nurse as the program's overall clinical coordinator. In such cases, the program coordination functions must be distinguished from those of director of the nursing care in the facility or on the unit. In NF-based units, the program clinical coordinator should ordinarily report to the facility DON rather than to the administrator. Another approach is to have two assistant nursing directors, one for the long-term care program and another for the subacute program, reporting to a single facility DON (Vaczek, 1994).

Many of the DON's functions and tasks parallel those of the medical director except that they are oriented primarily toward the nurse staffing and nursing care. Other tasks that are specific to a DON include the following.

- Manage nursing personnel, including staffing, recruitment, selection, position assignment, orientation, education, supervision, evaluation, and termination.
- Create and approve nursing staff job descriptions.
- Ensure effective mechanisms for the supervision and performance appraisal of all nursing personnel.
- Develop the nursing services philosophy and objectives.
- Educate nursing staff about standards of practice.
- Contribute the nursing perspective to patient care policy development.
- Help ensure that individual patient care plans and discharge plans are done appropriately.
- Coordinate nursing care with other patient care.
- Review and consult on specific aspects of nursing care in individual patients.
- Provide in-service education for nursing services personnel.

Like the medical director, the DON must also be willing and able to play a critical role as a manager, not just as a principal clinical person. This managerial role includes coordinating the nursing care with the overall interdisciplinary approach and helping to referee various differences in perspective and interpretation. In facilities with both traditional long-term care and subacute programs, many issues arise such as different regulatory and clinical requirements, different levels of staffing and pay, and the mutual misunderstandings between those on the different units. The DON must be able to deal with the reactions of existing staff in the long-term care program, and the conflicts between new and existing staff and between the long-term care and subacute nursing staffs (Vaczek, 1994).

Other Coordinating or Leadership Roles

Charge Nurse.   The program or facility DON should designate a charge nurse for each shift to supervise the direct nursing care. Charge nurses and supervisors in a subacute program should be registered nurses who are qualified by education, training and/or experience to care for the scope of patients in the subacute program. The charge nurse is responsible for:

- Supervising all nursing activities as assigned
- Reviewing patient status to ensure that appropriate care is being rendered

- Reviewing medication records for completeness and accuracy
- Assigning responsibility to the nursing staff for direct patient nursing care
- Supervising and evaluating the performance of nursing personnel on the unit
- Keeping the director of nursing and other appropriate individuals informed about the status of patients and related matters

Case Manager/Utilization Coordinator.   The Case Management Society of America defines a case management system as "a collaborative process that assesses, plans, implements, monitors, and evaluates options and services to meet an individual's health needs through communication and available resources to promote quality, cost-effective outcomes." (AHCA, 1994, p. 8) Case managers may work directly for an HMO, PPO, or managed care division of an insurer; for a case management or cost-containment company that then contracts with employers and insurers to handle their case management needs; or as independent case managers under arrangements with a number of insurers or employers.

Many subacute programs have an internal case manager or use someone to serve case management and utilization review functions in the subacute program. Valuable roles for this individual include coordination of assessments and problem identification, coordinating patient goal setting during interdisciplinary team conferences, support for cost-containment efforts, team building within the program, working with external case managers, and acting as a facility liaison with the patient, family, care team, and payers. This individual typically conducts initial and ongoing evaluations of the patient's stay to ensure that the care is timely and cost-effective, and to try to balance meeting patient needs against payer pressures to limit services.

The extent of a case manager's role in placing patients and negotiating rates varies considerably. But in a managed care era, case managers and utilization coordinators are increasingly important.

Department Heads/Service Directors.   Department head (housekeeping, social work, human resources, and so on) and service director functions will almost always be performed by those who already have broader organization-wide responsibilities. Their roles in the subacute program depend on how the program is structured and delegates various functions.

For instance, hospital physician department heads (such as the chief of surgery or head of the orthopedics division) may have much less of a role in overseeing the care in hospital-based subacute programs than they do with the acute-care portion because subacute programs are really a single service and because the subacute medical director should provide most major oversight functions. But whatever their level of direct contact with the subacute program, department heads should at least be familiar with the program's underlying principles, objectives, and needs, so that they can make appropriate business and clinical decisions.

Table 6–7, pp. 148–150, summarizes the roles and functions of subacute leadership.

PRACTITIONER ROLES IN SUBACUTE CARE

Common Practitioner Functions and Attributes

Subacute practitioners should have certain attributes which are both generally and clinically relevant.

General.   Because subacute care outcomes are the result of a total effort, sub-acute practitioners may help this effort in various ways (Table 6–8, p. 150). As discussed above, performance and attitude factors are important. Individuals must be skilled in their particular positions and must also be able to accommodate the overall strategy. On a sports team, even a skilled position player may be wrong for the team's overall strategy. For instance, a power hitter who is a slow runner and poor fielder may fit in well on a team where other players compensate for those weaknesses, but not for a team whose major strategies revolve around speed and defense. The team may change its strategy to fit the skills of an individual or require the individual to alter his or her performance to fit the team's strategy. In health care, the latter approach is much more feasible than the former.

Thus, technically proficient individuals are valuable but may also need additional training and feedback to provide the appropriate support. Although subacute programs are limited in the pool of available and interested practitioners and must accommodate some individual variability, they must be able to expect practitioners to adapt their skills and perspectives to the care and the care setting.

Direct care providers can help the program achieve its desired objectives more effectively by having certain other desirable attributes. They should be effective communicators and problem solvers, accept responsibility appropriately, be willing to be held accountable for their performance, give and accept feedback willingly, and support care quality improvement efforts. Although relatively few individuals have developed these skills fully, many practitioners and staff can improve their performance through appropriate coaching and feedback. Programs that recognize this and strive to optimize performance, rather than just accepting what they get, may be more likely to succeed.

Clinical.   Subacute programs must be able to deal with both the causes and the consequences of illness and functional impairment. Thus, subacute practitioners should be able to perform various relevant functions including assessing and treating acute and chronic illnesses and behavioral and functional impairments; helping patients and families cope with the psychosocial or economic consequences of these conditions; and managing a progressive decline possibly ending in death. They may do these things directly (by providing the care) or indirectly (by giving other practitioners appropriate support and guidance). Subacute practitioners must recognize their areas of expertise and willingly share the care with others who can complement their skills and services. For example, physicians have expertise in defining causes of illness and in selecting treatments, but they may benefit from a clinical pharmacist's input about medications or a physical therapist's or physiatrist's recommendations about choosing rehabilitation therapies.

Table 6–9, p. 151, lists desirable core functions and knowledge and skills for all subacute practitioners.

Specific Practitioners

Table 6–10, p. 151, lists the practitioners commonly involved in subacute care, and Tables 6–11, pp. 152–154, and 6–12, pp. 154–155, review their functions and desirable knowledge base. The following comments concern several of those disciplines.

Physicians.   As noted throughout this book, physicians have a vital role in subacute programs that differs in some important ways from other levels of the health care system. In subacute care, other disciplines may share or even assume some traditional physician functions such as problem identification, uncomplicated cause determination, and initiation of preventive measures. The supportive physician role is as important—or often more important—than the traditional active role as diagnostician, prescriber, and proceduralist. Physicians should value such participation, not reject it as invasion of their territory.

Physician involvement in the care of subacute patients is especially critical when new complications or condition changes arise; when patients, families, or staff need clarification of various medical issues; when complications or side effects of medications and treatments may be involved; when there are important issues about the intensity and scope of medical care desired by a patient or family; when payers question the length of stay or reason for continued treatment; to help clarify essential postdischarge services and support; to assess patient response to treatment; to identify and manage the causes of problems; and to provide documentation that helps enable appropriate reimbursement.

Qualifications.   Attending physicians for subacute patients may be either primary care physicians or specialists. Either one can potentially perform the functions, but each may have certain strengths and weaknesses. Specialists (for example, orthopedists, nephrologists, or cardiologists) may have a more in-depth understanding of the technical aspects of performing procedures or of managing complicated problems related to a single organ system. Generalists may have a better understanding of overall patient management, be better able to place the medical care in the context of the patient's overall treatment plan, appreciate the difference between treating an illness and solving a problem, and better understand how to help the staff, patients, and families deal with ethical and psychosocial issues. Regardless of their specialty, effective attending physicians must help manage the medical care in the proper context, integrate it with the services provided by other disciplines, and consider the wishes of patients and families.

Astute physicians will recognize that subacute care, like long-term care and other forms of nonacute care, offers a great opportunity to recapture a historical model of medical practice for a new era: that of medicine as a respected profession in which the physician has the opportunity to help care for patients rather than just manage illnesses, and where patient benefit is the primary consideration and medical care is a means to an end, not an end in itself. Physicians who can perform these roles effectively are just as skilled and valuable as those who can provide technically complex care and perform major procedures in acute care settings.

Physician Extenders.   Nurse practitioners (NPs) and physician assistants (PAs) also can play a valuable role in providing subacute care. Nurse practitioners are nurses whose training also includes the medical model of diagnosis and treatment. Physician assistants are individuals who are trained to perform the typical functions of physicians, diagnosing and treating illness and performing technical procedures consistent with their skills. Although there is considerable overlap between the skills and potential roles of NPs and PAs, there are some important differences. Besides being influenced by the nursing approach to patient care, NPs are trained to function as independent practitioners not requiring physician supervision, and PAs are more influenced by the medical approach and are trained to work under a physician's supervision.

In subacute programs, the potential roles of NPs and PAs are largely interchangeable. They may either be hired by the program or be employed by individual physicians with patients on the unit. Although they are not currently used much in these programs, they could be very beneficial. They can supplement the care where physicians are scarce, and they can perform many routine and episodic assessments that require expertise somewhere between that of a nurse and a physician. They can assess acute condition changes such as confusion or fever, and help a physician decide on the urgency and causes of the problem. Other useful functions include performing most of the initial history and physical, participating in interdisciplinary team conferences, verifying clinical information, reviewing drug regimens, and educating patients, families, and staff. By performing these functions, NPs and PAs can help improve the quality of the care, potentially shorten the length of stay, and reduce expensive, disruptive transfers out of the program to manage many acute illnesses.

Contractual Providers and Specialists.   As in long-term nursing care programs, many practitioners (physicians and nonphysicians such as speech therapists and psychologists) consult occasionally on subacute patients. They may be extremely helpful or they may actually inhibit effective care by making recommendations that are out of context. Their successful participation often depends on how they are guided and how they guide others.

Potential problems with any consultants (medical or otherwise) in any health care setting are that (1) they may lack the overall perspective of either the setting or the patient, (2) they may assume that the problem is in their domain just because they were called upon, and (3) they may feel that they have to recommend or change something to justify their presence on a case. Therefore, the attending physician and others familiar with the patient should ordinarily review consultant and specialist recommendations before they are implemented. The medical director should also clarify those who can write orders directly and have a means to evaluate all those who have such privileges. It may also help to provide consultants and specialists with written guidelines including a description of the program and its objectives, a discussion of the principles of subacute care medical practice, and an explanation of the role of consultants and the procedures for handling their recommendations.

TACTICS FOR ACCOMPLISHING DESIRED PERFORMANCE

Subacute programs and their leadership should recognize and act upon the principles discussed in this chapter. Trying to implement and operate a subacute program without the right attitudes, systems, and processes is like trying to build a house upon a makeshift foundation. It may stand for awhile, and may look good to unsuspecting outsiders, but eventually it will yield under stress.

Furthermore, there is ample evidence that good quality care can have a positive financial impact by enabling more consistent care, improving patient and payer satisfaction, permitting greater flexibility in service expansion, and reducing risk. Therefore, the time spent establishing a solid foundation for performance is preferable to subsequently having to repair a program weakened by confusion and disputes.

Effective programs need a system to integrate their various practitioners and staff to achieve the care objectives for this complex population with multidimensional problems. Outcomes are the bottom line, but for many reasons it matters how outcomes are achieved. Therefore, it is especially important to examine and relate both outcomes and processes (the basis for performance).

Even when people know what they are to accomplish or know the right thing to do, there are still many reasons why the right thing may not happen consistently or the objectives may not be achieved. The environment is a major influence on individual attitudes and performance (see Chapter 9).

Table 6–13, p. 155, lists some general tactics for strengthening individual participation and performance. Several of these are discussed in more detail below.

Define and Review Roles and Responsibilities Through Interdisciplinary Effort.

If allowed to define their roles and responsibilities unilaterally, people will typically focus on what they know and like. For instance, a football quarterback who likes to pass might consider his role to be throwing passes as often as possible. Although allowing the quarterback to have ample input, the smart head coach would not permit the quarterback to create the game plan by himself. Instead, his role must be defined in part around the team's strengths and weaknesses relative to the desired objectives. Others who must block for the quarterback or catch the passes should also have input, even if they do not have the final say.

Similarly, nurses, physicians, and others should not unilaterally define their own roles or determine policies relevant to other disciplines. Roles, job descriptions, and policies and procedures must be mutually compatible and relevant to patient care needs. For example, if nurses and clinical pharmacists can help monitor medications and recognize potential undesirable side effects, then physicians should not exclude them from performing these tasks. Or, the appropriate management of ethical issues may need to involve physicians, nurses, social workers, and others, each of whom has defined functions based on legal and regulatory requirements and facility policies. As another example, physicians serving as medical directors must review and sometimes correct physician performance. Therefore, administrators and DONs must clarify expectations, and the medical director must be prepared to meet them. If a physician is incapable or uncomfortable in performing some of these functions, and the administrator is unwilling or unable to get appropriate compliance, then problems may not be corrected, suboptimal care may continue, and others in the program may receive the wrong messages about accountability. It may help for each participant to put their interpretation of their roles and functions in writing to be compared with the expectations that others have of them (see Figure 8–1, p. 207).

Another important change is to broaden the scope of feedback about individual performance. Everyone needs frequent, timely, and specific feedback to change their behavior and improve their performance. But traditionally, feedback sources have usually been limited to an immediate supervisor or manager. Those with higher authority in organizations may strictly limit the content and scope of the feedback they receive. In contrast, effective feedback should be multidirectional. Without it, individuals tend to assume that their actions are appropriate and are likely to continue them. Every individual should be accountable to some degree to anyone who may be affected by his or her performance. This concept is discussed further in Chapter 9.

Identify Common Interests, Objectives, and Obstacles.　As discussed throughout this book, all players must appreciate their common interests and identify their common obstacles. For instance, everyone has a common interest in efficient, well-organized information systems, and everyone is adversely affected by inadequate communications and data.

Provide Essential Education to All Players.　Any setting using diverse individuals to deliver complex service must reinforce the proper foundations and continuously readjust that performance. For example, as new players join a basketball or football team, they must learn new approaches and understand their specific roles. No matter how much their experience and skill, they must perform together repeatedly before their roles become synchronized and complementary.

In subacute programs, all parties need opportunities to openly discuss problems, concerns, and issues related to specific cases. Team meetings, inservices, informal case-specific problem-solving activities, and feedback from the quality improvement program should all be used to reinforce and adjust individual and collective performance. Other useful opportunities for such discussion include interdisciplinary care conferences, quality assurance committee meetings, and management meetings between the administrator, DON, and medical director. Each program must provide participants with effective training and information about key issues such as the nature of subacute care and its relationships with other forms of care, the characteristics of the patients, the roles and relationships of various disciplines, how the program evaluates performance, and the procedures for resolving and preventing problems.

In summary, many disciplines and diverse individuals are involved in subacute care. Only some of the secrets to successful subacute care relate to the technical side of clinical practice. A proper team approach, correctly defined and repeatedly reinforced, can make a great difference in consistently providing effective and efficient care. All subacute participants need certain knowledge and skills and must identify and acknowledge their specific and common roles and responsibilities. Programs must identify participants' strengths and try to remedy their weaknesses through education, training, and consistent feedback that reinforces essential principles. The time and cost of prevention should repay itself by reducing the cost and time of having to deal with the consequences of inconsistent or incorrect performance.

References

Adams DC. False metaphors: Sports, competition, and the new leadership paradigm in health care. *Hosp Health Netw*. 1995; 69(21):42–44.

American Health Care Association. *Subacute Care: Medical and Rehabilitation Definition and Guide to Business Development*. Washington, DC: AHCA; 1994.

Joint Commission on Accreditation of Healthcare Organizations. *Survey Protocol for Subacute Programs*. Chicago: JCAHO; 1995.

Katzenbach JR, Smith DK. *The Wisdom of Teams*. Boston: Harvard Business School Press; 1993.

Levenson SA. *Medical Direction in Long-Term Care: A Guidebook for the Future*. Durham: Carolina Academic Press; 1993.

Lumsdon K. Mean streets: Five lessons from the front lines of reengineering. *Hosp Health Netw*. October 5, 1995:44, 46–50, 52.

Singleton G. Overcoming culture conflict. *Provider*. 1995; 21(4):27–30.

Turner S. Trustee tension: Can board members get their act together and build true system governance? *Hosp Health Netw*. 1995; 69(15):51–54.

Vaczek D. Who's in charge? DON's management skills are challenged when subacute units enter the picture. *Contemp Long-Term Care*. June 1994:75–76, 81.

FOR FURTHER READING

Bailis SS. The right stuff for subacute. *Provider*. February 1995:27–29.

Brown AD. Management perspectives. Trouble recruiting nurses as head nurse of our medical center's newly opened subacute care units. *Nurs Spectr*. 1995; 5(3):5.

Brown-Goebeler S. Subacute care: Nursing for the next century. *Medsurg Nurs*. 1994; 3(6):497–499.

Hegland A. LTC nurses go high tech. *Provider*. 1995;21(4):50–54.

Sherer J. Tapping into teams. *Hosp Health Netw*. July 5, 1995:32–35.

TABLE 6–1   OPTIONS FOR WORK TEAM MODELS

Model	Description	Comments
Choir model	• Team members share comparable skills. • Group focuses on completing a whole piece of work.	• Widely used in manufacturing settings. • Tends to break down when coordination among team members is minimal, or expertise required to do the whole job would take years of study and cross-training.
Symphony orchestra model	• Team composed of individuals with distinct, varied skills, all of which are integrated toward a common goal. • Teams must cross-coordinate.	• Requires strong leadership and coordination.
Football team model	• The success of individual players at many steps depends in part on the concurrent actions of other players.	• Requires finely tuned processes in which each person's performance is synchronized with that of others to complete a discrete process.
Home-care model	• Each team member independently contributes unique expertise. • Different team members perform functions at various times.	• May be appropriately used when individuals or groups function autonomously although coordination is needed.
Bowling team model	• Team members possess a set of common skills. • Very little coordination is necessary. • Each team member performs an action or job that requires no participation from any other team member for its successful completion.	• Not effective when activities need to be tightly integrated or closely coordinated.

TABLE 6–2   PARTICIPANTS IN MAJOR PROCESSES OF SUBACUTE CARE

Major Process	Principal Participants
Assessment (various phases)	Attending and specialist physicians, nurses, dietitians, rehabilitation and speech therapists, activities therapists, psychologists, social workers, nursing assistants, respiratory therapists, clinical pharmacists
Treatment of causes of primary and secondary problems	Nurses, physicians
Management of concurrent problems and functional limitations	Nurses, nursing assistants, dietitians, physicians, therapists, psychologists, social workers, respiratory therapists, activities therapists
Efforts to anticipate and prevent complications	Attending and specialist physicians, nurses, dietitians, rehabilitation and speech therapists, psychologists, social workers, nursing assistants, respiratory therapists, activities therapists, clinical pharmacists
Monitoring and follow-up	Attending and specialist physicians, nurses, dietitians, rehabilitation and speech therapists, psychologists, social workers, nursing assistants, respiratory therapists, activities therapists
Preparation for subsequent care	Social workers, case managers, nurses, physicians, therapists

TABLE 6–3	SOME FACTORS ESSENTIAL FOR A SUCCESSFUL TEAM APPROACH TO SUBACUTE CARE

- Participants with appropriate knowledge and skills
- Broad understanding of the rules of the game
- Clearly defined roles and responsibilities
- A consistent, rational problem-solving process
- Effective strategic planning
- Effective coaching and refereeing
- Recognition of common objectives
- Coordinated approach to identifying and removing obstacles to performance
- Fair assessment and feedback regarding responsibility and performance
- Appropriate incentives for effective performance

TABLE 6–4	FEATURES OF RELEVANT CULTURES THAT MUST BE BLENDED IN SUBACUTE CARE PROGRAMS

Care Type	Features
Acute medical	<ul><li>Quick, frequent, intensive interventions</li><li>Aggressively treatment oriented</li><li>Rapid response to any condition changes</li><li>Frequent testing</li><li>Patients relatively uninvolved in decision making</li><li>Physician-intensive</li><li>Plentiful resources as needed</li><li>Multiple practitioners with relatively little coordination</li><li>Few mandatory care standards</li><li>Mostly short-stay patients</li></ul>
Long-term nursing	<ul><li>Nursing- and nursing assistant-intensive</li><li>Primarily focused on activities of daily living support and supervision</li><li>Less aggressive treatment and testing</li><li>Individuals and families more involved in decision making</li><li>Interdisciplinary team approach</li><li>Many mandatory performance and care standards</li><li>Both long- and short-stay patients</li><li>Relatively slow response to changing conditions</li></ul>
Rehabilitative	<ul><li>Interdisciplinary team approach</li><li>Emphasis on managing consequences of illness and injury</li><li>Includes patients and families</li><li>Encourages patient participation and autonomy</li></ul>

TABLE 6–5	BASIC MEDICAL DIRECTION FUNCTIONS IN A SUBACUTE PROGRAM

- Be responsible for the overall coordination of the subacute program's medical care.
- Ensure adequate physician performance, both in patient management and in support of other pertinent disciplines.
- Ensure that the overall subacute care program provides safe, effective, and efficient care to the patients and those (such as families) who support them.
- Support the patient's rights.
- Define adequate systems, processes, and resources to support all those who provide care, and those who support them directly or indirectly.
- Help establish and ensure quality review to assess outcomes and improve care.
- Serve as a resource for education and training.

Adapted with permission from a position statement of the American Medical Directors Association, Columbia, MD, 1995.

TABLE 6–6	IMPORTANT KNOWLEDGE AND SKILLS FOR SUBACUTE MEDICAL DIRECTORS

- An understanding of quality indicators for the kinds of care and services provided in the subacute care program
- Skill and experience working in an interdisciplinary environment
- Knowledge of the various payment sources and systems for subacute care services
- Understanding the principles of long-term care
- Understanding the management of individuals with complex illness and associated medical and other conditions
- Understanding the continuum of care and the place of subacute care in that continuum
- Knowledge of long-term care regulations, especially those related to physician responsibilities
- General understanding of medical information systems
- Understanding the principles and processes of medical ethics
- Understanding the principles and methods of quality management
- Ability to develop and implement policies and procedures

TABLE 6–7   ROLES AND FUNCTIONS OF KEY GOVERNING AND MANAGEMENT PLAYERS IN SUBACUTE CARE

Roles and Functions	Knowledge and Skills
Owner/Board/CEO	

Owner/Board/CEO

- Adopt mission statement for program.
- Establish and reinforce appropriate organizational culture.
- Support the practitioners and support staff.
- Choose and support appropriate management.
- Ensure appropriate mechanisms to evaluate quality of care.
- Assess implications of quality reports.
- Ensure adoption of effective administrative and patient care policies.
- Appoint licensed administrator and define administrator's responsibilities and authority.
- Review administrative and clinical reports periodically.
- Approve the appointment or designation of a medical director.
- Approve bylaws of any organized medical staff.
- Approve budgets.
- Ensure effective quality, safety, and risk-management program.
- Specify authority for quality assurance, credentialing, other oversight.
- Define mechanism for physician privileges and oversight.

Knowledge and Skills (Owner/Board/CEO):

- Nature and components of subacute care
- Essential roles of key participants
- Health care reform/managed care trends
- Essential resources and attitudes needed for subacute care
- Basic understanding of quality criteria and methods
- Recognition of a governing body's roles in a health care organization
- How to evaluate implications of quality findings
- General care and operational standards
- Principles of optimizing individual performance

Administrator

- Coordinate business and clinical aspects of care.
- Support staff.
- Ensure adequate oversight of care.
- Establish system to anticipate and prevent problems.
- Help establish training and information systems to support care providers.
- Ensure enough appropriately trained professional and support personnel.
- Coordinate appropriate delegation of responsibilities and functions.
- Coordinate development and implementation of patient care, personnel, and other organizational policies.
- Obtain appropriate consultants to help develop and implement subacute program.
- Ensure that appropriate committees are established and operate effectively.
- Establish a system to review and improve performance.
- Establish and oversee systems to review quality, utilization, and risk management, and to solve and prevent problems.
- Ensure that patient care services are organized effectively.
- Help define qualifications, authority, and duties of those in key support and clinical functions.

Knowledge and Skills (Administrator):

- Principles of health care reform/managed care
- How to evaluate staff and practitioner needs
- Opportunities and risks of subacute care
- How to monitor facility's financial status
- Basic understanding of quality indicators and processes
- How to perform effective coaching and refereeing
- Principles and components of subacute care
- Broad understanding of TQM approach
- Temperament to allow TQM approach to flourish
- Principles of optimizing individual performance
- Ability to lead effective problem-solving efforts

Medical Director

- Coordinate program's medical care.
- Ensure adequate physician performance and support.
- Ensure program provides safe, effective, and efficient care.
- Support patient rights.
- Define adequate systems, processes, and resources.
- Help establish and ensure quality assurance mechanisms.
- Serve as resource for education and training.

Knowledge and Skills (Medical Director):

- Essential quality indicators
- How to work effectively in interdisciplinary environment
- Reimbursement sources and systems for subacute care services
- Principles of long-term care
- Continuum of care and place of subacute care within it
- Long-term care regulations, especially as they related to physician reponsibilities

TABLE 6–7   ROLES AND FUNCTIONS OF KEY GOVERNING AND MANAGEMENT PLAYERS IN SUBACUTE
CARE (CONTINUED)

Roles and Functions	Knowledge and Skills
	• Effective application of medical information systems • Concepts and principles of medical ethics • Principles and methods of quality management • How to develop and implement policies and procedures • Ways to optimize physician performance and influence their practices
Director of Nursing (DON) • Ensure provision of adequate, appropriate nursing care 24 hours a day, 7 days a week. • Organize appropriate, timely nursing services. • Coordinate nursing services with those of other disciplines and departments. • Help plan programs and services. • Ensure that regular and contract staff can care for subacute patients. • Develop a rational staffing plan consistent with the scope and acuity of the patients' conditions. • Ensure adequate documentation, maintenance, and distribution of nursing schedules. • Recommend staffing levels to the administrator. • Manage nursing personnel, including recruitment, selection, position assignment, orientation, in-service education, supervision, evaluation, and termination. • Create and approve nursing staff job descriptions. • Ensure effective mechanisms to supervise and appraise performance of all nursing personnel. • Establish nursing practice standards and ensure that all nurses are aware of them. • Coordinate nursing participation in quality management program both internally and with facility-wide program. • Help develop and implement patient care policies. • Ensure effective nursing participation in interdisciplinary care planning and discharge planning. • Ensure an adequate training program for nursing personnel. • Ensure availability of adequate references and information resources for nursing staff. • Participate in the budget process. • Ensure adequate supervision of nursing care on all shifts.	• Registered nurse with some background in acute and long-term care • Training or experience in relevant aspects of care • Some training or experience in at least one of the following: critical care, ventilator care, rehabilitation, complex medical care • Experience performing some technical nursing procedures • Knowledge of essential quality indicators • How to work effectively in interdisciplinary environment • Principles of long-term care • Continuum of care and place of subacute care • Long-term care regulations, especially as they relate to nurse responsibilities • Concepts and principles of medical ethics • Principles and methods of quality management • How to develop and implement policies and procedures • Ways to optimize individual performance
Case Manager/Utilization Coordinator • Perform preadmission assessment. • Help determine appropriate placement of prospective patients. • Help assess patient progress toward discharge. • Ensure that length of stay is appropriate and discharge plan is successfully implemented. • Facilitate communication regarding patients who may need change in service level. • Coordinate information transfer among various practitioners and between practitioners and referral and transfer sites. • Coordinate interdisciplinary team conference. • Help monitor quality-related issues.	• Payment sources for subacute care • Goals and objectives of subacute programs • Managed care concepts and practices • Documentation requirements of insurers • How to evaluate appropriateness of documentation for payment purposes • Roles and responsibilities of various practitioners in the program • Internal and external resources and programs available for patients during and after their stay

(continued)

TABLE 6–7   ROLES AND FUNCTIONS OF KEY GOVERNING AND MANAGEMENT PLAYERS IN SUBACUTE
CARE (CONTINUED)

Roles and Functions	Knowledge and Skills
• Help monitor compliance with pertinent laws, regulations, and payer requirements. • Help ensure that care plans and care-related documentation are consistent with internal policy and regulations, standards, and payer requirements. • Help educate relevant individuals about utilization issues. • Schedule home evaluations prior to discharge, if necessary.	
Charge Nurse • Supervise all nursing care-related activities on a unit or program. • Review care of individual patients as needed. • Screen or review patients with new onset of problems to ensure adequate assessment and timely reporting to physician. • Review medication and treatment records periodically as part of QA process. • Assign responsibilities to the nursing staff for direct nursing care. • Oversee and evaluate performance of all nursing personnel on the unit. • Inform DON of overall status, problems, needs on the unit.	• Registered nurse with training and/or experience in nursing management of transitional or long-term care patients • Some supervision, training, and/or experience in subacute, gerontological, rehabilitative, or psychiatric nursing or other relevant fields • Ability to resolve and referee disputes among individuals and disciplines • Ability to define and describe clinical problems, and triage symptoms and significant condition changes • Ability to show others correct techniques and procedures • Ability to help individuals optimize their performance

TABLE 6–8   HOW PRACTITIONERS MAY HELP ACHIEVE DESIRED RESULTS IN SUBACUTE CARE

- Perform a relevant assessment.
- Define a patient's problems correctly and completely in all dimensions.
- Evaluate a patient's overall condition.
- Help establish realistic care goals and prognosis.
- Correctly define service needs.
- Provide pertinent medical orders.
- Request pertinent support services and consultations.
- Manage associated illnesses and problems appropriately.
- Help maximize function and quality of life.
- Provide adequate, timely follow-up of problems until resolved.
- Periodically reassess the care plan and adjust treatments.
- Document the clinical rationale for decisions to treat or not to treat various problems.
- Clarify the treatment plan for staff, patients, and families.
- Help establish realistic patient and family expectations for the care and the outcomes.
- Try to prevent complications, and identify and treat those that arise.

Adapted with permission from Levenson SA. *Medical Direction in Long-Term Care: A Guidebook for the Future.* Durham, NC: Carolina Academic Press; 1993.

TABLE 6–9	FUNCTIONS, KNOWLEDGE, AND SKILLS DESIRED OF ALL SUBACUTE PRACTITIONERS

Functions

- Participate in interdisciplinary care planning and implementation
- Seek ways to improve the care
- Educate and train patients and families to enhance their participation in care processes
- Give and receive feedback on performance
- Follow appropriate policies, procedures, and protocols, or document reasons for variances
- Document pertinent assessments and other information

Knowledge and Skills

- Basic principles and concepts of subacute care
- Place of subacute care and its services in the care continuum
- Relevant aspects of assessment, problem identification, problem management, and follow-up
- Interdisciplinary approach to managing complex illness
- Individual's role in the care and in relation to others
- Ability to recognize personal limits of knowledge and skills and to get appropriate support
- Appropriate temperament to work in a collaborative environment
- General knowledge of the common conditions, syndromes, problems, complications, and needs of subacute patients
- Recognition of measures of progress and signs of condition change or complications
- Ability to optimize personal performance, and help optimize others' performance

TABLE 6–10	PRACTITIONERS PARTICIPATING IN SUBACUTE CARE

Core Practitioners

- Activities/recreation therapists
- Clinical pharmacists
- Dietitians/nutritionists
- Nurses
- Nursing assistants
- Physical and occupational therapists
- Physicians
- Social workers

Other Practitioners and Providers

- Clergy
- Ethicists
- Neuropsychologists
- Nurse practitioners/physician assistants
- Physician specialists/consultants
- Respiratory therapists
- Speech therapists

TABLE 6–11   FUNCTIONS, KNOWLEDGE, AND SKILLS OF SPECIFIC CORE DISCIPLINES

	Roles and Functions	Knowledge and Skills
Activities/ recreation therapist	• Help evaluate psychosocial and functional status. • Determine activities/therapeutic recreation needs. • Recommend appropriate programs. • Deliver effective services.	• Role of therapeutic recreation in improving and maintaining function • Means of delivering effective therapeutic recreation programs • Assessing patient needs for therapeutic recreation • Matching patient needs with appropriate programs
Clinical pharmacist	• Recommend optimal management of medications and treatments (e.g., routine medications, IV antibiotics, total parenteral nutrition, inotropics, chemotherapy, AIDS therapeutics). • Prepare medication profile/review completeness of medications list. • Review and recommend policies and practices to optimize medication usage and minimize drug misadventures. • Help establish a system to control drugs and biologicals. • Help establish a system to maintain organized drug records and scrutinize controlled drugs. • Help assure that all drugs are properly labeled and stored. • Review each patient's drug regimen and make appropriate recommendations. • Serve on pharmaceutical, infection control, and other relevant committees. • Consult to patient care conferences. • Help train staff for proper use of IV pumps and other infusion devices. • Help review and maintain contents of emergency medication kits. • Perform appropriate medication-related evaluations and studies. • Educate patient and family on drug regimen. • Monitor, document, report, and help manage adverse drug reactions.	• Common conditions treated, and medications used, in subacute patients • Preparation, delivery, storage, and administration of IV solutions and mixtures • Knowledge of regulatory requirements regarding medications • Knowledge of quality indicators for medication usage and pharmacy services • General knowledge of principles of fluid, electrolyte, and acid–base management • Principles and options for parenteral nutrition • Understanding of drug actions, interactions, indications
Dietitian/ nutritionist	• Assess nutritional status/needs of patients. • Advise on adequacy of patient diets. • Educate patients and families regarding relevant nutritional issues. • Educate dietary personnel and other staff. • Assess progress in nutrition based on lab values, medical condition, or other parameters. • Recommend and review special or restricted diets as indicated. • Help ascertain patient food preferences.	• Basic principles of nutrition in illness and preventive nutrition • Criteria for evaluating nutritional status • Options for managing nutritional deficiencies and excesses • Tactics for obtaining effective patient dietary compliance
Nurse	• Provide basic nursing care. • Assess and document condition, care	• Technical aspects of procedures and skills in performing them

TABLE 6–11   FUNCTIONS, KNOWLEDGE, AND SKILLS OF SPECIFIC CORE DISCIPLINES (CONTINUED)

	Roles and Functions	Knowledge and Skills
	needs, nursing problems. • Develop and implement nursing care plan. • Administer medications and treatments. • Document overall progress, condition changes, response to treatment, onset of complications or new conditions. • Help assess, define, and triage problems and condition changes. • Help assess and prepare patient for postdischarge needs. • Participate in ethical decision-making processes.	• Some training appropriate to services delivered to the types of patients admitted • Current knowledge of principles of care of low- and moderate-acuity patients • Ability to assess and triage condition changes • Basic physical assessment skills • Knowledge of potential complications of common acute illnesses and problems in these patients • Knowledge of rehabilitative approach to care • Pertinent OBRA '87 long-term care facility requirements
Nursing assistant	• Provide personal care and activities of daily living support. • Assist with rehabilitative and restorative care. • Monitor for and report progress and condition changes. • Help ensure adequate nutrition, hydration.	• Some special training for each type of subacute patient for whom they care. • Correct delivery of activities of daily living support and personal care • How to deal with basic patient and family questions and concerns • Basic recognition of signs and symptoms of conditions and condition changes
Physical and occupational therapist	• Help assess rehabilitative and restorative needs. • Recommend specific aspects of rehabilitative program. • Provide therapies. • Document and report patient progress in rehabilitative course. • Educate and train patients and families. • Assess postdischarge care needs and environment. • Help evaluate patient's overall condition and status.	• How to assess rehabilitative and restorative needs • Methods for providing rehabilitative services • Basic recognition of signs and symptoms of conditions and condition changes
Physician (attending)	• Provide diagnostic and treatment services. • Inform and educate patients and staff about condition, treatment options. • Define diagnoses and other problems. • Clarify and explain prognoses. • Manage acute illnesses in context of concurrent chronic conditions. • Determine proper scope and balance of medical interventions. • Coordinate care with other players. • Support staff decision making and patient management processes. • Educate and guide staff, patients, and families about treatment choices and decisions to limit treatment.	• Principles of subacute care • Relationship of subacute care to other parts of care continuum • Current and future environment for providing health care • How to communicate effectively with patients and staff • Management of complex illness and comorbidities • Understanding distinction between managing diagnoses and problems
Social worker	• Perform psychosocial and financial assessments. • Participate in care planning and	• Psychosocial, financial, and ethical issues in patient care • Family dynamics

(continued)

TABLE 6–11   FUNCTIONS, KNOWLEDGE, AND SKILLS OF SPECIFIC CORE DISCIPLINES (CONTINUED)

	Roles and Functions	Knowledge and Skills
	discharge planning. • Help ascertain patient preferences regarding extent of medical treatment. • Help families understand current illness, future prospects. • Assess patient and family strengths and weaknesses in resources, coping, communications. • Help ensure that families receive adequate training for postdischarge participation in problem management. • Ensure appropriate referrals/ follow-up postdischarge.	• Principles and practices of managed care • Awareness of available internal and external resources for current and subsequent care • Principles of managing patient/family problems, conflicts • Assessment of psychosocial problems and conditions

TABLE 6–12   FUNCTION, KNOWLEDGE, AND SKILLS OF OTHER DISCIPLINES INVOLVED IN SUBACUTE CARE

	Roles and Functions	Knowledge and Skills
Clergy	• Evaluate spiritual/religious needs. • Provide psychosocial support to patients and families. • Help mediate conflicts among family members or between patients/families/ staff. • Help other staff deal with psychosocial aspects of patients and families. • Participate in ethical decision-making processes.	• Relationships between illness and psychosocial well-being • Medical ethics principles and processes • Options for ethics decision making in health care • Principles of family roles • Patient and family support/counseling tactics
Ethicist	• Help discuss and recommend approaches to issues of extent and duration of medical treatments, patient rights, etc.	• Psychosocial influences on illness and recovery • Principles of ethical issues • Options for ethics decision making in health care • Concepts of ethics decision-making process • Legal factors influencing ethical decision making • General principles of subacute care
Neuropsychologist	• Assess nature and degree of impairment of those with significant head injury or other neurological and psychiatric impairments. • Perform psychological testing. • Recommend specific interventions to manage such impairments. • Authorize or provide specific treatments.	• Basic principles of neurology and psychology • Assessment of neuropsychological capabilities and deficits • Options for managing cognitive and behavioral disturbances due to illness or injury
Nurse practitioner/ physician assistant	• Perform basic histories and physical examinations. • Write medical orders under physician's supervision.	• Understand relationships of transitional care to other components of care continuum • Communicate effectively with patients

TABLE 6–12	FUNCTION, KNOWLEDGE, AND SKILLS OF OTHER DISCIPLINES INVOLVED IN SUBACUTE CARE (CONTINUED)	
	Roles and Functions	**Knowledge and Skills**
	• Assess acute condition changes. • Review test results and discuss with physician. • Educate staff, patients, and families about specific aspects of a patient's condition and prognosis. • Supplement the physician's role as needed.	• How to assess acute illness, function, chronic impairment • At least some training and/or experience in dealing with the care of those with complex illness and comorbidities
Physician specialist/ consultant	• Assess specific aspects of a patient's medical condition, as requested. • Recommend specific aspects of diagnosis and management to the attending physician.	• Expertise in specialty for which consulted • Understanding of nature of subacute care • Recognition of attending physician's primary role in approving treatment recommendations • Appreciation of the interdisciplinary care environment • Understanding distinction between managing diagnoses and problems
Respiratory therapist	• Provide specific respiratory treatments to patients as ordered. • Recommend specific treatment modalities and parameters for delivering various treatments. • Recognize and report possible complications or condition changes related to respiratory conditions or treatments. • Ensure proper operation of respiratory equipment. • Recommend appropriate equipment/ supplies for the program. • Perform quality monitoring of respiratory services.	• Operation, maintenance, and repair of ventilators and other respiratory therapy equipment • Knowledge of respiratory physiology • Ability to recognize possible complications or condition changes related to respiratory conditions or treatments • Quality indicators for respiratory services
Speech therapist	• Help assess nature and extent of linguistic and swallowing deficits. • Recommend specific aspects of rehabilitative program in these areas. • Provide speech therapies. • Document and report patient progress in rehabilitative course.	• How to assess and manage speech and swallowing disorders • Methods for providing speech therapy services • Recognition of measures of progress and signs of condition change or complications

TABLE 6–13	SUMMARY OF TACTICS TO ACHIEVE DESIRED PERFORMANCE FROM SUBACUTE CARE PARTICIPANTS

• Define and review individual and discipline-specific roles and responsibilities through interdisciplinary effort.
• Identify the common interests and concerns of all parties.
• Help players at all levels understand proper roles and relationships.
• Evaluate and supplement current knowledge and skills.
• Provide ample opportunity for conceptual debate and discussion.
• Provide all parties with means for continuing personal education and improvement.
• Have all parties explain in writing their perspectives on appropriate attitudes and roles.
• Ensure frequent feedback to all participants about their performance of their roles and functions.

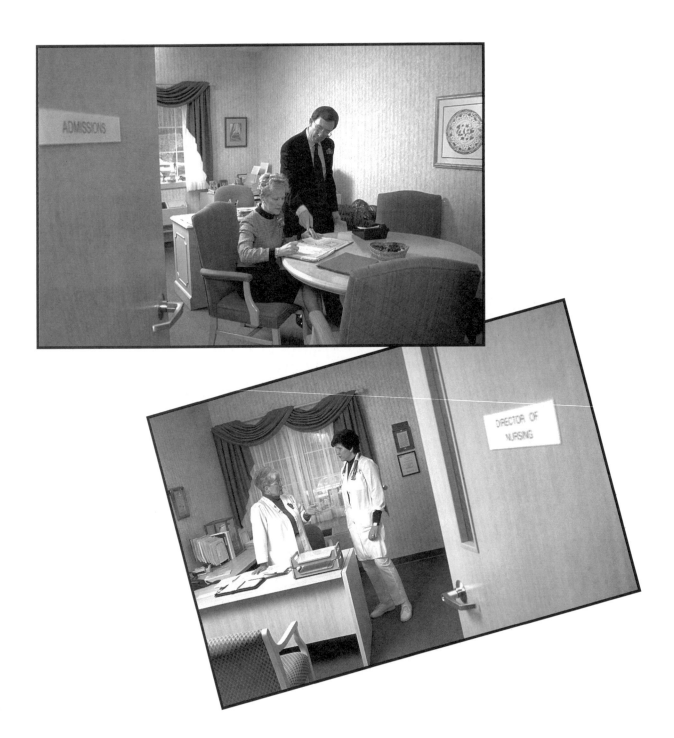

THE PROCESSES OF CARE

CHAPTER 7

Subacute care is given by individuals who are organized into various clinical departments or services. Frequently, the care is centered around specific syndromes or treatments, such as pain management or orthopedic rehabilitation, that are the focus of the individual's admission to the program.

Regardless of the reasons for admission or the care objectives, all subacute care involves processes that must consistently be done effectively and efficiently. The processes are performed sequentially, as are many of their associated tasks. Although these processes are similar to those in other settings such as the acute care hospital, they have some important differences in scope and components. This chapter will discuss those processes of care at length, and explain how understanding those differences is essential to successful provision of subacute care.

ESSENTIAL PROCESSES

Processes of care are identifiable collections of functions and tasks performed by appropriately trained and skilled individuals, to achieve an overall care objective for individuals with illness, injury, or disturbed function. They require effective, consistent individual performance. The processes, and many of the tasks within each process, must be performed sequentially to achieve those goals. For example, the process of assessment partially precedes that of problem identification. But it is less important whether the assessment itself is done in any particular order. Every patient's care involves the same processes, although not necessarily to the same degree. For instance, every patient needs some problem identification, but some patients may have had most of their problems identified previously and others may have new problems develop after admission.

The processes of subacute care are listed in Table 7–1, p. 181. They begin with preadmission assessment and selection and continue through postdischarge follow-up. Figure 8–1, p. 207, illustrates the relationship of these processes as building blocks of a systematic approach to care.

Patient Selection

The first step, patient selection, occurs before admission. Most patients are referred by hospital discharge planners or case managers, but sometimes they are referred directly by physicians, nursing facilities, or other sites. To date, the Medicare reimbursement system has been a major influence on where people have received care prior to their referral. For instance, the requirement for a 3-day prior hospital stay to qualify for Medicare skilled has limited the use of subacute programs for direct admission of those with mildly or moderately unstable acute conditions who need short-term care but not necessarily hospitalization. Some pilot programs have been allowed to bypass this restriction (Zimmer, 1993) in attempts to provide a more cost-effective continuum.

The primary objectives of the preadmission selection process are to decide if the patient needs admission to a subacute program and if the program can provide the essential care and services for that individual. Table 7–2, pp. 181–182, lists the items that should be covered by a preadmission assessment.

Although programs sometimes accept patients who later turn out to be unsuitable, a systematic approach should make such occurrences the exception rather than the rule. If the preadmission assessment is mistaken, then the program must either be able to adjust to meet the newly identified needs or be able to transfer the person elsewhere.

General Selection Criteria.   Each program needs general selection criteria. These may be based on the services offered and the conditions that can be handled (inclusion criteria) or those that are not offered or cannot be managed (exclusion criteria), or some of each. Table 7–3, p. 182, lists examples of some general inclusion and exclusion criteria found in many subacute programs. Exclusion criteria may be relative (exceptions will be considered in some cases) or absolute (the program cannot handle the situation under any circumstances).

The program should delineate the scope of services and the types of patients who will be admitted to the unit, such as ventilator patients, brain injury patients, or rehabilitation patients. In addition, each program must recognize that patients come not just with service or treatment needs, but also with other associated problems that cut across programs and treatment categories, such as fluid volume deficits, depression, activity intolerance, skin impairment, and altered breathing patterns. There is evidence that the existence of these other problems affects outcomes, costs of care, and lengths of stay (Rosenthal et al., 1992, 1995).

Another important distinction for the subacute program is that of problem correction versus secondary or tertiary prevention. Sometimes, prevention of further decline is a more realistic objective than substantial recovery. For example, a patient with major deficits from a recent major stroke may recover only partially, and may also need prevention of skin breakdown, improvement of nutrition and hydration status, or prevention of contractures. The planned patient management must consider all of these issues, so that the staff can be adequately prepared and the patient and family can have more reasonable expectations.

Elements of the Screening Process. Subacute programs commonly receive referrals through an admissions or marketing office. Many programs use a case manager or other liaison person to collect information about prospective admissions. This individual would see if the prospect broadly meets financial and clinical criteria. This requires communicating with the patient's current nurses, social workers, and physicians, and may also necessitate visiting current care sites for direct patient assessment and chart review. The case manager would assess severity of illness and look in greater depth at other relevant issues (Table 7–2, pp. 181–182).

Many programs also use an admissions team, consisting of nurses, physicians, social workers, administrators, and sometimes a case manager or UR coordinator. This team determines the appropriateness of admissions based on the above information. It must also consider the abilities, limits, and concerns of those who will provide the care. For example, a patient may be acceptable medically but may present complex nursing problems such as a frequent need for respiratory treatments or the management of difficult behavior. The nursing staff must be able to handle those problems so that the patient may be accepted. Whether or not the program uses this team approach, there must be a means by which the care providers assess the appropriateness of admissions and the quality of accompanying information and give the admissions liaison person or team feedback about these things.

A nurse, physician, or other individual may need to contact the referring site for additional clarification. A physician may need to be consulted when there are possible complications, when additional communications with physicians at the referring site are needed, when there are questions about continuing service needs, when it is unclear whether the patient meets the criteria for the program, or under other circumstances. For example, a patient with an infectious complication such as TB or hepatitis may need a review to determine the appropriate management and precautions. Usually, the program medical director will be the consultant, although it could be the attending physician or a specialist such as a pulmonologist. This reviewer may desire or need the input of other consultants.

Having adequate information about patients upon admission is essential. Although the patient's condition may change between the time of acceptance and the actual admission, it has traditionally often been very difficult to get all the desired or essential information in a timely fashion before having to make a decision, or the information from referral sources may be incomplete or inaccurate. In a managed care environment, these processes must become more consistently reliable. The need to discharge or accept a patient in a hurry should not be used to excuse transfers without relevant information. Inefficiencies in compiling and providing such information consistently and in a timely fashion must be addressed by all levels of the health care system.

Each subacute program should provide its usual referral sources with a list of essential information it needs to be able to make effective admission decisions. A program that is part of a network should have its information needs integrated with other portions of the network, so that vital information can be shared effectively.

Postselection, Preadmission Preparation.   After the review group has decided to accept a patient, the case manager or admissions coordinator should inform various individuals (administrator, billing office, and so on) of the severity of illness, level of service need, care objectives, and the like. The payer should be informed of the relevant factors involved in the proposed cost of the care (Table 7–4, p. 183). In dealing with managed care arrangements, this information should be included in a referral agreement, which is completed after reaching verbal agreement.

After admission is confirmed, the case manager or coordinator should verify the admission date with the discharging and admitting facilities, confirm transportation arrangements, meet with the family and give a tour, coordinate any preadmission team meeting, and confirm that all necessary equipment, supplies, pharmaceuticals, and personnel will be available upon admission.

Assessment

Assessment is the process by which various practitioners assemble a database on an individual by evaluating multiple dimensions of the individual's physical and mental condition and social and functional status. Assessment may include direct observation, examination, testing (X-rays, blood tests, and so on), and review of past or current information about the individual (consultant reports, hospital discharge summaries, and the like).

Assessments of subacute patients should address those areas that are relevant to their conditions and their care (Table 7–5, pp. 183–184). Gathering this information begins prior to admission, but accelerates upon admission. The preadmission assessment can be supplemented by additional evaluation after admission. For example, the referring program may report that the individual has pain and needs pain management. Upon admission, a pain assessment must characterize the pain further according to its origin, location, severity, alleviating and exacerbating factors, current treatment, and response to treatment.

There is considerable debate about the necessary scope of assessments. Assessments are the principal route to appropriate, complete problem definition, which is in turn the foundation for effective care planning and management. Therefore, they are a means to an end. They need to be broad and thorough enough to enable complete problem definition. Unfortunately, because of the great variation in the scope and accuracy of the problem identification done prior to admission to subacute programs, it may be easy to miss significant problems by assuming that an assessment can be limited to what has already been identified. Therefore, although the scope and content of the assessment should be flexible, there is a core of information relevant to almost all subacute patients that may be broader than many practitioners recognize. Managing problems in psychosocial and functional dimensions is as essential to the care of medical and surgical patients as managing health-related issues is to the care of rehabilitation and psychiatric patients.

Relationship of the Minimum Data Set to the Assessment.   Many subacute patients receive care in skilled nursing facility (SNF) beds. The OBRA '87 federal regulations covering nursing facility (NF) care mandate the use of a Resident Assessment Instrument (RAI) consisting of two parts: a Minimum Data Set (MDS) and the resident assessment protocols (RAPs). For patients who are covered by Medicare and who stay longer than 14 days, the facility must complete the MDS, which is a collection of information regarding patient function, psychosocial status, medical conditions, and other relevant parameters (Table 7–6, p. 184). The MDS sections most relevant to the care of subacute patients are cognitive patterns, communication/hearing patterns, physical functioning and structural problems, disease diagnoses, health conditions, oral/nutritional status, skin condition, and special treatments and procedures. The RAPs are a set of 18 evaluation and care protocols that may be triggered by individual or combined findings on the MDS. For example, recording an observation of abnormal cognitive function may trigger the RAP for further evaluation of causes of delirium (acute confusional state).

Many of the MDS data items overlap those used in other assessment tools, although the terminology and rating scales may vary. For example, MDS coding for mobility is on a scale of 0 (independent) to 4 (totally dependent), and it is broken down into "walk in room," "walk in corridor," locomotion on unit," and "locomotion off unit." The same item in the Functional Independence Measure (FIM) scale—often used in rehabilitation programs—is called "locomotion" and is divided into "walk/wheelchair" and "stairs," each coded from 1 (total assistance) to 7 (complete independence).

Each subacute program must decide if it must complete the MDS, if it wants to use the MDS even if it does not have to, what other data collection instruments it might use instead of or in addition to the MDS, and how to avoid duplication of effort. The best approach may be to view all the patient-related information as one database, with various pieces of information being needed for care-related and other purposes. In a paper-based system, it is very difficult to avoid extra work, or to readily combine the data elements from different sources to meet different output requirements. Computerization is likely to be the most effective approach because it enables any data element to be entered only once and then retrieved and used readily for different reporting purposes.

Another reason that the MDS has been required in subacute programs is because of its additional use as a source of information for a prospective case-mix payment system (see Chapter 12). Programs should familiarize themselves with this application so they understand the multiple uses of a common database. Additionally, the accompanying RAPs can help the staff assess acute condition changes.

Additional Responsibilities for Assessment.   Some aspects of the assessment are discipline-specific, and others are cross-disciplinary. For instance, although physicians assess all patient organ systems, both nurses and physicians should assess a patient's breathing patterns and skin condition, and social workers or nurses may do more detailed assessments of cognitive function.

The assessments done by various disciplines must be closely coordinated. Each program should work out the various responsibilities (Table 7–5, pp. 183–184). Although the order of assessment is generally unimportant, the various portions should be complementary so that the total assessment enables appropriate problem definition. Descriptions of problems should consider both the current status and changes in status over time; for example, recent decline or improvement in function, cognition, or medical condition.

Based on these pre- and postadmission assessments, various kinds of information—also reflecting analyses and conclusions—should be documented in the patient's medical record (Table 7–7, p. 185). For example, a Mini-Mental Examination Score is a measurement of a patient's cognitive function and attention span. A diagnosis of dementia is a conclusion based on that information plus other observation and testing.

The organization of the data can make a difference in the ease with which the information is used and the ability of staff to make sense of it. Although the arrangement and location of this information will vary among programs, it is important that it be accurate, accessible, and interpretable by those needing it to help them make care decisions.

Programs should help and expect physicians to provide timely, complete, and relevant information. For example, this might include a standardized history and physical form (Figure 7–1) or, eventually, computerized documentation including voice-activated input. A medical diagnosis list (Figure 7–2) is also very helpful in allowing many disciplines, covering physicians, and others to rapidly review the nature and current status of the causes of a patient's problems.

Time Frame for Assessment.   Each subacute program should indicate the time frames for completing assessments. Within 48 to 72 hours of admission, most of the important information about an individual should be known. To some extent, the time frame will be influenced by regulations or accreditation requirements. For instance, the Joint Commission on Accreditation of Healthcare Organizations (JCAHO) standards require the initiation of assessments within 24 hours and completion within 48 hours; completion of each patient's assessment within 14 days of admission, except for the medical assessment, which must be completed within 72 hours; and subsequent reviews within 30 days or in response to changes in the patient's condition.

During the stay, most of the database will remain constant but some will change. Patients should be reassessed periodically, both after specified intervals and for condition changes. As discussed more fully in Chapter 10, some of these changes are relevant to assessing outcomes and quality of care.

Problem Definition

The next step is to define each patient's problems correctly and completely. As noted throughout this book, doing so for the subacute patient—as with the long-term care patient—differs from other phases of medical care.

Patients' problems must be distinguished from their medical diagnoses. Diagnoses are definable medical syndromes or conditions representing disruptions of the body's normal structure or function, which may cause or contribute

FIGURE 7–1   HISTORY AND PHYSICAL FORM RELEVANT TO SUBACUTE CARE

Admission History and Physical

Patient Name: **ID #:**

Exam Date:

PRESENT MEDICAL HISTORY

This is the _____ admission for this   y.o.   .

Transferred From:

Recent Medical Course:

Symptoms related to current problems:

PAST MEDICAL HISTORY

Major previous illnesses:

Allergies:

Family History:

　　Pertinent positive FH:

SYSTEMS REVIEW

　　☐ Systems review unattainable because of _____.

　　☐ Systems review completely negative.

　　☐ Systems review positive for the following significant problems or conditions (describe positive finding in
　　　space provided):

General	☐ Chronic pain ☐ Recent weight loss ☐ Overall decline in condition
Skin	☐ Pruritus ☐ Excessive dryness
EENT	☐ Visual disturbance ☐ Hearing disturbance ☐ Loss of smell ☐ Loss of taste ☐ Difficulty chewing/swallowing
Respiratory	☐ Dyspnea ☐ Cough ☐ Dyspnea on exertion
Cardiovascular	☐ Hypertension ☐ Chest pain ☐ Palpitations ☐ Dizziness/syncope/falling ☐ Dyspnea/orthopnea ☐ Edema ☐ Claudication
Gastrointestinal	☐ Bowel incontinence ☐ Abdominal pain ☐ Heartburn ☐ Change in bowel habit ☐ Melena/hematochezia
Gynecological	☐ Abnormal vaginal bleeding ☐ Discharge
Genitourinary	☐ Frequency/nocturia ☐ Urgency ☐ Incontinence ☐ Hematuria ☐ Voiding difficulty (☐ hesitancy, ☐ straining, ☐ intermittent stream)
Musculoskeletal	☐ Joint pain ☐ Swollen joints ☐ Recent fracture/dislocation ☐ Limited range of motion

(continued)

Neurological   ☐ Headaches   ☐ Dizziness   ☐ Falling   ☐ Balance problem   ☐ Gait disturbance
               ☐ Pain   ☐ Paresthesias   ☐ Tremor

Psychiatric   ☐ Memory disturbance   ☐ Paranoia/delusions   ☐ Behavioral disturbances

Endocrine   ☐ Increased urination   ☐ Increased thirst   ☐ Lethargy

OTHER RELEVANT HISTORY

PHYSICAL EXAMINATION

General

Hydration   ☐ Well hydrated   ☐ Moderate dehydration   ☐ Severe dehydration

Nutritional status   ☐ Well nourished   ☐ Moderately well nourished   ☐ Poorly nourished

Level of consciousness   ☐ Alert   ☐ Lethargic   ☐ Stuporous   ☐ Comatose

Overall   ☐ In no acute distress   ☐ Acute distress due to:

Vital Signs

Pulse Rate: ☐ Regular   ☐ Irregular

BP: ☐ Postural changes in BP

Resp Rate: ☐ Labored   ☐ Unlabored

Temp:

Skin: ☐ Normal moisture, color, texture for age.   ☐ No pressure sores.   ☐ Nails WNL.
          ☐ No rashes.   ☐ <u>Abnormalities:</u>

Head: ☐ Normocephalic.   ☐ No evidence of trauma.   ☐ Normal hair and scalp for age.
          ☐ <u>Abnormalities:</u>

Eyes: ☐ Eyelids WNL for age.   ☐ Corneas clear.   Pupils ☐ equal ☐ regular ☐ reactive to
light.   ☐ Sclerae nonicteric.   ☐ Conjunctivae WNL.   ☐ No cataracts.
          ☐ Ophthalmoscopic WNL.   ☐ Vision: glasses/contact lenses.   ☐ <u>Abnormalities:</u>

Ears: ☐ External ears WNL.   ☐ Canals clear.   ☐ TMs appear intact.   ☐ Can hear normal
conversation   ☐ with a hearing aid.   ☐ <u>Abnormalities:</u>

Nose: ☐ External nose WNL.   ☐ Septum midline.   ☐ No masses.   ☐ No nasal discharge.
          ☐ No sinus tenderness.   ☐ <u>Abnormalities:</u>

Mouth: ☐ Lips and tongue WNL for age.   ☐ Mucous membranes intact.   ☐ Palate WNL.
          ☐ No growths.   ☐ <u>Abnormalities:</u>

Teeth/gums: ☐ Has most of own teeth.   ☐ Little or no periodontal disease.   ☐ No dental caries.
          ☐ Uses dentures.   ☐ <u>Abnormalities:</u>

Pharynx: ☐ Uvula midline.   ☐ Throat unremarkable.   ☐ <u>Abnormalities:</u>

Neck: ☐ No JVD.   ☐ Thyroid unremarkable.   ☐ Normal range of motion.
          ☐ <u>Abnormalities:</u>

FIGURE 7–1   HISTORY AND PHYSICAL FORM RELEVANT TO SUBACUTE CARE (CONTINUED)

Lymph nodes: ☐ No adenopathy.   ☐ Abnormalities:

Chest: ☐ Shape and symmetry WNL for age.   ☐ Bony thorax unremarkable.   ☐ Abnormalities:

Lungs: ☐ Clear to P&A.   ☐ No rales, rhonchi, wheezes.   ☐ Normal breath sounds.
☐ Abnormalities:

Heart: ☐ Regular rate, rhythm.   ☐ 1st and 2nd sounds WNL.   ☐ No murmurs or rubs.
☐ PMI not enlarged.   ☐ No S3 or S4.   ☐ Abnormalities:

Peripheral vascular: Normal and equal   ☐ carotids,   ☐ brachials,   ☐ radials,   ☐ femorals,   ☐ popliteals,
dorsalis pedis.   ☐ No bruits.   ☐ Abnormalities:

Breasts: ☐ Normal for sex and age.   ☐ No masses or discharge.   ☐ Abnormalities:

Abdomen: ☐ Symmetrical.   ☐ Soft.   ☐ Not tender.   ☐ No scars.   ☐ No rebound, guarding.
☐ Not distended.   ☐ No masses.   ☐ Percussion WNL.   ☐ Bowel sounds heard
throughout.   ☐ Liver, spleen not enlarged.   ☐ No bruits.   ☐ No hernias.
☐ No ascites.   ☐ No aortic aneurysm.   ☐ Abnormalities:

Rectal: ☐ No pain or masses.   ☐ No bleeding.   ☐ No hemorrhoids.   ☐ Sphincter tone WNL.
☐ Prostate WNL.   ☐ No impaction.   ☐ Abnormalities:

Genitalia: ☐ Normal for sex and age.   ☐ No discharge or bleeding.   ☐ No uterine prolapse.
☐ Abnormalities:

Extremities: ☐ Full active/passive ROM upper and lower.   ☐ No edema, clubbing, cyanosis.
☐ No deformities.   ☐ Abnormalities:

Musculoskeletal: ☐ No evidence of fractures.   ☐ Muscle tone and strength normal for age.
☐ No contractures.   ☐ No joint deformity.   ☐ No missing limbs.   ☐ Abnormalities:

Neurological: ☐ Motor function intact.   ☐ Sensory function WNL for age.   ☐ CNs II-XII WNL.
Gait   ☐ normal for age   ☐ not tested.   ☐ Cerebellar function WNL.   ☐ No paralysis/
paresis.   ☐ Speech normal.   ☐ Reflexes normal.   ☐ Pathological reflexes.
☐ Abnormalities:

Psychiatric: ☐ Oriented × 3.   ☐ Affect appropriate.   ☐ Attention span good.   ☐ Communication
WNL.   ☐ No abnormal ideation.   ☐ Appropriate response to questions.
☐ Abnormalities:

Miscellaneous:

OVERALL MEDICAL ASSESSMENT

SUGGESTED PATIENT GOALS (check all that apply/describe as needed):

Short-Term   Long-Term

General Objectives

____	____	Restore previous level of health/function
____	____	Improve current level of health/function short of previous level
____	____	Stabilize medical condition (prevent further decline or death)
____	____	Supportive care for terminal condition

(continued)

FIGURE 7–1   HISTORY AND PHYSICAL FORM RELEVANT TO SUBACUTE CARE (CONTINUED)

Short-Term   Long-Term

Other Goals

Short-Term	Long-Term	
____	____	Increase mobility and function
____	____	Relieve pain
____	____	Reduce dysfunctional behavior
____	____	Improve independence
____	____	Improve mobility
____	____	Improve nutritional status
____	____	Discharge home
____	____	Others:

Rehabilitation Potential

To what extent might Rehab be beneficial to this individual?

☐ Very much   ☐ Somewhat   ☐ Not at all

If Rehab is appropriate, to what extent could this patient potentially participate in some Rehab program?

☐ Very much   ☐ Somewhat   ☐ Not at all

Need for Special Programs and Services

Which, if any, of the following special treatments, programs, or services might benefit this individual?

☐ Special diet ☐ Feeding tube ☐ Parenteral feedings ☐ Intravenous fluids ☐ Suctioning ☐ Oxygen
☐ Special dressings or appliances ☐ Protective skin care ☐ Turning/repositioning program ☐ Pressure
relieving measures ☐ Special bed ☐ Wound care/treatment ☐ Therapeutic activities ☐ Social services
intervention ☐ Others

Miscellaneous

Are there any other noteworthy things about this individual, from a physician's perspective?

Signed: _____

Date: _____

to problems. Problems are circumstances, signs and symptoms, or conditions that significantly disrupt an individual's life.

Primary problems are the main consequences of a current episode of illness or those requiring the most or the most immediate attention. Secondary problems are those of lesser magnitude or urgency to the current need for care.

Not all problems have a directly discernible cause, and not all of a person's diagnoses cause a problem. Some problems have one or more identifiable causes, and for others only some or no causes can be identified. Many of the same problems can be caused by different diagnoses and the same diagnosis can cause any number of different problems. Only some problems are the consequences of medical illness, and nonmedical problems (for example, family-related, mood, and personality disturbances) have been shown to impact outcomes. Treating medical causes may result in (1) full resolution of problems, (2) partial resolution of problems, (3) no effect on problems, or (4) worsening of problems.

FIGURE 7–2   A FORM FOR DOCUMENTING A MEDICAL PROBLEM LIST

MEDICAL DIAGNOSIS LIST

ICDA Code	Diagnosis	Present on Admission	Onset During Stay	Recurrent During Stay	Present on on Discharge
	Principal diagnosis:				

For example, a patient may have chronic obstructive lung disease with blood gases showing a pH of 7.33 and a pCO_2 of 44, but may not have altered breathing or need any specific treatments. Someone with a sodium level of 131 mg/dl may have volume overload needing medical management, or may have no discernible or treatable cause. A transient decline in blood pressure may reflect gastrointestinal bleeding or may return to normal spontaneously.

Hospital-based care is oriented toward managing discrete diagnoses. By the end of the hospital stay, the major diagnosis has usually been defined and some treatment initiated, but the broader consequences or coexisting conditions may have only been addressed partially, necessitating additional posthospital care. Although patients may be referred to subacute programs primarily because of their service needs (ventilator care, wound management), the unit must further define and address all relevant problems as much as possible, even when the underlying causes cannot be fully corrected. Missing some of the important co-existing problems can result in a prolonged and more costly stay, less complete recovery, more complications, and poorer outcome.

One way to understand these distinctions is to compare typical physician and nonmedical problem lists. For example, nursing diagnoses are problem oriented, not disease centered. They are most often used by nurses to help define their care plans. However, they are not just the domain of nurses. Their importance lies in the fact that they reflect the consequences rather than the causes of illness and injury. This problem-oriented approach more appropriately reflects the overall care needs of those with multidimensional problems.

Table 7–8, pp. 186–189, is based on 34 nursing diagnoses that have been found to be related individually and collectively to morbidity, mortality, and length of stay in acute care patients (Rosenthal et al, 1992, 1995), and the criteria for determining their presence. These diagnoses and criteria also apply to subacute patients, as shown in Table 7–8. Figure 7–3 is a sample format for documenting these problems in each patient. As discussed at length in Chapter 10, this information is not only relevant to the care, but can provide an important foundation for measuring outcomes and risk-adjusted reimbursement. Therefore, both medical diagnoses and nursing diagnoses (problems) should be documented for each patient.

A successful subacute care program should appreciate the implications of these concepts for the care and for the responsibilities of various disciplines. Problem definition, like assessment, must be an interdisciplinary process, with disease-related problems being only one component. All dimensions of problems, including functional and psychosocial, are important. Addressing each problem requires performance of numerous tasks in the areas of assessment, monitoring, management, and follow-up. For instance, Table 7–9, pp. 190–198, shows the tasks involved in managing the problems listed in Table 7-8. This information can be used to help construct critical pathways to guide the management of various patients.

Subacute programs may differ in who performs which functions, but must ensure that all the functions are performed consistently. For example, nurses may be responsible for recognizing the onset of an infection (fever, increased respirations, change in sputum, and so on), physicians may be responsible for identifying the cause of the infection and ordering treatment, nurses for administering treatments, both physicians and nurses for monitoring the responses to treatment, and dietitians for assessing the patient for nutritional deficits caused by, or predisposing to, complications of the infection. Whatever the division of responsibilities, the information must eventually be aggregated and interpreted to properly define each individual's problems.

Physicians obviously play a critical role in defining and managing a patient's problems. They must be flexible enough to recognize that they may have more than one role for the same patient and various roles in different patients. Physicians are skilled at identifying the causes of medical illnesses, but they may not be as adept at defining and managing other nonmedical problems or consequences related or unrelated to those illnesses. Because most subacute patients arrive with their major diagnoses already established, the physician may not need to play as much of a diagnostician role unless new problems arise during the stay. A physician may also need to authorize or modify medical orders to deal with problems identified by other disciplines (for example, ordering re-

FIGURE 7–3   A TOOL FOR RECORDING NURSING PROBLEMS TO ENABLE A SEVERITY-OF-ILLNESS SCORE

PATIENT PROBLEM/CONDITION LIST

Condition/Problem	Present on Admission	Onset During Stay	Recurrent During Stay	Present on Discharge
Group 1. Overall Health	------	------	------	------
Risk for injury				
Infection/contagion				
Prolonged disease/disability				
Instability				
Impaired life-support systems				
Group 2. Nutrition and Metabolism	------	------	------	------
Fluid volume excess				
Fluid volume deficit				
Bleeding				
Altered nutrition				
Impaired skin integrity				
Altered oral mucous membranes				
Altered body temperature				
Group 3. Urinary and Fecal Elimination	------	------	------	------
Urinary incontinence				
Altered urinary elimination				
Constipation				
Diarrhea				
Bowel incontinence				
Group 4. Activity and Exercise	------	------	------	------
Activity intolerance				
Ineffective airway clearance				
Ineffective breathing pattern				
Impaired gas exchange				
Decreased cardiac output				

(continued)

FIGURE 7–3   A TOOL FOR RECORDING NURSING PROBLEMS TO ENABLE A SEVERITY-OF-ILLNESS SCORE (CONTINUED)

PATIENT PROBLEM/CONDITION LIST

Condition/Problem	Present on Admission	Onset During Stay	Recurrent During Stay	Present on Discharge
Altered health maintenance				
Impaired physical mobility				
Self-care deficit				
Group 5. Psychosocial Concerns	------	------	------	------
Self-esteem disturbance				
Hopelessness/depression				
Dysfunctional grieving				
Altered family processes				
Social isolation				
Impaired verbal communication				
Ineffective individual coping				
Family coping: potential for growth				
Spiritual distress				
TOTAL SEVERITY OF ILLNESS SCORE[a]				

[a]Total score is derived by adding up the total number of problems checked as active at any one time.

habilitation therapies or psychological testing, or stopping a medication that may be causing confusion or depression).

Each program also needs a system to effectively coordinate the processes of problem identification/assessment, monitoring, management, and follow-up. The interdisciplinary approach should overcome the tendency to compartmentalize or "own" various aspects of the assessment or of the care. There must be flexible assignment of responsibility and a sense of mutual accountability that crosses disciplinary boundaries.

The case examples in Chapter 11 distinguish diagnoses and problems, and should help clarify how the problems must be addressed for the care to succeed fully.

Identifying Care Objectives

Based on assessment and problem identification, practitioners must establish care objectives, that is, "What is expected to be accomplished by treating this individual?" There are several levels of issues here: (1) what will be treated or managed, (2) what is the likely impact of such treatment on an individual's problems, and (3) what is the likely impact on the person's overall level of functioning? Each of these objectives is distinct and has different implications for treatment decision making.

The goals of treatment may include recovery to at least the status prior to the episode of illness or injury, partial recovery toward that status, stabilizing the condition (that is, preventing further decline or death, as in respiratory failure due to pneumonia in a person with chronic obstructive lung disease), preventing or managing the complications caused by those conditions, or supporting an expected decline or dying process. For example, an individual transferred to subacute care after an extended bout with cancer and recent chemotherapy might receive pain management and continuing chemotherapy. The impact of these treatments on the cancer may range from curative to negligible. Ultimate effects on function may include reducing pain, enabling functional improvement and return home, or causing complications and accelerating decline.

Therefore, care objectives must be pertinent and realistic. Previously in health care, there had been more emphasis on providing service than on accomplishing something by giving that service. But in the future, the impact of treatment on the overall condition and the extent to which an overall objective is achieved, must be considered just as important as the rendering of treatment. The results should be compared to the predicted results to help measure outcomes.

Establishing care objectives must be an interdisciplinary process involving the patient and family as well as practitioners. If a person's significant problems can be resolved fully, then the care objective will probably be straightforward. But when problems are unlikely to be resolved fully, criteria are needed for determining the appropriate goal of the treatment and the point at which the subacute care package is no longer needed or useful to achieve those goals.

If anticipated care objectives are not being achieved, then the objectives must be reassessed. They may have been unrealistic to begin with, or they might require more time or a change in treatment. This should lead to other discussions of whether the care should continue until the objectives are achieved, the care should continue but at another site, or a reduction in level of care is desirable because the objectives cannot be achieved.

Despite progress in predicting outcomes and risks, there are still many patients who fall into a gray area, where it is hard to predict consistently who can benefit the most from specific treatments and services, and when it is not worth giving someone a treatment or service. Thus, treatment may still be given despite the likelihood of negligible impact because of the remote possibility of doing some good. Important issues for subacute care include deciding how much treatment to give for how long, how long it should take to achieve certain care objectives, and when to stop delivering services at that level and transfer a patient elsewhere. Further research is needed to develop criteria for predicting more consistently who can benefit from what level of care, and when care may be considered medically ineffective. But enough information exists currently to allow this to be done effectively in many cases. One way to help this effort is to use the data collected during the care of subacute patients to analyze the factors that are most helpful to accurate predictions.

Care Planning

When diagnoses and problems are clarified and the care objectives are established, then it is possible to create a care plan. A care plan is a detailed road map to achieve the care objectives based on defining a person's problems, determining causes, managing and preventing problems, and determining the results of management.

As with the other steps in the processes of care, the overall care plan should be primarily interdisciplinary and problem-oriented, and only secondarily diagnosis- or discipline-specific. A unified care plan for each patient should describe the overall objectives and approaches. The plan should at least identify patient needs; realistic, measurable patient goals; the care and services intended to meet those goals; the disciplines responsible for performing essential functions; the expected time frame for achieving the goals; the anticipated disposition; and contingency plans for significant condition changes.

Although the roles of individual disciplines may vary among subacute programs, ultimately the same tasks must be performed to accomplish the functions that can help achieve the care objectives. All relevant disciplines should have input into the care planning, regardless of whether they have their own discipline-specific written care plan. Physicians must still contribute to the discussion and ensure that medical orders are relevant to overall care objectives, even though they may not be present for an interdisciplinary care planning meeting.

To some extent, the processes involved in achieving the care objectives affect the efficiency of the care. Therefore, the care plan must be viewed from the perspectives of how well and how efficiently the subsequent processes achieve the care objectives. As discussed in Chapter 10, this can be related to process quality indicators.

The Process.   Care plans are usually established and reviewed through interdisciplinary meetings, although this is not required. An initial or interim care plan should be developed as soon as possible (but no later than 72 hours) after admission, and used to initiate care until a more formal plan based on an interdisciplinary review is developed. A specific individual (a nurse, case manager, or physician) may be identified to coordinate the care planning process and to verify the care plan, which should be updated at least weekly or when there is a significant condition change.

Even though making their own assessments, subacute care staff must still depend to some extent on the information provided by the prior care site. This reinforces the need to improve and coordinate information management among various providers and regions. Practitioners are seriously handicapped by insufficient or inaccurate information because their care plan may then miss addressing some important problems.

Management of Known Problems

A system is needed to manage each patient's known problems, that is, those that are identified prior to or at the time of admission. Each patient has a primary reason for admission to the subacute program (respiratory insufficiency, multiple pressure ulcers, general deconditioning), and also may have any number of secondary problems.

Treatment is done to try to correct the causes of problems where possible and to manage the resulting functional and physical deficits. It should also address the effects of chronic conditions and try to prevent or limit the extent of damage from complications. For instance, a patient who is accepted with multiple coexisting conditions, laboratory evidence of severe undernutrition, or significant volume depletion either acquired or not fully treated during the hospital stay may have a prolonged postacute stay. The case manager should use a list of red flags to check for the presence of these issues during the initial screening. Similarly, a physician advisor or other member of any admissions committee who recognizes those flags may need to check further into their origin and severity.

Table 7–10, p. 199, lists the various categories of origins of problems in subacute patients. As discussed earlier, secondary problems may have considerable influence on outcomes. Certain problems such as nutritional deficits and alterations in cardiac output tend to be common to many subacute patients. Because most of these problems can be identified, anticipated, prevented, and managed effectively when they arise, each subacute program should have relevant protocols. For example, delirium is common in acutely ill, institutionally treated (hospital, NF, subacute care) patients and often reflects treatable conditions, such as infections, medication side effects, and metabolic disorders. Because the presence of delirium is unquestionably associated with increased morbidity and mortality, it is important to assess and manage it effectively (Levkoff et al, 1988).

In managing these common problems, subacute programs should try to use practice guidelines and protocols as much as possible. These can help ensure that certain processes of problem identification, workup, and follow-up are done, while still allowing for practitioner flexibility to choose among treatment options. Figure 7–4 gives an example of guidelines for addressing delirium in the subacute and long-term patient.

Each program should ensure that the various individuals and disciplines understand their roles in managing these problems (Table 7–9, pp. 190–198). At different points, these roles may diverge or converge. For instance, various disciplines perform assessments independently, they begin to identify problems separately but should define them jointly; the physician authorizes care and treatment through the medical orders, the different disciplines then deliver specific components of the care and separately monitor the individual's response to the care, but should then jointly consider progress and possible care plan adjustments.

Prevention and Management of New Problems/Complications

During the subacute patient's stay, problems and condition changes may arise that are either related or unrelated to existing ones. Related problems may either be complications of existing conditions or different conditions associated with existing ones. For example, intestinal obstruction or bleeding stomach ulcer may be complicated by perforation, or pneumonia may be complicated by septicemia. On the other hand, skin breakdown is associated with—but not caused directly by—strokes or other conditions that result in immobilization. Also, the same problem may be due to various causes. For example, rectal bleeding may be caused by conditions as diverse as medications, hemorrhoids, antibiotic-induced colitis, and major gastric hemorrhage. An example of unrelated problems would be the occurrence of pneumonia in a patient admitted for follow-up care after knee replacement surgery.

FIGURE 7–4

GUIDELINES FOR MANAGING ALTERED MENTAL STATUS AND BEHAVIOR IN THE SUBACUTE AND LONG-TERM PATIENT

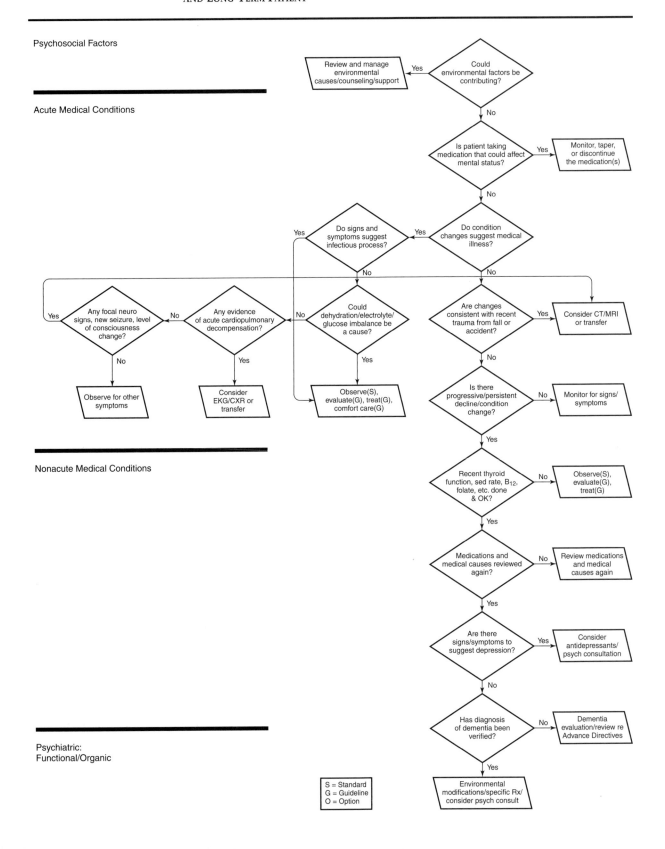

One of the most difficult challenges in the care of those with multiple concurrent conditions and problems is to determine the cause of an acute condition change. Any set of signs and symptoms could be caused by an exacerbation or complications of existing conditions, new onset of an unrelated condition, medication side effects or complications, or some combination of the above. Or, the signs and symptoms may be transitory or may not represent any significant or detectable problem. Because their causes and consequences may at first be unclear, these new-onset problems may require a higher level of diagnostic and decision-making support (including communications and information management, laboratory, and radiology) than managing known problems.

Especially in a managed care environment, subacute programs must minimize and carefully scrutinize their hospital transfers. Thus, each program needs a mechanism for anticipating and trying to prevent complications; for identifying, defining, and determining the severity of new problems and condition changes; for managing these problems; and for determining whether they should interrupt the treatment plan or even whether they require patient transfer to another setting. Table 7–11, p. 199, lists factors influencing decisions about possible transfer of patients for condition changes.

Responsibility.   Physicians and other skilled clinicians (clinical nurse specialists, RNs, nurse practitioners, or physician assistants) are especially important for this function because of their training and experience at recognizing and defining such problems. But all disciplines involved in the care—including nursing assistants, social workers, and physical therapists—may have a role in screening for the onset of new problems or changes in current condition. They should all be aware of the potential risks and complications of each patient so that they may help identify their onset, understand why the care plan might change, and help explain the situation to the patient and the family. For instance, even nonphysicians should be able to identify altered breathing patterns or changes in mentation and attention span so that they can at least bring them to the attention of others who can determine the significance and identify causes. Each program should make the clinical guidelines and protocols accessible for all team members and include instructions about their use as part of any orientation and training program.

Handling Condition Changes.   Each program needs procedures for handling significant changes in patient status. These changes should be documented and reported to the attending physician in a timely fashion (which may vary depending on their severity). Unexpected changes should be reported promptly, especially if the patient is more unstable. Anticipated changes may be reported more routinely, unless otherwise requested. For example, a dialysis patient may become mildly hypotensive several hours after dialysis, but because that is a known problem it may be handled by using a relevant protocol for managing postdialysis patients, without physician input. However, if the vital signs become very unstable or the symptoms do not subside after instituting the measures listed in the protocol, then a physician should be contacted and may need to assess and manage the situation promptly. Policies and procedures should identify the nature and scope of changes to be identified and reported (for example, complications of IV therapy, peritoneal dialysis, wound healing). Table 7–12, pp. 200–201, gives an example of guidelines developed for triaging condition changes common to subacute and long-term care patients. A mechanism is also needed for reporting information about condition changes to patients and families, and explaining the situation and the treatment options. For instance, some individuals who enter the unit substantially stable may suddenly have a complication, a rapid decline, or even die. Explaining the reasons for decisions and minimizing surprises to the care recipients are both important risk-management approaches. Therefore, medical record documentation should explain the basis for decisions to do or not to do things. This is important to show that a relevant process was followed in case a situation turns out to be different than assessed or anticipated.

Prevention of Nosocomial/Iatrogenic Problems

For reasons discussed throughout this book, subacute patients are at relatively high risk for nosocomial (associated with being in a health care facility) and iatrogenic (associated with medical diagnostics and treatments) illnesses and injuries. These are significant problems in much of health care, causing and complicating many hospitalizations, increasing costs of care and lengths of stay, and contributing to death and disability (Leape et al, 1993; Lefevre et al, 1992; Palmer, 1995). Common iatrogenic conditions include medication complications, altered mental status, and the complications of devices and treatments. Common nosocomial problems include falls, pressure sores, infections, and altered mental status.

Despite extensive discussions in the health care literature for several decades and the recognition that many of these problems are preventable, the public is often unaware of the problems and some practitioners have tended to overlook them. Patients are rarely capable of recognizing when their problems may be due to their treatments or care, rather than to their illnesses. Partially because of physician resistance, care sites have been reluctant to initiate protocols and practice guidelines, and accrediting bodies such as the JCAHO have had few standards related specifically to responsibility for preventing or recognizing these problems. Therefore, every subacute program must recognize the potential for these problems and have protocols for trying to prevent them and for recognizing their possible onset. All quality-assurance and risk-management programs should include a review of the care for possible instances of these problems and should reinforce measures to try to prevent them.

Preparation for Completion of Treatment Course

Discharge Planning.   Because subacute care emphasizes limited (short- to intermediate-term) duration of stays, preparation for completion of the treatment course and the discharge process itself are both very important and remarkably time consuming. Discharge planning is not just a matter of finding someone else to care for the patient whose time and money is about to run out. The program must prepare the patient for a safe and orderly transfer or discharge.

Therefore, every subacute program needs a systematic approach to preparing for discharge and managing the discharge process. Especially in a managed care environment, facilities and practitioners should not cut corners in these processes or ignore problems that may result from inadequate transition. Doing so tends to pass the problems off on someone or someplace else.

Early Preparation. Discharge planning must begin as early as possible. Realistic discharge options should be evaluated as part of the preadmission assessment. When a patient is first referred to a program, there should be some indication of the goals for discharge and the factors that could inhibit achieving those objectives.

The interdisciplinary team should assess discharge potential as part of the care planning process. Objectives of care, based on specific functional and behavioral goals, should be developed. Discharge criteria may fall into one of several categories: (1) completion of a preplanned stay, (2) care objectives have been achieved, (3) further progress toward achieving care objectives is unlikely, or (4) the patient's condition worsens to the point that the facility cannot provide the care adequately. Care objectives must be related to criteria for deciding when they are accomplished, such as "Patient will ambulate 150 feet with no more than minimal assistance," "Cardiac rhythm will be stable," or "Wound site will be drainage free and patient's family will be able to change dressings." These guidelines may be included in critical pathways.

For example, a joint replacement patient may be admitted with the expectation of an 11-day postoperative stay, based on knowledge of the usual time needed for sufficient functional improvement to permit a return home. But the stay could be prolonged by medical (such as evidence of thrombophlebitis) or psychosocial (inadequate support at home to help with transfers, dressing, or shopping) factors. Or, a patient admitted after a prolonged hospital stay with multiple problems might be ready for discharge when her fluid and electrolyte imbalance is corrected, the anemia has improved enough to permit ambulation without easy fatigue, and there are no further episodes of aspiration pneumonia. A ventilator patient in a persistent vegetative state might be discharged as soon as the blood gases are stable and another care site is available, even though there are periodic pulmonary infections requiring antibiotics. A patient with chest pain may be able to stay on the unit pending a workup, but persistent EKG evidence of myocardial ischemia could imply the need for transfer to a monitored bed in a hospital.

One part of discharge planning is choosing the appropriate site for subsequent placement. After the initial interdisciplinary team conference, there should be communication with potential discharge sites. Each program should use a systematic approach, such as that discussed in Chapter 3 and outlined in Figure 3–1, p. 45.

The program should identify and discuss community resources so the patient and family can understand the options. Managed care organizations should be aware of the range of options and their strengths and weaknesses so that they can assemble a cost-effective package of services that will help restore function and minimize problem recurrences. Efforts to arrange those resources must consider cost, transportation, waiting lists, and eligibility requirements. A home visit (usually by rehabilitation therapists or social workers) may help evaluate and prepare the home environment and family support.

Identifying and Addressing Factors Influencing Discharge. After admission, ongoing monitoring is done to evaluate the course of the illness and the person's response to treatment and care, and to detect the occurrence and nature of any complications of the current problems or treatments. Based on monitoring, treatment is modified, discharge is planned, and the prognosis is adjusted.

Table 7–13, p. 201, lists issues that should be identified and clarified in discharge planning. As with care management, a key to effective discharge planning is to identify the patient's problems anticipated after discharge and to devise a plan to address them. Chapter 10 discusses some factors associated with longer-term maintenance of functional gains and morbidity and mortality.

Information Transfer.   The subacute program should be able to expect adequate informational support from a referring program. Similarly, because of the need for greater continuity of care and reduced duplication of services, the planning must take into account preparing both the next care site and the care recipients.

A discharge summary of essential information about the patient should be provided at or close to the time of discharge (Table 7–14, p. 202). Alternatively, a format such as that used to present the cases in Chapter 11 may give a clearer overall picture.

There are ways in which subacute programs can help their practitioners prepare discharge summaries more expeditiously, especially by setting up a patient database and various reports on computer to generate much of the summary automatically. Although a physician still needs to summarize the clinical course of the stay, there is no compelling reason to have separate medical, nursing, and other summaries. A single composite summary could save time and duplication, and still provide the essential information. This is another example of an area where a change in traditional approaches may improve care efficiency.

Responsibilities.   Discharge planning is often coordinated internally by an individual such as a social worker, utilization coordinator, or case manager. Parts of it may also involve a managed care organization case manager or an outside health, social, or welfare agency. These roles may be flexible as long as the essential functions are performed.

Patient/Family Education

Because patients must often continue to receive additional care after discharge and families must often continue to participate in the care, they need information and training. Particularly important is the impact of the condition and any residual deficits on an individual's family, work, and social roles (Gleckman & Brill, 1995). Every subacute program should have processes to accomplish these objectives. Table 7–15, p. 203, lists important areas of education and training.

The responsibility for educating patients and families should be shared by multiple players, not just practitioners. Providing verbal instruction is time consuming and often not very efficient, and listeners may not retain very much information. To the greatest extent possible, computer-based, video, and audio technologies should be used to relieve practitioners of the time involved in detailed one-on-one instruction. The practitioner's time may be best spent addressing specific questions and reinforcing information after the patient and family have received and reviewed audio, video, or computer-generated information. This is an area where computer-based self-instruction and interactive video may be enormously helpful. Although discussion and interpretation of information may be the role of practitioners, the management should spearhead the development and implementation of processes and systems to help facilitate the provision of information. The program administrator should help practitioners gain access to some of the many patient education materials already available and identify educational areas needing further development.

Follow-Up

Effective subacute programs cannot stop with discharge. Follow-up is essential for the program to obtain information to help improve its services and give consistently effective and efficient care. This can be divided into two categories: review of outcomes, and review of problems and concerns related to the patient's stay (Table 7–16, p. 203). In turn, the outcomes can be divided into those related to the stay (short- and intermediate-term) and those subsequent to it (long-term). The problems and concerns can be divided into those related to the patient and family, those related to the staff, and those of outsiders such as managed care organizations and referral sites.

Outcomes. It is important to evaluate the results achieved for each patient to see if these were optimal and whether the program achieved them effectively and efficiently. It is also valuable to examine the potential avoidability of adverse events such as complications and side effects that occurred during a patient's stay, and if they were detected and addressed promptly.

Problems and Concerns. During the stay, both the recipients and the providers of care may have had certain issues. For example, the patient may have questioned the way that some treatments were administered, the family may question the timeliness of the information they received or the ultimate care outcomes, and staff may have issues about the ready availability of supplies, the functioning of equipment, or the effective participation of other disciplines or departments.

These issues should be addressed as part of an overall quality management program. The program manager or administrator and the case manager are the most likely individuals to coordinate such assessments. The DON, medical director, and other department heads and clinical leadership should participate in these problem solving activities and take appropriate corrective actions to improve subsequent performance or prevent problems.

REFERENCES

Gleckman AD, Brill S. The impact of brain injury on family functioning: Implications for subacute rehabilitation programmes. *Brain Inj.* 1995; 9(4):385–393.

Leape LL, Lawthers AG, Brennan TA, Johnson WG. Preventing medical injury. *QRB Qual Rev Bull.* 1993; 19(5):144–149.

Lefevre F, Feinglass J, Potts S, et al. Iatrogenic complications in high-risk, elderly patients. *Arch Intern Med.* 1992; 152(10):2074–2080.

Levkoff SE, Safran C, Cleary PD, et al. Identification of factors associated with the diagnosis of delirium in elderly hospitalized patients. *J Am Geriatr Soc.* 1988; 36:1099–1104.

Palmer RM. Acute hospital care of the elderly: Minimizing the risk of functional decline. *Cleve Clin J Med.* 1995; 62(2):117–128.

Rosenthal GE, Halloran EJ, Kiley M, et al. Predictive validity of the nursing severity index in patients with musculoskeletal disease. *J Clin Epidemiol.* 1995; 48(2):179–188.

Rosenthal GE, Halloran EJ, Kiley M, et al. Development and validation of the Nursing Severity Index. *Med Care.* 1992; 30(12):1127–1141.

Zimmer JG. Needed: Acute care in the nursing home. *Patient Care.* 1993; 27:59–68.

TABLE 7–1   THE ESSENTIAL PROCESSES OF SUBACUTE CARE

Process	Objectives
Patient selection	• Decide whether individual needs subacute services. • Determine whether the program can meet the patient's needs.
Postselection/ preadmission	• Provide relevant and required information to the patient/family. • Inform and prepare appropriate staff to accept the admission.
Assessment	• Collect information about the individual that allows proper definition of the problems.
Problem definition	• Correctly and completely define the individual's problems and needs so that the appropriate care plan can be developed.
Identifying care goals and objectives	• Correctly and completely define the purpose of giving care and the criteria that will be used to determine when the objectives have been met.
Care planning	• Create a plan to address the individual's problems, including the responsibilities of various individuals and disciplines.
Management of known problems	• Identify and implement appropriate treatment alternatives to address the individual's primary (main reason for admission) and secondary (coexisting) problems.
Management of new problems/complications	• Identify and manage problems that arise as a result of existing conditions or that did not exist previously.
Prevention of nosocomial/ iatrogenic problems	• Identify areas of high risk and potential problems that may arise as a result of medications and treatments or by being in a health care facility, and institute measures to try to prevent those problems and to recognize them if they arise despite precautions.
Preparation for completion of treatment course	• Monitor responses to treatment and progress toward discharge. • Plan for discharge and transfer by ensuring appropriate transfer site, follow-up of problems, and communication of information to the patient, family, and others who will be providing continuing care.
Follow-up	• Review care outcomes for the subacute stay and for a period of time after discharge. • Review problems, concerns based on input of the providers and recipients of care.

TABLE 7–2   IMPORTANT INFORMATION IN A PREADMISSION ASSESSMENT

Category	Related Issues
Referral source	• Is the referral source known to the program? How reliable and complete is the information they typically provide about the patients they refer?
Patient problems	• What are the individual's problems? What is the level of medical stability? Is this subacute program able to handle them?
Medical diagnoses	• What are the medical diagnoses? Which are clearly defined and which are still speculative? Which need further testing and clarification?
Relevant lab tests/ findings	• What are significant test results that help define the patient's situation? What abnormalities need ongoing monitoring?
Current treatments/ services/medications	• Does the individual require treatments, equipment, supplies, or other care that may not be readily available, that are not customarily given here, or that might require special staff preparation or training?
Care objectives	• What are the objectives of care? What problems are foreseen in achieving them? How realistic are they? What is the anticipated time frame for achieving them?
Anticipated treatments/ services	• Does the individual have unusually complex behavioral or medical problems that might require special staff preparation or training? Would consultation or support for

(continued)

TABLE 7–2	IMPORTANT INFORMATION IN A PREADMISSION ASSESSMENT (CONTINUED)
Category	**Related Issues**
	the staff from the referral site or referring practitioner be available if they had subsequent problems or questions regarding the treatment?
Special precautions	• Does the individual have a problem requiring special monitoring, precautions, isolation, etc?
High-risk/likely complications	• What complications have occurred so far? What problems and complications are likely to occur?
Significant decision makers	• What is the patient's decision-making capacity? If the patient is the primary decision maker, is anyone else often involved in making decisions? If the patient is not the primary decision maker, then who is?
Limits on medical care/directives	• Are there advance directives or other statements about wishes regarding medical care? Are there any significant or absolute limits on certain care measures?
Patient/family expectations	• What have the patient/family been told about the problems and their likely outcome? What have they been told to expect in the subacute program? What questions and concerns have they raised? What is their level of understanding of what is happening? How have they responded so far to the situation?
Financial status/insurance coverage	• What is the patient's financial and insurance status? Who will be covering reimbursement for the subacute stay? What are the expectations for length of stay? What processes must be followed to obtain authorization for various tests and treatments that the patient is expected to need?

TABLE 7–3	EXAMPLES OF ADMISSION INCLUSION AND EXCLUSION CRITERIA

Inclusion

- Mostly and usually medically stable
- Continues to require frequent nursing intervention because of needs for monitoring, assessment, and treatment
- Requires one or more forms of rehabilitation therapies for a variable time with a goal of improvement
- Reimbursement is available for the essential services and care
- Reasonable expectation for discharge
- Individual and/or support systems (families, community resources, etc.) are available and willing to participate in the care plan

Exclusion

- More than moderate medical instability
- Fever over 101°F without an identified cause or active management plan
- Recovery is not anticipated, or there are stringent limits on medical interventions by choice of patient or substitute decision maker
- Individual and/or support system unwilling or unable to participate in the care plan
- Multiple, active problems are frequently unstable or that do not have a readily identifiable cause
- New hip fractures requiring acute management and possible surgery
- Severe head injury accompanied by high degree of instability
- Severe cardiac decompensation requiring a high level of monitoring and complex management
- Severe respiratory failure requiring acute ventilator care
- Psychiatric problems that represent a danger to the patient or to others

TABLE 7–4	**RELEVANT FACTORS TO INFORM PAYER RELATED TO PROPOSED COST OF CARE**

- Acuity level
- Therapy level/cost of therapy
- Pharmacy cost (estimate based on current prescriptions)
- Supplies (estimate for those not included in per diem)
- Durable medical equipment (recommendation for rent or purchase)
- Initial plan of care
- Payment terms
- Cost of nursing care

Used with permission from Barbara A. Marte, Multicare, Hackensack, NJ.

TABLE 7–5	**ITEMS TO BE ASSESSED IN THE SUBACUTE PATIENT UPON ADMISSION**

Category	Specific Items	Responsibilities
Physical status	• Vital signs • State of nutrition and hydration • Level of discomfort and distress • Height and weight/basal metabolic index • Cardiorespiratory status • Gastrointestinal status • Musculoskeletal status • Condition and function of extremities	• Physician/nurse • Physician/dietitian/nurse • Nurse/physician/PT/OT/nursing assistant • Nurse/dietitian/physician • Physician/nurse • Physician/nurse • Physician/nurse/PT/OT • Nurse/physician/PT
Neurological status	• Evaluation of neurologic system • Sensorimotor, proprioception, muscle tone, reflexes • Coordination, motor skills • Pain status • Speech, phonation, swallowing	• Physician • Physician/nurse/PT • OT/physician/nurse • Physician/nurse/nursing assistant • Nurse/speech therapist
Dentition	• Status of teeth, gums, oral mucosa • Condition and problems of any dentures • Ability to chew, swallow, and any limitations	• Nurse/nursing assistant/physician/dentist • Nurse/nursing assistant • Nurse/physician
Skin integrity	• Color, moisture, rashes, wounds, ulcers, bleeding sites, abnormal growths	• Nurse/physician/nursing assistant
Bowel and bladder status	• Elimination pattern	• Nurse/nursing assistant
Behavior and mental functioning	• Behavior and cognitive status • Sleeping patterns • Memory • Communications ability • Decision-making capacity	• Nurse/social worker/nursing assistant/physician • Nurse/nursing assistant/physician • Social worker/nurse/physician • Nurse/social worker/PT/physician/ activities therapist • Social worker/nurse/physician
Functional capabilities	• Ability to perform activities of daily living and instrumental activities of daily living • Mobility • Bowel and bladder continence • Activity/exercise patterns, capabilities	• Nurse/OT/PT/physician • Nurse/PT • Nurse/physician • Activities therapist/OT/nurse

(*continued*)

TABLE 7–5   **ITEMS TO BE ASSESSED IN THE SUBACUTE PATIENT UPON ADMISSION (CONTINUED)**

Category	Specific Items	Responsibilities
	• Transfer capabilities	• Nurse/PT/OT
	• Joint range of motion	• Nurse/PT/OT
	• Strength and endurance	• Nurse/PT/OT
	• Posture	• Nurse/PT/OT
	• Gait	• Nurse/PT/OT
	• Social functioning	• Social worker/nursing assistant/activities therapist
Mood/attitude	• Reactions to illness, disability	• Social worker/nurse/nursing assistant/ physician
	• Health perception	• Social worker/nursing assistant/nurse
	• Self-perception	• Social worker/nursing assistant/nurse

PT = physical therapist; OT = occupational therapist.

TABLE 7–6   **CATEGORIES OF INFORMATION FOR THE MINIMUM DATA SET FOR NFS AND SNFS**

- Identification and background information
- Cognitive patterns
- Communication/hearing patterns
- Mood and behavior patterns
- Psychosocial well-being
- Physical functioning and structural problems
- Continence in last 14 days
- Disease diagnoses
- Health conditions
- Oral/nutritional status
- Oral/dental status
- Skin condition
- Activity pursuit patterns
- Special treatments and procedures
- Discharge potential and overall status

TABLE 7–7	INFORMATION THAT SHOULD BE DOCUMENTED UPON ADMISSION TO SUBACUTE CARE PROGRAMS

Category	Examples
Admitting diagnoses	• Primary: left hip fracture with total hip replacement • Secondary: coronary artery disease/depression/urinary tract infection
Nursing diagnoses/problems	• Volume overload; bowel incontinence; altered breathing pattern
Current medical findings	• Rales both lung fields; irregular pulse; erythema over incision site without drainage; pain to palpation of hip
Diet	• Regular with no added salt; nutritional supplements
Medication and treatment orders	• Physician orders for standing and PRN medications; nature and frequency of treatments; special services and equipment
Functional status	• Capacity to perform daily life functions (ADLs and IADLs) • Status of self-care in bathing, dressing, grooming, toileting • Human and mechanical assistance needed • Rehabilitation potential • Ability to participate in structured individual or group activities
Code status and ethical considerations	• Resuscitation status • Wishes regarding any limitations on aggressive medical interventions in case of condition change
Mental and emotional status and decision-making capacity	• Mini-Mental Status Examination score; assessment of decision-making capacity; emotional and mood disturbances
Medication and other allergies	• Known and possible allergies, with description of actual problem (rash, anaphylaxis, nausea, etc.)
Precautions/contraindications	• Restricted mobility or weight bearing; cardiac precautions
Anticipated problems/high risks	• Anticoagulated patient who tends to fall has high risk of bleeding; patient who has been in bed has high risk of skin breakdown
Current diagnostic test results	• Results of EKG, lab tests, X-rays, special studies
Contingency plans	• Do Not Resuscitate; send to hospital for recurrence of bleeding; notify orthopedist if surgical site is painful
Current treatments and services	• PT and OT; turn and position; dressing changes twice daily
Psychosocial information	• Personality/behavioral profile • Use/abuse of drugs or alcohol • Personal preferences and habits: food, clothing, schedules, bathing, sleeping • Education, occupation, hobbies, activities, religious preferences, and habits • Cultural influences and language • Social and environmental setting • Family circumstances • Current living situation • Other social, ethnic, cultural, emotional, and health factors • Financial resources • Availability of support at home
Significant others	• Names, addresses and phone numbers of significant others (relatives, friends)
Current and previous care providers	• Names, addresses, phone numbers, and specialties of physicians, other practitioners

ADLs = activities of daily living; IADLs = instrumental activities of daily living; OT = occupational therapy; PT = physical therapy.

TABLE 7–8   **COMMON PROBLEMS IN SUBACUTE PATIENTS, BASED ON NURSING DIAGNOSES (WITH EXAMPLES)**

Group 1. Overall Health

Risk for Injury

- Patient who feels light-headed when getting up or has balance problems
- Patient with impaired judgment who climbs out of bed frequently to go to bathroom without getting assistance or does not remember safety instructions or cues
- Patient with recent history of recurrent falling

Infection/Contagion/Risk for Infection

- Patient with aspiration pneumonia
- Patient with wound site infection or peritonitis
- Patient with AIDS who has been getting opportunistic infections
- Patient with recent cancer chemotherapy who is now immunosuppressed

Prolonged Disease/Disability

- Patient with chronic heart disease or rheumatoid arthritis resulting in disability

Clinical Instability

- Patient with unstable vital signs
- Patient with an active infection or respiratory difficulty that causes fluctuations in conditions requiring daily nursing monitoring and physician availability to assess

Impaired Life-Support Systems

- Patient requires some external life-support mechanisms to keep from deteriorating or dying
- Patient requiring ventilator support

Group 2. Nutrition and Metabolism

Fluid Volume Excess

- Patient with congestive heart failure, valvular heart disease, or other cardiac problem has 3+ pitting edema of both legs to the knees [Do not include patients with stasis dermatitis or similar conditions]

Fluid Volume Deficit

- Patient who appears dehydrated, has had decreased oral intake
- Patient has been on diuretics, has had recent diarrhea, vomiting, fever, or continuous gastric suctioning; has not been drinking enough recently; becomes confused, more lethargic
- Patient with oliguria or polyuria

Bleeding

- Patient has rectal bleeding, internal bleeding, hematemesis, or hemoptysis

Altered Nutrition

- Patient who has recently been hospitalized for several weeks, was on IVs for a week after surgery, and since then has not been eating well
- Patient who has been losing weight despite adequate food intake
- Patient who is eating sporadically; lab work on admission shows albumin 2.9, cholesterol 145
- Patient who requires hyperalimentation because of inability of oral intake

TABLE 7–8	COMMON PROBLEMS IN SUBACUTE PATIENTS, BASED ON NURSING DIAGNOSES (WITH EXAMPLES) (CONTINUED)

Impaired Skin Integrity

- Patient with one or more pressure ulcers
- Patient with draining or unhealed postoperative wounds requiring care
- Patient with ulceration due to tumor metastases

Altered Oral Mucous Membrane

- Patient with ulcerations of oral cavity
- Patient with oral candidiasis after chemotherapy

Altered Body Temperature

- Patient with hypothermia
- Patient with fever

Group 3. Urinary and Fecal Elimination

Urinary Incontinence

- Patient with multiple sclerosis who has overflow incontinence
- Patient who is comatose who has no control over urination
- Patient on diuretics who leaks urine

Other Altered Urinary Elimination Pattern

- Patient with prostatic obstruction who has trouble voiding or gets distended bladder
- Patient with oliguria or anuria
- Patient who has painful urination

Constipation

- Patient who has decreased bowel motility because of medications
- Patient who needs regular laxatives, enemas, or stool softeners because of difficult or painful bowel movements

Diarrhea

- Patient who has been on antibiotics for several weeks who has several days of loose stools
- Patient with peptic ulcer disease or diverticulitis who has loose stools as a symptom of the disease's activity
- Patient on tube feeding who has persistent osmotic diarrhea

Bowel Incontinence

- Patient who cannot control bowel movements

Group 4. Activity and Exercise

Activity Intolerance

- Patient who cannot tolerate exercise because of a pulse that is too slow or too fast
- COPD patient whose exercise tolerance has declined markedly because the lung function is no longer stable
- Patient who is too weak to tolerate activity because of long, debilitating illness or prolonged immobility
- [Do not include patients who are stuporous or comatose]

Ineffective Airway Clearance

- Patient who is unable to cough effectively enough to remove airway secretions (whether or not requires suctioning)

(continued)

TABLE 7–8   COMMON PROBLEMS IN SUBACUTE PATIENTS, BASED ON NURSING DIAGNOSES
                  (WITH EXAMPLES) (CONTINUED)

Ineffective Breathing Pattern

- Patient with respiratory rate or pattern that is different from baseline
- Patient who is in respiratory distress
- Patient with COPD who has cough, dyspnea, orthopnea, cyanosis

Impaired Gas Exchange

- Patient requiring ventilatory support
- Patient with dyspnea on exertion
- Patient with decreased oxygen content, decreased oxygen saturation, increased pCO_2, as measured by blood gas analysis
- Patient with confusion, lethargy, or somnolence secondary to hypoxia or CO_2 retention

Decreased Cardiac Output

- Patient with hypotension or shock
- Patient with confusion, dyspnea, or restlessness due to congestive heart failure
- Patient with reduced left ventricular ejection fraction after recent myocardial infarction
- Patient in cardiogenic shock
- Patient with persistent congestive heart failure or recurrent pulmonary edema

Altered Health Maintenance

- Patient who has a recent history of alcohol or substance abuse
- Patient with overeating disorder, morbid obesity
- Patient who is unaware of or incapable of seeking help from individuals or community agencies and programs to support in-home health care

Impaired Physical Mobility

- Patient with impaired bed mobility, transfers, ambulation
- Patient requiring assistive devices for mobility, ambulation, transfers

Self-Care Deficit

- Patient who needs at least some support in eating, bathing, dressing, toileting

Group 5. Psychosocial Concerns

Self-Esteem Disturbance

- Patient who denies or has difficulty accepting or coping with a limitation, deformity, or disfigurement
- Patient who refuses appropriate rehabilitation program
- Patient who frequently tries to direct own treatment, constantly challenges medical and nursing care
- Patient who refuses to participate in own care or to take responsibility for self-care (self-neglect)

Hopelessness/Depression

- Patient who expresses feelings of hopelessness, despair, extreme anger, or guilt
- Patient who shows marked decrease in physical activities, eating, sleeping secondary to mood alteration

Dysfunctional Grieving

- Patient focused on a significant actual or perceived loss (person, object, function, status, relationship)

TABLE 7–8	COMMON PROBLEMS IN SUBACUTE PATIENTS, BASED ON NURSING DIAGNOSES (WITH EXAMPLES) (CONTINUED)

- Patient who expresses suicidal thoughts, anger, despair
- Patient crying frequently about current illness
- Patient preoccupied with recent or impending death of someone close
- Patient who feels rejected, useless, worthless, unable to make decisions

Altered Family Processes

- Patient with a dysfunctional family situation where family appears unable to adapt or communicate effectively
- Patient whose spouse has recently been diagnosed with a major illness, making spouse less available to deal with the patient's concerns and less able to focus on information about patient's condition

Social Isolation

- Patient who expresses feelings of aloneness or loneliness
- Patient who lives alone with little or no social contact

Impaired Verbal Communication

- Patient who cannot speak words but can understand others
- Patient with dysarthria or difficulty in articulation
- Patient with aphasia after a stroke
- Patient with multiple sclerosis, Parkinsonism, or other chronic neurological condition affecting speech

Ineffective Individual Coping

- Patient verbalizing inability to cope
- Patient who has difficulty dealing with facing own problems, situation, or conduct because of denial, rationalization, or other inappropriate use of defense mechanisms
- Patient with history of destructive behavior toward self or others
- Patient who is unable to meet own basic needs
- Patient who gets very agitated every time he or she is asked to make a decision about treatment options or when a nurse or physician tries to discuss his or her current condition and prognosis
- Patient who is very manipulative, asking same questions repeatedly of many individuals, apparently not hearing the answer but claiming that no one is willing to answer the question
- Patient with long-standing history of substance abuse and personal neglect, failure to take medications or follow through with treatments or other care
- Patient who shows signs and symptoms of depression

Family Coping: Potential for Growth

- Family member expresses desire for help in managing current illness, condition

Spiritual Distress

- Patient who expresses current experiencing of disturbance in belief system because of condition or situation
- Patient who expresses that he or she has no reason for living
- Patient who expresses anger, resentment, fear over meaning of life, suffering, death

TABLE 7–9   TASKS INVOLVED IN MANAGING COMMON PROBLEMS IN SUBACUTE PATIENTS

GROUP 1. OVERALL HEALTH

	Assessment/Problem Identification	Monitoring	Management	Follow-Up
Risk for injury	• Assess potential for injury. • Identify risk factors for injury. • Identify and assess causes of those risk factors. • Assess cardiovascular, musculoskeletal, and neurological systems. • Assess mobility, strength and endurance. • Assess cognitive function. • Evaluate environmental factors (furniture, call bell, etc.).	• Observe patient attempts at mobility. • Monitor vital signs after any falls. • Observe for unsafe behaviors.	• Provide supervised progressive mobilization program as appropriate. • Modify medications to reduce any medication-related risks. • Identify and implement preventive measures. • Identify and provide appropriate assistive devices.	• Instruct patient in preventive measures and use of assistive devices. • Instruct patient/family in postdischarge risk reduction. • Review and compare pre- and postintervention mobility and falls occurrence.
Infection/contagion	• Define infection by site(s). • Identify causes of infection. • Evaluate for nutrition and hydration deficits.	• Monitor vital signs. • Evaluate for signs/symptoms of complications of illness (lethargy, decreased oral intake, confusion). • Monitor for side effects of treatments.	• Select appropriate treatments of infection. • Treat significant complications. • Correct any nutrition and hydration deficits. • Institute relevant preventive measures/precautions. • Review and adjust medications that might be contributing to greater infectious risk or severity of complications.	• Evaluate response to treatment. • Assess impact of any complications. • Instruct patient/family in postdischarge follow-up, continuation of antibiotics.
Prolonged disease/ disability	• Identify the nature, severity, duration, and functional impact of chronic conditions. • Identify treatable conditions that might be confused with irreversible problems.	• Monitor signs/symptoms that might give further clue to nature/causes/severity of problems.	• Order relevant treatments • Implement relevant rehabilitative/restorative services. • Review and adjust	• Compare pre and post-intervention functional status. • Instruct patient/family in postdischarge preventive measures and

	Assessment/Problem Identification	Monitoring	Management	Follow-Up
	• Assess functional and cognitive status. • Assess need for rehabilitative/restorative services.		medications that might be increasing functional or cognitive problems. • Identify and implement appropriate preventive measures.	• Evaluate response to treatment. • Discuss situation with patient/family.
Instability	• Assess cardiac and pulmonary status. • Assess and define causes of instability. • Assess fluid/electrolyte balance.	• Monitor vital signs. • Monitor for onset of additional problems/complications. • Monitor course of underlying conditions.	• Treat causes of instability. • Review and adjust medications that might be contributing to instability. • Develop contingency plan if instability becomes immediately life-threatening.	• Monitor response to treatment. • Review situation with patient/family.
Impaired life-support systems	• Assess cardiac and pulmonary status. • Assess impact of problem on organ systems.	• Monitor vital signs. • Monitor for onset of additional problems/complications.	• Treat causes of instability. • Review and adjust medications that might be causing or contributing to instability. • Develop contingency plan if instability becomes immediately life-threatening.	

GROUP 2. NUTRITION AND METABOLISM

	Assessment/Problem Identification	Monitoring	Management	Follow-Up
Fluid volume excess	• Review causes of volume excess. • Assess causes of significant alterations in vital signs. • Assess fluid/electrolyte balance. • Assess for organ systems complications of volume overload: confusion, dyspnea, weakness, change in level of consciousness (LOC), stasis dermatitis. • Evaluate diet. • Assess strength and endurance.	• Monitor vital signs. • Monitor for medication side effects.	• Treat significant fluid/electrolyte imbalances. • Modify diet orders as needed. • Review and adjust medications that might be causing or contributing to volume excess. • Order and modify medications to correct excess volume.	• Reassess fluid/hydration status after attempts at correction.

(continued)

TABLE 7-9

TABLE 7-9   TASKS INVOLVED IN MANAGING COMMON PROBLEMS IN SUBACUTE PATIENTS (CONTINUED)

	Assessment/Problem Identification	Monitoring	Management	Follow-Up
Fluid volume deficit	• Review possible causes of volume deficit. • Assess causes of significant alterations in vital signs. • Evaluate fluid/electrolyte balance. • Assess for signs/symptoms of organ end-complications of volume deficit: confusion, lethargy, falling, orthostatic hypotension, weakness, change in LOC. • Evaluate food and fluid intake. • Assess strength and endurance.	• Monitor vital signs. • Monitor hydration-related signs and symptoms.	• Correct significant fluid/electrolyte imbalances. • Modify diet orders as needed. • Review and adjust medications that might be causing or contributing to volume deficit.	• Reassess fluid/hydration status after attempts at correction.
Bleeding	• Define nature, frequency, scope, site, amount of bleeding. • Identify site of bleeding. • Assess possible end-organ complications of decreased blood volume. • Define urgency of need for any intervention. • Assess for possible treatable causes of bleeding. • Assess need for transfusions. • Assess for signs/symptoms of hypotension: confusion, tachycardia, dyspnea, weakness, change in LOC.	• Monitor vital signs. • Assess bleeding sites.	• Manage bleeding site as needed. • Order and implement blood replacement as needed. • Identify and adjust medications that might be causing or contributing to bleeding. • Develop contingency plan if bleeding becomes immediately life-threatening.	• Evaluate for recurrent bleeding. • Evaluate response to any treatment, including transfusions.
Altered nutrition	• Assess possible causes of nutritional deficit. • Review management of nutrition and hydration during any preceding hospital stay. • Identify nature, scope, and components of nutritional deficit. • Evaluate calorie intake and current diet. • Assess causes of significant	• Measure nutritional intake periodically. • Monitor signs/symptoms related to nutritional status.	• Identify and implement options for addressing nutritional deficit. • Review any invasive treatment options with patient/family. • Order increased portions, supplements, or other measures to improve nutritional status.	• Instruct patient/family in adequate diet.

	Assessment	Planning / Intervention	Evaluation
	nutritional deficit. • Assess for signs/symptoms of nutritional deficit: skin color and condition, confusion, lethargy, weakness, change in LOC.	• Modify diet orders as needed. • Review and adjust medications that might be causing or contributing to anorexia or weight loss.	• Instruct patient/family in postdischarge risk reduction for further skin impairment. • Instruct patient/family in continuing treatment (dressing changes, identification of new infection, etc.) and follow-up.
Impaired skin integrity	• Assess potential for skin impairment. • Identify and define any current skin impairments (ulcers, abrasions, dryness, etc.). • Identify risk factors for skin impairment. • Identify and assess causes of any current skin impairments. • Assess mobility, cognitive function, and LOC.	• Observe patient positioning, turning, mobility. • Evaluate skin condition periodically. • Modify medications to correct any medication- or nutrition-related risks. • Identify, order, and implement appropriate preventive measures. • Identify and implement treatment options for existing skin impairment.	
Altered oral mucous membranes	• Identify any alterations in oral mucous membranes. • Identify causes of any alterations in oral mucous membranes. • Evaluate nutrition and hydration status.	• Monitor oral pain, discomfort, food intake. • Review and adjust medications that might be causing or contributing to any alterations in oral mucous membranes. • Order and implement measures to relieve symptoms. • Order and implement measures to treat causes.	• Evaluate and document response to treatments.
Altered body temperature (ABT)	• Define nature, frequency, duration, scope of ABT. • Identify cause(s) of ABT. • Assess for signs/symptoms of life-threatening ABT: hypotension, confusion, cardia arrhythmia, weakness, change in LOC, neurological signs.	• Monitor vital signs. • Review temperature trends. • Order and implement treatments for defined or suspected causes of fever. • Identify and adjust medications that might be causing or contributing to ABT. • Develop contingency plan if ABT becomes immediately life-threatening.	• Evaluate temperature trends and responses to treatments.

(continued)

TABLE 7–9   TASKS INVOLVED IN MANAGING COMMON PROBLEMS IN SUBACUTE PATIENTS (CONTINUED)

GROUP 3.   URINARY AND FECAL ELIMINATION

	Assessment/Problem Identification	Monitoring	Management	Follow-Up
Urinary incontinence	• Describe patterns of urinary continence. • Define type of incontinence. • Identify cause(s) of incontinence. • Order urinalysis, renal function, and other relevant tests.	• Monitor urinary output.	• Initiate symptomatic or cause-specific measures. • Review and adjust medications that might be causing or contributing to urinary incontinence.	• Compare pre- and post-intervention continence.
Other altered urinary elimination pattern	• Describe pattern of urinary output. • Order urinalysis, renal function, and other relevant tests.	• Monitor urinary output and characteristics.	• Review and adjust medications that might be causing or contributing to altered renal function or urination.	• Compare pre- and post-intervention urinary and renal function.
Constipation	• Describe pattern of bowel function. • Identify any treatable causes of constipation. • Assess GI system. • Review diet.	• Monitor bowel movements (frequency, characteristics).	• Review and adjust medications that might be causing or contributing to constipation. • Manage other causes.	• Assess postintervention response, compare to pre-intervention status.
Diarrhea	• Describe pattern, characteristics of bowel movements. • Identify any treatable causes of diarrhea. • Order relevant tests of pathogenic organisms, toxins, etc.	• Monitor bowel movements. • Observe for development of dehydration.	• Treat any specific causes. • Review and adjust medications that might be causing or contributing to diarrhea. • Manage any complications.	• Document symptomatic improvement or progression.
Bowel incontinence	• Describe pattern, characteristics of bowel movements. • Identify any treatable causes of fecal incontinence. • Order relevant tests of pathogenic organisms, toxins, etc.	• Monitor bowel movements. • Observe for development of dehydration/skin breakdown.	• Treat any specific causes. • Review and adjust medications that might be causing or contributing to bowel incontinence. • Manage any complications.	• Document symptomatic improvement or progression. • Check impact of treatment on complications such as skin breakdown or excess fluid loss.

	Assessment/Problem Identification	Monitoring	Management	Follow-Up
Activity intolerance	• Assess current activity level. • Identify functional limitations. • Identify and assess causes of functional limitations. • Assess strength and endurance. • Assess cognitive function. • Evaluate cardiovascular function. • Assess musculoskeletal problems.	• Monitor activity at various times over several days.	• Provide appropriate human and mechanical assistance. • Treat medical factors limiting activity tolerance. • Initiate measures to prevent complications of inactivity.	• Evaluate and document results of treatments and support.
Ineffective airway clearance, ineffective breathing patterns, impaired gas exchange	• Describe character of respiratory problem (frequency, sputum characteristics). • Assess possible predisposing factors and causes. • Assess nutrition and hydration status. • Assess cardiopulmonary function. • Assess oxygenation status. • Order lab tests to evaluate hematocrit and overall hematologic status. • Obtain X-rays as indicated. • Assess for signs/symptoms of hypoxia or CO_2 retention: confusion, lethargy, weakness, change in LOC, respiratory distress.	• Monitor vital signs. • Monitor sputum characteristics. • Monitor blood gases or pulse oximetry. • Monitor cardiopulmonary function. • Monitor operation of any mechanical ventilatory equipment.	• Treat pulmonary infection. • Give supplemental gases as needed. • Treat significant complications. • Provide relevant mechanical treatments (chest PT/inhalation therapy/suctioning). • Correct any nutrition and hydration deficits. • Review and adjust medications that might be causing or contributing to respiratory distress or drying of secretions.	• Obtain follow-up radiologic, blood, and blood gas studies.
Decreased cardiac output	• Identify causes of decreased output. • Assess stability of vital signs. • Evaluate fluid/electrolyte balance. • Assess for signs/symptoms of organ end-complications of in-	• Monitor pulse, blood pressure, functional status, signs and symptoms.	• Address specific causes. • Correct significant fluid/electrolyte imbalances. • Review and adjust medications that might be causing or contributing to decreased output.	• Reassess cardiac and functional status during and after correction efforts.

(continued)

TABLE 7-9

TABLE 7-9   TASKS INVOLVED IN MANAGING COMMON PROBLEMS IN SUBACUTE PATIENTS (CONTINUED)

	Assessment/Problem Identification	Monitoring	Management	Follow-Up
	adequate cardiac output: confusion, lethargy, falling, orthostatic hypotension, weakness, change in LOC. • Evaluate food and fluid intake. • Assess endurance and activity tolerance.		• Prevent complications.	
Altered health maintenance	• Assess extent of impact on deficits in personal care and health maintenance.	• Monitor conditions and problems related to inadequate health maintenance.	• Identify and use services, programs, or individuals who can provide effective support.	• Assess impact of auxiliary services on individual's overall health status.
Impaired physical mobility	• Identify type and scope of mobility impairment. • Identify level of support/assistance needed because of impairments. • Define causes of deficits.	• Observe and document level of function under various conditions (steps, room, etc.).	• Address treatable causes of mobility limitations. • Prevent complications of prolonged immobility. • Provide appropriate devices and human support. • Provide appropriate rehabilitative and restorative services.	• Observe and document changes in mobility over time.
Self-care deficit	• Identify type and scope of functional deficits. • Identify level of support/assistance needed because of deficits. • Define causes of deficits.	• Observe and document level of function under various conditions.	• Address treatable causes of self-care deficits. • Provide appropriate devices and human support. • Provide appropriate rehabilitative and restorative services.	• Observe and document changes in functional status and self-care capacities over time.

GROUP 5. PSYCHOSOCIAL CONCERNS

	Assessment/Problem Identification	Monitoring	Management	Follow-Up
Self-esteem disturbance, depression, grieving, spiritual distress	• Describe and define nature of problem. • Identify and assess causes. • Assess cognitive function and mood.	• Monitor participation in daily routine. • Monitor changes in mood, cognition, and behavior.	• Provide individual and group interventions as indicated. • Select and administer medications as indicated	• Evaluate progress in relation to treatments and interventions.

	Assessment	Monitoring	Intervention	Evaluation
	• Evaluate decision-making capacity. • Assess family and other support systems. • Assess neurological system function and deficits.	• Monitor effectiveness of actual decision making in various situations.	for more incapacitating symptoms. • Arrange for appropriate support services.	• Evaluate changes in family and patient functioning, participation, understanding, responsiveness, cooperation.
Altered family processes	• Assess strengths and deficits in family and other support systems. • Describe and define nature of specific patient problems possibly related to family situation. • Identify and assess causes of problems. • Assess patient problems that may contribute to family process alterations. • Evaluate decision-making capacity.	• Monitor patient participation, mood, cognition, and behavior. • Monitor family behavior and patient/family interactions.	• Provide individual and group interventions as indicated. • Identify and access internal and external organizations, programs, or services that may help provide support.	
Social isolation	• Describe and define nature of problem. • Identify and assess causes of isolation. • Assess cognitive function and mood. • Assess neurological system function. • Evaluate decision-making capacity.	• Monitor participation in daily routine. • Monitor changes in mood, cognition, and behavior. • Monitor patient interactions with others such as staff and family.	• Provide individual and group interventions as indicated. • Try medications as indicated for more incapacitating symptoms. • Identify and access internal and external organizations, programs, or services that may provide support.	• Evaluate shifts in patient attitude, participation, mood, responsiveness. • Observe for progression to full-blown depression. • Measure changes in level of functioning over time.
Impaired verbal communication	• Describe and define nature of problem. • Identify and assess causes. • Assess cognitive function. • Assess neurological system functioning. • Evaluate decision-making capacity.	• Monitor communication efforts by and to individual. • Monitor changes in mood, cognition, and behavior.	• Arrange rehabilitative and restorative services as indicated. • Ensure adequate means of alternate communication where feasible.	• Evaluate changes in communications capability in relation to treatments and interventions.

(continued)

TABLE 7-9   TASKS INVOLVED IN MANAGING COMMON PROBLEMS IN SUBACUTE PATIENTS (CONTINUED)

	Assessment/Problem Identification	Monitoring	Management	Follow-Up
Ineffective individual coping	• Describe and define nature of coping difficulty. • Identify and assess causes. • Evaluate and define cognitive function and mood. • Assess neurological system function. • Evaluate decision-making capacity.	• Monitor participation in daily routine. • Monitor changes in mood, cognition, and behavior. • Observe patient reactions and responses to various situations.	• Provide individual and group interventions as indicated. • Try medications as indicated for more incapacitating symptoms.	• Evaluate changes in mood, coping, performance in relation to treatments and interventions.
Family coping: potential for growth	• Describe and define areas of family interest/deficits.	• Monitor family behavior and interactions with patient and staff.	• Provide information and support, or individual and group interventions as indicated.	• Evaluate progress in family functioning and support in relation to various interventions.

TABLE 7–10   ORIGINS OF PROBLEMS IN SUBACUTE PATIENTS

Category	Description	Examples
Illness-related risks and complications	Identifiable potential or recurrent problems not currently active but which could arise during the stay	Bleeding in someone with a history of peptic ulcer disease; pulmonary embolism after knee surgery
Chronic illnesses	Conditions causing long-term or progressive symptoms and complications, for which there is no known cure	Dementia, osteoarthritis, osteoporosis
Nosocomial and iatrogenic conditions	Conditions known to be associated with institutional care or with medical treatments and diagnostics	Undernutrition, general deconditioning, medication side effects, falls, incontinence, delirium
Aging-related problems	Conditions associated with normal aging that may affect response to treatment, recovery from illness, or risk of complications	Slower internal drug metabolism, thinning of skin, lower maximum heart rate, decreased visual acuity
Cognitive and functional limitations	Problems associated with decreased ability to perform activities of daily living and instrumental activities of daily living	Confusion, decreased mobility
Psychosocial circumstances	Social and personal problems and situations that affect a person's mood, function, participation, cooperation, finances	Depression, limited family support, inability to cope with illness

TABLE 7–11   IMPORTANT CONSIDERATIONS IN DECISIONS TO TRANSFER PATIENTS WITH CONDITION CHANGES

Category	Issues
Ability to manage instability on site	Widely or frequently fluctuating vital signs may represent a condition that requires a greater frequency and intensity of monitoring and management than can be safely handled on the unit.
Ability of program to assess causes	Some conditions (e.g., pneumonia, dehydration) can be detected by easily available, uncomplicated tests, but others might have more obscure causes requiring more complex or frequent testing.
Proximity of alternate care site	A hospital- or SNF-based program may have resources in close proximity, but a free-standing rural program may not have another site readily available for transfer.
Advance directives	Advance directives may limit hospital transfers or specific categories of testing and intervention.
Ability of those on site to perform and report detailed assessment	The presence of those who can evaluate and triage a condition (correctly define its urgency) may facilitate keeping someone on site by making it more likely that the urgency or causes of the problem have been identified correctly.
Likelihood of seriousness of complication	Conditions with a higher potential to be life-threatening (shock, myocardial infarction) may be better treated elsewhere.
Influence of payer or managed care organization (MCO)	The policies of the patient's MCO may require approval of the attending physician, or may expect the MCO's attending physician to try to manage the patient on the unit before any transfer is attempted.

TABLE 7–12   **EXAMPLES OF GUIDELINES FOR NOTIFYING ATTENDING PHYSICIANS OF CONDITION CHANGES**

Condition	Immediate (Notify the attending or on-call physician as soon as possible)	Nonimmediate (Notify the attending or on-call physician no later than the next office day)
Abdominal pain	Abrupt onset severe pain or distension; OR with fever, vomiting	Moderate diffuse or localized pain, unrelieved by antacids or laxatives
Bleeding	Uncontrolled, or repeat episode within 24 hours (e.g., bloody emesis, bloody stools not from hemorrhoids, profuse vaginal bleeding, grossly bloody urine)	Controlled; no further episodes; bleeding from hemorrhoids
Blood pressure, high	Persistent BP over 2-hour span > 210 systolic and/or > 110 diastolic; OR recent increased BP with headache, chest pain, change in level of consciousness (LOC), abnormal neurological signs	BP fluctuations 10% or more above usual range
Blood pressure, low	BP systolic < 90 or diastolic < 50 or more than 20 points below usual; OR accompanied by chest pain, altered LOC, falling, dizziness, diaphoresis	BP remaining 10% or more below normal range, but without symptoms
Chest pain, pressure, or tightness	New or abrupt onset; OR recurrent that is not relieved in 20 minutes by previously ordered nitroglycerin × 3; OR accompanied by diaphoresis, change in vital signs, nausea and vomiting, or new EKG changes	Known history of chest pain with increased frequency of episodes
Confusion	Abrupt significant change from usual, associated with fever, new-onset abnormal neurological signs	Persistent change in confusion or LOC from usual with no other significant symptoms
Consciousness, altered	Sudden change in LOC or responsiveness	Gradual but persistent recent change in LOC or responsiveness
Diarrhea	Acute onset of multiple loose stools with change in vital signs (e.g., temperature > 101°F)	Intermittent loose stools with stable vital signs
Dyspnea	Acute onset of change from usual pattern; OR with chest pain, labored respirations, cyanosis, or unstable vital signs	Recent intermittent change from usual pattern; OR only partial response to previously ordered treatment; recurrent episodes now more frequent
Edema	Abrupt-onset unilateral leg edema; OR abrupt onset with tenderness, redness, or dyspnea	Progressive unilateral or bilateral edema
Emesis	Repeat episodes with blood or coffee grounds, pain; OR associated with changes in vital signs	One episode
Fall	With obvious deformity; OR hip pain to palpation or inability to walk; OR head injury; OR abnormal neurological status; OR new-onset confusion; OR laceration with uncontrolled bleeding	No bleeding; no injury or minor injury (e.g., bruise or skin tear); increased frequency of falls in 24- to 72-hour period

(continued)

TABLE 7–12	EXAMPLES OF GUIDELINES FOR NOTIFYING ATTENDING PHYSICIANS OF CONDITION CHANGES (CONTINUED)	
Condition	**Immediate** (Notify the attending or on-call physician as soon as possible)	**Nonimmediate** (Notify the attending or on-call physician no later than the next office day)
Family request	Requesting or demanding to speak to physician now	Persistent, recurrent concern that may need physician attention
Medication error	Causing any new symptoms; OR involving a cardiac, psychotropic, or other drug with potential for significant toxic side effects	
Pressure sore	Stage II, III, or IV receiving no treatment and no treatment protocol to cover situation	New-onset grade II or higher pressure sore with available treatment protocol initiated; OR progression of pressure sore despite interventions
Seizures	Any new-onset seizure activity; OR status epilepticus	Self-limited seizure in someone with known seizure activity who is already on an anticonvulsant
Suicide, potential	Makes a suicidal gesture; OR discusses a detailed plan for carrying out suicide	Persistent or progressive depression, but not making any specific suicidal threats
Weakness, general	Abrupt-onset general weakness with fever, change in LOC, or other acute symptoms	Gradual- or progressive-onset general weakness without fever, change in LOC, or other acute symptoms
X-ray, abnormal	New or unsuspected finding of clinical significance, such as fracture or pneumonia	Old or long-standing finding, or no change from previous study

TABLE 7–13	IMPORTANT CONSIDERATIONS IN DISCHARGE PLANNING

- Individual's anticipated level of independence in self-care and overall living
- Structural and functional aspects of the potential discharge environment
- Possible impediments to discharge (home situation, environment, family support, confusion, frailty)
- Ongoing need for monitoring and treatment
- Plans for providing necessary treatments, services, and assistance after discharge
- Patient and caregiver understanding of the situation and the essential postdischarge care, and their ability to perform relevant functions (make appointments, give medications, provide treatments, recognize complications, etc.)
- Support available at home or outside the organization
- Patient and/or family's financial resources
- Available community resources

TABLE 7–14   IMPORTANT COMPONENTS OF DISCHARGE SUMMARIES FOR SUBACUTE CARE

Component	Explanation	Examples
Diagnoses	Acute and chronic medical illnesses and conditions present at discharge or that resolved during the stay	• Diabetes mellitus • Post-partial bowel resection • Left-sided pneumonia
Problems	List of problems active at the time of discharge	• Self-care deficit • Intermittent confusion • Impaired verbal communication • Social isolation
Summary of the course of treatment	Treatments, complications, progress, special tests, and assessments during the stay	• Therapies given • Results of X-rays • Significant lab abnormalities • Intermittent infections
Behavioral and functional status	Level of functioning at discharge, compared to admission and during the stay	• Functional measurement/activities of daily living scores on discharge • Evidence of depression, cognitive impairment, behavior problems
Continuing medication and treatment orders	Medications and treatments that must be continued after discharge	• Discharge medication list • Dressing changes • Injections
Indication of needs for follow-up and continuing care	Appointments or arrangements made or that need to be made	• Home health care • Outpatient rehabilitation • Follow-up testing
Supply and equipment needs	Items needed by the patient and family to enable continuing care	• Wheelchairs, braces, walkers • Ventilators • Cleansing solutions • Bandages and dressings
Patient/family instructions	List of any patient and family education and instructions provided	• Who and when to call for follow-up appointments • How to give breathing treatments • How to recognize possible complications

TABLE 7–15   IMPORTANT AREAS OF PATIENT AND FAMILY EDUCATION AND TRAINING

Area	Examples
Condition and prognosis	• Major diagnoses and problems • Plan for managing problems • Anticipated course (improvement, stabilization, complications) • Likely longer-term outcomes and residual deficits • Possibilities for new or recurrent problems
Treatments and care	• Procedures for managing colostomy, dressings, insulin injections, etc. • Medications: purpose of each, proper usage, potential problems • Anticipating and discussing compliance with treatments, medications, follow-up • Contingency plans if unexpected problems arise
Essential follow-up care	• Appointments for follow-up care • Specific problems that must be monitored, tested • Means for maintaining and monitoring adequate nutrition and hydration
Options for subsequent care management	• Alternatives for subsequent care, based on cost, service package, patient and family wishes • Impact of reimbursement
Safety and injury prevention	• Precautions to prevent high-risk complications such as falls, wound site infection
Fears and concerns	• Trying to address specific patient and family fears and concerns (chances for full recovery, risk of further decline, coping with residual disabilities)

TABLE 7–16   ITEMS FOR FOLLOW-UP AFTER A PATIENT'S SUBACUTE STAY

Area	Specific Issues
Review of outcomes	**For Stay** • Achieved versus predicted result • Occurrence of complications of illness • Occurrence of iatrogenic or nosocomial conditions • Assessment of unanticipated transfers (e.g., hospital) **Subsequent** • Functional status maintained • Rehospitalization • Recurrence of condition that was corrected during stay
Review of problems/concerns	• Problems/concerns raised by patient and family • Issues raised by staff • Issues raised by payers, other outsiders

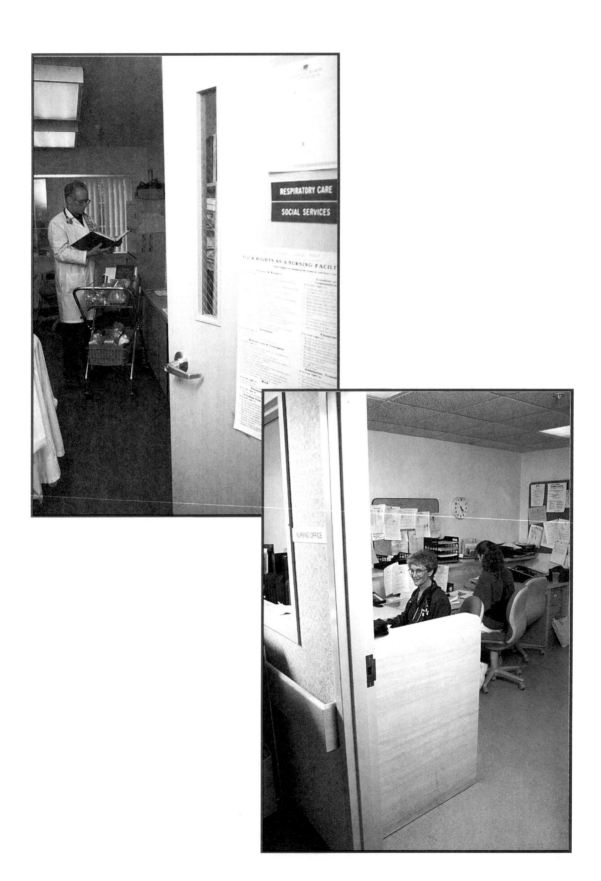

THE ORGANIZATION AND SUPPORT OF CARE AND PRACTITIONERS

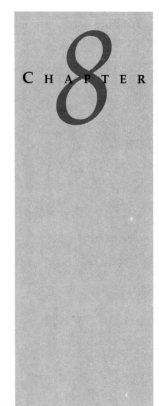

CHAPTER 8

*A*s a complex program involving many individuals and disciplines, subacute care must be systematic. Various individuals and disciplines must coordinate their activities so that the care can be harmonized and their performances can be appropriately assessed and improved.

To ensure that those processes are done effectively and efficiently and that the right individuals are involved in managing problems of diverse origin, the care should be organized around care management and planning systems. This chapter addresses the systems that organize and coordinate various aspects of the care and the practitioners providing the care.

CARE MANAGEMENT SYSTEM

As discussed throughout this book, the delivery of complex care requires an effective system. Otherwise, it is quite difficult to ensure that processes will occur consistently and correctly and that individuals will perform appropriately and reliably. Having defined the essential care processes, it is possible to identify their associated components, participants, and relationships. Figure 8–1 illustrates how the various processes form the foundation for subsequent ones, and how, taken together, they provide the basis for achieving care objectives.

A care management system is an orderly approach to accomplishing the processes involved in providing care to meet individual and programmatic care objectives. Table 8–1, p. 233, lists the essential components of such systems. They should incorporate and reflect appropriate philosophies, as discussed throughout this book, such as the interdisciplinary approach to care, effective interpersonal communication, and sound problem solving. They should ensure that the care is consistently given correctly and efficiently by identifying ways to facilitate and improve pertinent processes and the performance of those involved in those processes. And they should organize related functions such as defining patient needs and problems, organizing and delivering vital services, and establishing and reinforcing appropriate roles and relationships. Systems must be structured enough to ensure that desired processes always occur, but flexible enough to allow for individualized care.

The care management system should be organized by the management and clinical staff, implemented via an interdisciplinary approach, and evaluated and improved by all participants including care recipients, practitioners, and providers. It should identify the roles and relationships of the various disciplines involved in the processes of care. These disciplines must function independently at times, and jointly at other times. They perform their own assessments and deliver treatments using their own skills and methods. But the same disciplines must jointly define problems, determine the care objectives, and assess the results of care.

For instance, many patients who come into subacute programs have some undernutrition. The physician, nurse, and dietitian would assess for signs of nutritional deficiency. The physician would order tests that reflect nutritional status. If oral intake is inadequate, the dietitian would recommend alternatives such as oral supplementation. The physical and occupational therapists might become involved to determine if use of adaptive devices and set-up assistance to improve functional independence could help. The nursing assistants would provide that assistance and also document the extent of meal consumption. A speech therapist would be involved if there was a swallowing problem, and might recommend altered consistency of food and fluids. The patient and family would need to be involved if there was consideration of tube feeding or other artificial nutrition or hydration. At any time, the director of nursing (DON) or medical director may need to consult on the case if these individuals could not agree on the extent of the nutritional problem, the appropriate interventions, or the duration of using various alternatives. Eventually, these individuals must decide whether and when the problem has resolved, whether changes in the approach are indicated if it is not improving, and what should be done to prevent its recurrence.

Coordination.   A typical core team for overseeing and refining the care management system would include the program administrator, case manager, med-

FIGURE 8–1   RELATIONSHIPS OF THE PROCESSES INVOLVED IN SUBACUTE CARE

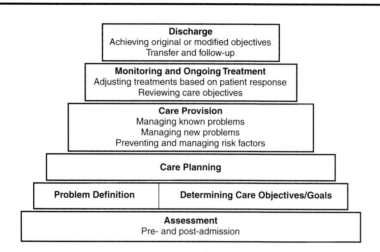

ical director, program nurse manager, rehabilitation manager, and other department or service leadership such as a principal social worker and dietitian.

Other Tactics.   To help promote a common understanding of subacute care, programs should consider providing each participant with a reference manual. This might include a statement of the program's core principles (Figure 8–2); information about the program's objectives and scope of services; a summary of the backgrounds, training, and experience of different individuals; relevant quality indicators and performance standards for various disciplines and departments; and important general policies.

ORGANIZING THE CARE PROCESSES

Consistent processes should be used to deliver care to each patient even though the scope of these processes will vary among different patients. Responsibilities should be assigned for both the coordination of the care and verification of the completion of each of the care processes. By discharge, the program coordinators should feel confident that each process was performed effectively and efficiently. It may help to have a formal verification document (Table 8–2, pp. 234–235) similar to the checklist that every airplane flight must complete before takeoff. Someone should sign off for each step even though several individuals or disciplines might have been responsible for carrying them out. This not only shows that things were done, but also provides a trail for retrospective quality review. Additionally, it can help ensure that no steps are overlooked and that responsibility is assumed appropriately in the absence (due to vacation, illness, or other assignments) of the principal coordinator.

Systematic Approach to Assessment

There should be a systematic approach to assessment. The scope of the assessments may vary among patients (for example, a more detailed functional as-

FIGURE 8–2   AN AGREEMENT FOR SUBACUTE CARE PARTICIPANTS

I am a practitioner or other care provider in this facility's subacute care program. Certain attitudes, systems, and processes are essential for the program to succeed. Therefore, I have read and agree to the following:

- I understand that subacute care is a complex system intended to care for people with complex problems.
- I recognize that I have an important role in providing that care, along with many other disciplines and individuals.
- I recognize that my role may vary depending on the condition and needs of different patients.
- I agree to participate in a truly interdisciplinary process as part of a collection of individuals with common goals and objectives.
- I will try to make decisions in light of the overall program objectives of optimal care, good quality, and cost-effectiveness.
- I recognize that the things I do, and the ways in which I do them, may help or inhibit the performance of others and the success of the program.
- I will accept my responsibilities and will participate in defining and refining them, consistent with the patients' needs and the program's goals.
- I will offer feedback about my participation in the program, and will accept feedback regarding my performance in the program.
- I will help prevent problems, especially in high-risk situations, and will help effectively identify and manage problems that arise.
- I recognize my role in effective communications, and will try to do things to improve the effectiveness of such efforts throughout the program.

Signed _____

Date _____

---

sessment would be done in a rehabilitation patient with good potential than in a vegetative comatose patient), but the core components and the roles of various disciplines in that assessment should be consistent.

The program should consider ways to streamline and coordinate these assessments. For example, appropriate roles can be defined for the various tasks of assessment, monitoring, treatment, and follow-up for those with different problems (see Table 7–9, pp. 190–198). Typically, several disciplines will assess the same patient characteristic and each discipline will assess multiple items. All the disciplines should use comparable data-collection instruments and criteria. In the interest of efficiency, individual items should be assessed by just one discipline primarily and reviewed or interpreted by others as needed, unless redundancy is essential to improve the accuracy or reliability of the data.

For example, nurses, physicians, social workers, rehabilitation therapists, and activities therapists may all assess a patient's cognitive and emotional status. They should use the same instruments (Mini-Mental Status Examination, depression scale, and so on) or agree to use comparable scales that effectively enable comparison. It might be most efficient for one discipline, such as social services, to perform a Mini-Mental Status Examination and a screening test for depression, while the nurses document observations and the physicians consider medical causes of altered mood or cognition. At the team conference, the various disciplines would discuss their respective observations and reach a consensus on whether altered cognition or depression are problems, and on how to assess causes and select appropriate treatment. Subsequently, the nurses, social workers, and activities therapists would observe and document the patient's relevant signs and symptoms and the physician would coordinate treatments, medications, and further testing with the interdisciplinary care team.

Each program should establish policies for the completion of initial assessments and their subsequent review. These may be influenced by regulatory or accreditation requirements. For instance, the Joint Committee on Accreditation of Healthcare Organizations (JCAHO) requires an initial assessment to be initiated within 24 hours and completed within 48 hours, and reassessments to occur when patient condition changes significantly but at least every 30 days (Joint Commission, 1995, p. 48).

Systematic Approach to Care Planning

Subacute care focuses on managing a collection of patient problems. Therefore, the care plan process should be problem-oriented and should include specific objectives and measurable criteria for knowing when those objectives have been achieved. Both the care providers and care recipients should be involved.

The format of the care planning process should ensure that relevant disciplines have input into defining problems and care objectives. All care plans should use a similar core format and be supplemented based on each patient's needs. For example, care plans should identify the responsibilities for the related tasks unless these are predefined by more general protocols (for instance, the same discipline is always responsible for suctioning or nutrition education).

Care plans should always be included as part of the patient record. They can provide a valuable basis for an interdisciplinary team conference (ITC) or other collective discussion about the patient's course and treatments. To improve efficiency, programs should consider using computer-based and generated care plans linked to comprehensive assessments, such as those now being created for long-term care.

Systematic Approach to Care Delivery and Reassessment

Although many treatments and care are delivered independently by various disciplines, they must be coordinated and based on a common game plan. The players must understand their roles in the care of each patient and all essential tasks for each patient must be performed. Some of these tasks are common to all patients (for example, monitor vital signs, assess response to treatment), some are common to a category of patients (for example, change dressings in those with wounds, monitor IVs in those receiving infusion therapies), and some are patient-specific (for example, manage dysfunctional patient/family dynamics, evaluate the home setting in preparation for discharge). An effective care management system ensures that all these processes are done appropriately and in a timely fashion given the different combinations of service needs in different patients.

Team Meetings.   Some regular interdisciplinary review of the care and the problems of individual patients is essential. This is most often achieved via an ITC, which serves multiple functions (Table 8–3, p. 236).

The initial ITC differs in some important ways from subsequent ITCs. Its principle objectives are to define or to confirm the individual's actual and potential problems and to establish or refine a blueprint for managing them. Participants must create a care plan based on events prior to the admission and on preliminary assessments.

Subsequent ITCs are typically scheduled weekly or biweekly, although only some patients may be discussed that frequently. These ITCs focus on patient progress toward improvement and discharge, recognition of the onset of complications and new conditions, refining the problem list, assigning responsibility for dealing with various problems or fulfilling certain functions, dealing with payers and utilization review issues, reviewing the results of various tests and consultations, and addressing staff, patient, and family issues. It may be necessary to modify the discharge plan, for example, because of limited progress or new complications. Such changes should be reviewed with the patient, treatment team, and (as appropriate) the payer before being finalized.

Review and Revision of the Care Plan.   An interim care plan should be developed by the core interdisciplinary team within 72 hours of completing the initial assessments. A more definitive care plan should be developed by the end of the first ITC and reviewed subsequently. Reasonable time frames for such review are biweekly for the first quarter, monthly for the second quarter, and then quarterly, with more frequent reviews dictated by changes in condition (JCAHO, 1995, p. 67).

Typically, a clinical care coordinator or internal case manager coordinates this process and facilitates review of issues where various disciplines may have different perspectives or interpretations. For example, a speech therapist or dietitian may suggest nutritional supplements or tube feedings, although the nurse feels that the patient could eat more but does not like the food.

Participants.   All disciplines caring for the patient should contribute to the ITC review. Either the direct care provider or a representative who knows about the patients and their problems should be present. For instance, the social worker at the ITC may have the responsibility for all the patients, and the medical director may represent some or all of the attending physicians. If unable to be present, the attending physician should answer important questions either before or soon after the ITC. Either routinely or as needed, the patient and/or family may be present for a portion of the ITC, especially as discharge approaches.

The ITC coordinator should document the discussions and conclusions from the meeting as a reference in case questions or problems arise later. Some follow-up of items discussed at the ITC may be more urgent than others. For example, if the nurses are concerned about the timely availability of blood for transfusion from the local blood bank or of IV fluids from the pharmacy, the ITC coordinator may need to address the problem and then inform the practitioners of any actions. Or, if a patient's family is very upset about the lack of information from the attending physician, the medical director may need to address this promptly with the attending physician and report some resolution to the ITC coordinator, who then informs the nursing staff.

Systematic Approach to Planning and Processing Discharges

There should be a systematic approach to discharge planning and processes. First, preparation for discharge should confirm that the processes of care have been completed satisfactorily and the objectives of care achieved (Table 8–2, pp. 234–235). The case manager or care coordinator is a likely individual to do this. A discharge summary should provide the important information to the next care site. It should be produced efficiently by combining appropriate existing documentation with a succinct summary of the patient's course rather than repeated documentation of existing information on different forms. The cases in Chapter 11 are presented in a format that might be used for this purpose.

Mechanism for Patient Participation and Choices

There should be a systematic approach to obtaining patient and family participation, and a system for providing essential patient and family support. This system should emphasize education, training, and explanation of the rationale for various decisions. In conjunction with this, the program should vigorously evaluate and pursue ways to improve the effectiveness of patient and family participation in decision-making processes, including analyzing the various causes (Table 8–4, p. 237).

Enhancing Communication.   Patients and families are unlikely to absorb or understand all of the information that they receive in health care settings. Sometimes the care may be complicated by gaps in their participation, knowledge, and understanding. The practitioners and staff should not assume that care recipients comprehend the information they provide or their answers to various questions. To help the process, policies and other information should be offered in writing, in laymen's terms. Patients and families should be able to voice their questions and concerns and designated staff should be accessible to answer any questions. These and related measures (Table 8–5, p. 237) are vital to reduce risks and help improve the care.

Patient Care Principles and Rights.   Because each patient has a unique combination of problems, needs, wishes, and values, the care should be individualized as much as possible. During the assessment process, the wishes and expectations of the patient and family (or designated surrogate) should be discussed and considered in formulating the care plan. For example, a patient may desire some medical treatment but not resuscitation or return to the acute hospital. Limits on the rights of families to override the wishes of a competent individual or to reverse an advance directive must be clarified based on applicable law and regulation. Other patient rights issues may arise when the individual's or family's needs, wishes, or behaviors conflict with those of other patients or with the staff's or facility's legal and ethical responsibilities.

Systematic Approach to Managing Ethical Issues

A large body of medical literature and case law now affirms the rights of individuals to participate in health care decision making and supports alternative decision making for those whose participation is limited by choice or by illness or disability. Every subacute program needs a systematic process to managing ethical issues because these issues are complex, options for care or limits on care vary, and practitioners and care recipients often have diverse perspectives.

As in long-term care settings, subacute programs have an additional challenge because of the limited time for discussions and decision making during hospital stays. Prior to the subacute admission, the issues may have been addressed only partially and the patient's progress and prognosis may not yet have been clarified. Therefore, all subacute programs should initiate discussion as soon as possible after admission or even before admission if necessary. For example, a program's ability to provide care for a comatose ventilator-dependent patient may depend on expectations for intervention in case of continuing instability or further decline.

These decisions should be made by the patients and families in conjunction with the appropriate care providers, which may include the physicians, nurses, social workers, and clergy, and sometimes dietitians or therapists. Any limited treatment plans should address each aspect of care to be implemented or altered when the plan takes effect. Treatment options should be considered for both the treatment of acute illness and the plan regarding possible resuscitation. It is often helpful to have the patient or substitute decision maker choose specific treatment directives (for example, about use of IVs, artificial nutrition, hospital transfers, and the like). Other pertinent discussions, decisions, and conclusions should be documented nearby in the medical record. Table 8–6, p. 238, gives an example of policies and procedures related to managing these issues, and Figure 8–3 is a consolidated documentation form for various issues related to ethical decision making to be supported by more detailed documentation of such things as the basis for conclusions about a person's decision–making capacity or a Do Not Resuscitate order.

Table 8–7, p. 239, lists important issues involved in these processes. The references at the end of the chapter may be consulted for further details about the philosophies of, legal and regulatory influences on, and process for managing medical ethical issues.

Systematic Approach to Providing Health-Related Support Services

Health-related support services (laboratory, radiology, nuclear medicine, and so on) should either be organized internally or available by contract, or some of each. Either way, a mechanism is needed to ensure that they are timely, effective, and cost-effective. Both the administrative and clinical management staff should be involved in making and overseeing external arrangements.

Transfer Agreements.   Each program needs a transfer agreement with local hospitals and other facilities, and procedures in case a patient needs immediate transfer for services that the program cannot provide. The written agreement may be general but it should be based upon an understanding of each party's roles and needs. In an integrated delivery system, each organization and level of care must be concerned about what happens to patients both before and after their stay. For instance, a hospital to which a subacute program transfers its patients must be prepared to handle limited treatment plans and manage those with comorbidities.

FIGURE 8–3   CERTIFICATIONS OF HEALTH CARE DIRECTIVES AND SUBSTITUTE DECISION MAKING

Patient Name _____

Place date at top of column; initial each applicable item; enter later items or changes in new column

	Admission			
Decision-making capacity				
Patient currently *capable* of making informed health care decisions				
Patient currently *incapable* of making informed health care decisions				
Existence of directives				
Written directives exist (date of directive)				
Oral directives made and documented (record date of relevant progress note)				
Triggering of directives				
Directives in effect by choice of competent patient				
Directives are triggered by patient's lack of capacity (see above)				
Primary decision maker				
Primary decision maker is *patient*				
Primary decision maker is *surrogate decision maker* (Name/Relationship:)				
Primary decision maker is *court-appointed guardian* (Name:)				
Qualifying conditions				
Patient is *terminally ill*				
Patient is in *persistent vegetative state*				
Patient has *end-stage condition*				
Specific care plan elements in effect				
Do Not Resuscitate (No CPR)				
Do Not Hospitalize				
No Lab Tests or Other Workup				
No Intravenous Fluids				
Do Not Use Antibiotics				
No Artificial Nutrition or Hydration				
Other directives, as follows:				

See reverse for clarifications and definitions of the above items

(continued)

FIGURE 8–3   CERTIFICATIONS OF HEALTH CARE DIRECTIVES AND SUBSTITUTE DECISION MAKING
(CONTINUED)

Reverse Side

Explanations of Specific Items

Date (Write in date in current or new column)	
Patient currently *capable* of making informed health care decisions	Can communicate choice; understands enough of implications of decision to act in own interest
Patient currently *incapable* of making informed health care decisions	Incapable of communicating choice; unable to understand enough to act in own interest
Written directives exist	There is some form of written advance directives, statement of wishes, etc.
Oral directives made and documented	Attending physician and one other witness must document in medical record
Directives in effect by choice of competent patient	A still competent patient can choose to implement directives or have agent make decisions
Directives are triggered by patient's lack of capacity	Patient cannot make informed health care decision; physician must certify as incapable if patient is conscious or able to communicate by any means
Appropriate decision maker is *patient*	Patient can be partially impaired and still have enough cognitive function to make some decisions
Appropriate decision maker is *surrogate decision maker*	Order of authority is spouse, adult child, parent, adult sibling, close friend
Appropriate decision maker is *court-appointed guardian*	Guardian takes precedence over any surrogates
Patient is *terminally ill*	Death imminent; condition incurable by any known measures; using a life-sustaining procedure will not make an appreciable difference in outcome
Patient is in *persistent vegetative state*	Unconscious; physically dependent; certified by the attending physician and one other physician specializing in cognitive function
Patient has *end-stage condition*	Severe, permanent deterioration; incompetent; dependent in ADLs; treatment of irreversible condition is medically ineffective
Specific care plan elements in effect are:	Initial all of the following that apply:
Do Not Resuscitate (No CPR)	No mechanical ventilation or chemical or mechanical efforts to restart pulse or respirations
Do Not Hospitalize	No transfer to acute care hospital
No Lab Tests or Other Workup	No workup of condition changes, no lab tests
No Intravenous Fluids	Do not use IVs for hydration or medications
Do Not Use Antibiotics	Treat infections symptomatically only
No Artificial Nutrition or Hydration	No tube feedings or parenteral nourishment or hydration
Others	Write in any other specific instructions

CLINICAL SERVICES

Clinical services are discrete collections of practitioners and other direct care providers with common characteristics, functions, and backgrounds. For instance, in the hospital, physicians are organized into various departments and their functions are further classified into services such as the medical service, neurosurgical service, or intensive care unit (ICU) service. Subacute programs have activities, nursing, medical, and other services. Some of these (nursing, for example) are based in internal departments, and others (physicians, for example) are usually nondepartmental. In subacute programs, clinical services should also be the means for organizing, training, and overseeing the performance of individual practitioners to harmonize those performances with the desired processes of care.

In either hospital- or nursing facility-based settings, many of the appropriate departments and clinical services may already exist. For instance, hospitals already offer respiratory therapy, but most nursing facilities do not. Nursing and skilled nursing facilities already have activities therapists, but hospitals usually do not. It is unnecessary to duplicate existing arrangements for the subacute program. However, the roles and tasks of these players in subacute care may differ from those in other programs and settings despite any overlap in the problems managed and treatments or care rendered. Therefore, it is worth reconsidering and clarifying these responsibilities and relationships specifically for the subacute program.

Each clinical service needs defined objectives and roles and appropriate oversight. Essential services must be available or accessible as needed. Each service should define its purpose, the responsibility for coordination and oversight, its availability, its component individuals and disciplines and their primary functions and tasks, essential education and training for its members, important policies and procedures, and any special needs, issues, and concerns.

Occasional Practitioners and Staff.   Health care organizations nationwide often have problems finding enough staff who will perform capably and consistently for each patient, from day to day, and even during different parts of the same day. Nursing and physician services must try to achieve consistency and predictability among their staff. Great variance among individuals or between shifts is likely to increase the risk of errors and avoidable complications. Covering physicians must assume the same functions as the attending physician while they are on call.

Many programs use part-time and registry staff of widely varying skills and performance, especially to provide nursing care. Despite these limitations, programs still should deal systematically with their contract and other outside and occasional staff. Their lapses and mistakes cannot be rationalized by simply noting that everyone has similar problems. Although outsiders may not be under the same level of control as employees, it should be possible to improve their performance and reduce the risks caused by their lapses.

To help deal with these situations, performance expectations of all disciplines should be developed and essential functions clearly defined. Protocols should cover desired approaches to common situations that the staff of any program are likely to face at different times (for example, handling family complaints or managing condition changes at night and on weekends). Patient care plans should be as explicit as possible to minimize personal variations in interpretation. Table 8–8, p. 240, lists other possible tactics for improving reliability and performance of any occasional practitioners and staff, including registry nursing.

ORGANIZATION OF SPECIFIC CLINICAL SERVICES

Table 8–9, p. 240, lists the various clinical services involved in subacute care. These services are discussed in the following sections. Principles for the organization and oversight of various services, which can also serve as an organizational basis for even nonaccredited programs, may be found among the CARF and JCAHO subacute accreditation standards (JCAHO, 1995).

Activities Service

The activities service (Table 8–10, p. 240) should coordinate the efforts of those providing therapeutic and recreational activities to individuals who may benefit from them. Besides being a common component of the rehabilitative/restorative approach to each patient, therapeutic activities may be helpful in those affected by psychosocial and activity-related deficits such as disturbed self-concept, depression, grieving, social isolation, impaired verbal communication, ineffective individual coping, and spiritual distress. For example, music therapy and pet therapy can help both acutely and chronically ill individuals with cognitive impairments or depression. As appropriate, subacute patients should be assessed by the activities staff. The activities staff should also participate in the interdisciplinary team conference, discharge planning, and patient and family education.

Oversight.   The services may be coordinated by a certified activities therapist who is primarily in the subacute program or works throughout the organization, or via an outside contractual arrangement with a part-time activities therapist.

Dietary Service

The dietary service (Table 8–11, p. 241) is responsible for meal preparation and delivery, and for coordinating the nutritional assessment, management, and education of the patients. It should work with other disciplines, including nursing and occupational therapy, to assess nutritional status and try to find reasons for inadequate nutritional intake. Whether employees or consultants, clinical dietitians should consult regarding patients' dietary needs, help educate patients and families, assist with menu planning, and review and approve all regular and therapeutic menus.

For those with undernutrition, the dietitian should recommend alternatives such as oral supplementation, additional portions, and assessment and use of adaptive devices and set-up assistance to improve functional independence. Parenteral nutrition should be used judiciously. Patients with swallowing or other intake problems should be assessed appropriately, in conjunction with a physician or speech therapist. Additional studies of swallowing or special food preparation (such as texture alteration) may be indicated. Appropriately trained nursing assistants should assist patients with swallowing difficulties.

Policies and procedures for dietetic care should include methods for providing and supervising dietetic services; participation of dietetic staff in patient care management; methods for planning, preparing, and serving meals and for ordering, receiving, and storing food and supplies; and safety and sanitation practices, including employee health, food handling, and documentation requirements.

Oversight.   A dietary services supervisor should participate, or assign responsibility for participation, in the patient management processes. This person should also help develop and implement dietary policies and procedures; coordinate menu planning and ordering of food and supplies; direct the receipt, storage, preparation, and service of food; and ensure safe and sanitary kitchen areas and equipment, consistent with applicable regulations and standards. A clinical dietitian should oversee the dietitians involved in care management.

Laboratory and Other Testing Services

Every subacute program needs adequate laboratory, radiologic, and other diagnostic support (Table 8–12, p. 241). Common situations in which these are helpful include the following.

- Defining the nature, scope, and severity of a patient's problems
- Evaluating the response to various treatments and progress toward discharge
- Determining the causes or sources of problems
- Monitoring the course of problems that began prior to, and which persist upon admission to, the subacute unit
- Monitoring for potential or actual complications of treatments, illnesses, and medications
- Assessing condition changes or new onset of signs and symptoms

Laboratory, radiologic, and other core diagnostic services should always be accessible. They may be provided within the program, within the facility, by another facility, by an outside provider, or by some combination. Any STAT services should be able to make results available within 2 to 4 hours of the test (blood draw, X-ray, and the like). However, in contrast to high-acuity care, subacute programs are generally not intended to provide intensive, complex, or frequent diagnostic testing other than blood work. A patient whose condition is sufficiently unstable or complex to warrant such testing may need other placement, especially if frequent transfers to another site for testing are needed. However, for less intensive nursing and medical care needs, it may be more cost-effective to provide the care at the less costly subacute site and transport the patient occasionally for testing.

Most subacute programs either use contract lab services or the existing hospital lab service. Hospital-based subacute programs use the hospital's radiologic services, and non-hospital-based programs may have basic on-site radiology capabilities and use a portable service or transport patients to another setting for more complex radiologic studies.

The subacute program itself is unlikely to have anyone directly responsible for overseeing technicians or others giving these services. However, the program must ensure that any contract services meet appropriate licensure and accreditation qualifications. Often, the medical director serves as the liaison between the program and the clinical aspects of these services, and an administrator is the liaison to the business and management side. Also, the subacute program must assess the appropriateness, timeliness, and reliability of any outside service, and give the service relevant feedback about its performance.

Examples of such quality oversight within the program include (1) a laboratory's consistency in returning STAT results within an agreed-upon time; (2) the number of redraws needed because of problems such as lost or inadequate samples or hemolysis; (3) whether changes in routine lab results are generally compatible with clinical condition changes; and (4) the timeliness with which radiology reports are returned and the helpfulness of their content.

The impact of internal processes on these services should also be scrutinized. For example, there should be adequate support for blood drawing during off-hours and a means should exist to triage results and notify physicians appropriately based on clinical urgency.

Medical Service

As discussed in Chapter 6, the vital role of physicians in caring for subacute patients (Table 8–13, p. 242) differs in some important respects from their roles in other settings. Table 8–14, p. 243, lists ways in which physicians can help or hinder subacute programs. The principal purposes of a medical service are to give adequate and competent medical coverage to directly and indirectly help achieve the overall care objectives, including health-related ones. Physicians must help correctly define and manage treatable conditions, help identify and achieve reasonable medical outcomes, and not cause or exacerbate complications and preventable problems.

Organization of Physicians.   In hospitals, physicians have been organized into medical staffs—independent associations of a diverse collection of practitioners with widely varying backgrounds, specialties, skills, and interests. The hospital is ultimately held responsible for the care delivered to its patients and for the practices and performance of those delivering the care. The medical staff organization has assumed the responsibility for overseeing the performance of the physicians practicing therein.

The nonorganized, or informal, staff is simply a group of individuals who practice in the same setting. This is more typical of subacute and long-term care programs. In subacute programs, a relatively few physicians provide the care in a small unit. Those participating in a hospital-based subacute unit may already be part of the hospital's organized medical staff. In a unit based in a nursing or skilled nursing facility, they may simply be one of several independent practitioners who practice elsewhere in the facility or at another facility.

The organization of hospital physicians is specialty-oriented, as are many of the units and programs providing care. Although all subacute patients need attending physicians, only some of them need specialist or subspecialist attention. Some subacute physicians will serve as both attending physicians and as consultants at various times. For example, the generalist may be able to handle all but the most complex services (a general internist may handle uncomplicated ventilator care) and the specialist may be able to serve effectively as an attending physician (the orthopedist may be able to manage the orthopedic rehabilitation patient with stable congestive heart failure but will need medical consultation if the heart failure worsens).

Therefore, although subacute programs do not need formal medical staff organizations, some structure is essential. The physicians should at least be organized enough to ensure adequate primary and consultative physician coverage as needed, accountability for performance, and sufficient support for the overall care being provided. Table 8–15, p. 244, lists essential elements to enable successful subacute physician performance, which are discussed in the following sections.

Open Versus Closed Staffing.   Medical staffs may be classified further as either open or closed. Membership on an open staff is available to any practitioners who meet certain basic requirements and wish to admit and attend the patients. In contrast, closed staff membership is only available to physicians and others who can meet certain more stringent criteria, such as those in a particular group or those who are salaried by a facility. Patients admitted to a facility with closed staffing are frequently assigned to, or select, a physician who will remain as their attending physician as long as they are in the facility.

Subacute programs may have either of these arrangements. But because it is hard for a program to find enough of the right kinds of physicians, the optimal arrangement may be a limited staff, something in between closed and open. That is, the staff is open to any interested physicians, but they must meet certain qualifications and agree to abide by certain policies and guidelines such as those discussed in this chapter.

Models of Physician Coverage.   Medical coverage for subacute care may involve a combination of private practitioners, hospital medical staff, medical school faculty, and residents under facility supervision; shared staff from other long-term care facilities; and nurse practitioners (NPs) or physician assistants (PAs) under physician supervision. Among other things, these physician extenders (NPs and PAs) can do routine assessments, assess and monitor condition changes, review and modify medication and treatment regimens (with a physician's support or input), and perform basic procedures.

Basic Expectations.   The medical director should inform the physicians of basic performance expectations. These include participation in a cooperative team approach, tailoring the medical role to the phase of the patient's illness and their overall care objectives, and direct and indirect ways in which physicians can help support and improve the care.

Because the mere provision of such information cannot ensure its effective use, other follow-up mechanisms must exist. To some extent, bylaws can provide the ground rules for physician participation as part of an organized medical staff. However, they are not always needed (for example, if the physicians in the subacute program are not a formal medical staff organization). An alternative would be to use a written statement of principles such as that given in Figure 8–2, supplemented by more detailed performance expectations at the level of policies and procedures.

Assurance of Requisite Knowledge and Skills.   A subacute staff must be organized enough to allow for evaluation of physicians' essential knowledge and skills. Some of this evaluation is common to every level of care and some of it is program- or level-of-care specific. Technical knowledge of diagnosis and treatment of disease is important but not sufficient for optimal role fulfillment. Credentialing and privileging have evolved as the principal means for health care facilities and organizations to oversee physician practices.

Physician credentialing is a process by which health care organizations collect and document information about physicians to help ensure that they have the potential to provide a desired level of care and services. **Privileging** is a process by which health care organizations define the circumstances under which someone is allowed to practice their profession or specialty and the scope of that practice. Credentialing is a prerequisite to, but not the same as, a privileging process.

Credentialing for Subacute Physicians.

The medical service should have some mechanism to investigate and document relevant credentials of the physicians providing care to its subacute patients. JCAHO-accredited programs are required to have credentialing and privileging processes for this purpose. These processes must be combined with some mechanism for performance evaluation to be able to compare actual to desired or required performance.

Table 8–16, p. 244, lists types of physician credentials including knowledge, skills, training, experience, licensure and certification, and general performance characteristics. Table 8–17, p. 245, lists categories of information that would be useful on an application form for physicians who wish to provide subacute care. The categories are basically identical to those included in applications for membership in organized medical staffs in hospitals and some nursing facilities. Figure 8–4 gives an example of a privilege request form for physician participation in a subacute program, or where the physician is not adequately credentialed in another setting.

For facilities having or seeking JCAHO subacute accreditation, the standards permit the use of existing credentials wherever possible. However, the program is responsible for reviewing those credentials and should grant relevant privileges.

Granting Privileges to Subacute Physicians.

Some physicians may feel that their hospital privileges are sufficient to automatically qualify them to provide subacute care. If the same knowledge and skills were needed to care for patients at all levels of need, then possessing them should be enough to ensure that they apply to all situations. But credentials usually demonstrate a physician's qualifications in relation to their specialty, not their role. A colonoscopy may be the same whether it is done in a physician's office or a hospital. The postoperative orthopedic care for a knee replacement may be identical at any site. But the consequences of illnesses and the care needed to manage individuals suffering from those various consequences are often different for various phases.

Although the subacute credentialing process may be similar to that in the acute hospital, the privileging criteria should differ in some important ways. Instead of the specialty- and procedure-specific privileges typical in hospitals, subacute privileges should be problem- or syndrome-specific (head-injured patients, cardiac rehabilitation, pulmonary care patients, and so on), based on the typical combination of syndromes and service needs for these patients. Where appropriate, criteria should also consider specific age groups, such as pediatrics.

FIGURE 8–4   PHYSICIAN PRIVILEGE REQUESTS, SUBACUTE PROGRAM

Category of Care	Sources of Relevant Training/Experience	Privileges Granted
_____ **Complex medical care** Assessment and management of complicated or multiple concurrent medical illnesses (e.g., unstable diabetes; general metabolic instability; enteric and parenteral feedings; complex pressure sores, vascular ulcers; cardiac decompensation/arrhythmias)	_____ **Residency** _____ **Advanced training/fellowship** _____ **CME** _____ **Special workshops/seminars** _____ **Practice experience**	_____ **No conditions** _____ **Conditional:**
_____ **Complicated infections** Assessment and management of complicated infections (e.g., HIV; multiple organisms; opportunistic infections; colonization of wounds, indwelling tubes, catheters, etc.)	_____ **Residency** _____ **Advanced training/fellowship** _____ **CME** _____ **Special workshops/seminars** _____ **Practice experience**	_____ **No conditions** _____ **Conditional:**
_____ **Oncology** Managing cancer and cancer therapy; prescribing and monitoring chemotherapy; pain management and rehabilitative care for cancer patients	_____ **Residency** _____ **Advanced training/fellowship** _____ **CME** _____ **Special workshops/seminars** _____ **Practice experience**	_____ **No conditions** _____ **Conditional:**
_____ **Pulmonary care** Weaning patients from ventilator, rehabilitation and management of complications of those with major primary pulmonary illnesses, respiratory instability, and secondary causes of ventilatory failure	_____ **Residency** _____ **Advanced training/fellowship** _____ **CME** _____ **Special workshops/seminars** _____ **Practice experience**	_____ **No conditions** _____ **Conditional:**
_____ **Renal/dialysis** Managing patients with advanced renal failure; overseeing dialysis; managing any complications of illness and dialysis	_____ **Residency** _____ **Advanced training/fellowship** _____ **CME** _____ **Special workshops/seminars** _____ **Practice experience**	_____ **No conditions** _____ **Conditional:**
_____ **Pain management** Managing pain related to medical, surgical, or other conditions by medication and/or mechanical modalities	_____ **Residency** _____ **Advanced training/fellowship** _____ **CME** _____ **Special workshops/seminars** _____ **Practice experience**	_____ **No conditions** _____ **Conditional:**
_____ **Terminal care** Managing terminal/hospice care; pain management; instituting limited care plan; making ethical decisions regarding withholding/withdrawing of treatment	_____ **Residency** _____ **Advanced training/fellowship** _____ **CME** _____ **Special workshops/seminars** _____ **Practice experience**	_____ **No conditions** _____ **Conditional:**
_____ **Postsurgical care** Postoperative medical and surgical complications; surgical wound management	_____ **Residency** _____ **Advanced training/fellowship** _____ **CME** _____ **Special workshops/seminars** _____ **Practice experience**	_____ **No conditions** _____ **Conditional:**
_____ **Rehabilitation** Supervising rehabilitation of patients with injuries, stroke, fractures, general deconditioning; ordering	_____ **Residency** _____ **Advanced training/fellowship** _____ **CME**	_____ **No conditions** _____ **Conditional:**

(continued)

FIGURE 8–4   PHYSICIAN PRIVILEGE REQUESTS, SUBACUTE PROGRAM (CONTINUED)

Category of Care	Sources of Relevant Training/Experience	Privileges Granted
physical therapy, occupational therapy, speech-language pathology services, neuropsychological services for patients with such disabilities as head and spinal cord injuries _____ **Cardiac rehab** _____ **Orthopedic rehab** _____ **Traumatic brain injury rehab**	_____ **Special workshops/seminars** _____ **Practice experience**	
_____ **Psychiatric care** Managing major depression; acute organic psychosis; complex or fluctuating behavioral, cognitive, or mood disturbances	_____ **Residency** _____ **Advanced training/fellowship** _____ **CME** _____ **Special workshops/seminars** _____ **Practice experience**	_____ **No conditions** _____ **Conditional:**
_____ **Other** (list and describe)	_____ **Residency** _____ **Advanced training/fellowship** _____ **CME** _____ **Special workshops/seminars** _____ **Practice experience**	_____ **No conditions** _____ **Conditional:**
PROCEDURES _____ **Chest tube insertion** _____ **Electroconvulsive therapy (ECT)** _____ **Hemodialysis** _____ **Lumbar puncture** _____ **Paracentesis** _____ **Percutaneous catheter insertion** _____ **Minor surgery (wound debridement, suturing, etc.)** _____ **Peritoneal dialysis** _____ **Thoracentesis**	_____ **Residency** _____ **Advanced training/fellowship** _____ **CME** _____ **Special workshops/seminars** _____ **Practice experience**	_____ **No conditions** _____ **Conditional:**

Additional information regarding qualifications

Where applicable, describe below those specific aspects of training or experience that you feel are relevant to the requested privileges:

Internship/residency

Advanced training/fellowship

Continuing medical education

Special workshops/seminars

Practice experience

Privileges Requested By (signature):

                                                                    Date Requested:

Privilege Request Reviewed/Approved By:

(Physician)   **Date Approved:**

(Administration)   **Date Approved:**

(Governing body [where applicable])   **Date Approved:**

The few procedures that might be performed by a physician could be listed as in Figure 8–4, as part of a privilege delineation form.

In conjunction with the medical staff, the medical director should determine those circumstances when physicians should be encouraged or required to obtain consultation. Physicians who only consult in the subacute program and do not write any orders directly or assume primary care of patients do not need privileges.

Privilege Review Mechanism.   In departmentalized hospital medical staffs, physician credentials are usually reviewed by a department chairman (and sometimes also by the head of a division or service) and by the medical executive committee, and then presented to the governing body to approve formally and to grant privileges. But facilities with subacute programs may not have governing bodies or may have the administrator function as the governing body's on-site representative. Therefore, the facility administrator and program medical director may be the principal individuals involved in granting privileges. Clinical medical directors of distinct subacute services (pulmonary, orthopedic rehab, and so on) should help review physician privilege requests and develop relevant qualifications for providing different kinds of care. In facilities where subacute care is part of a broader network of services, subacute privilege reviews may be added to existing privileging and credentialing mechanisms.

Table 8–18, p. 246, summarizes important steps in credentialing and privileging physicians for subacute care programs. Those seeking or having JCAHO accreditation should consult the subacute standards for the specific requirements (JCAHO, 1995, p. 118).

Coordination of Physician Practice With Patient Need.   A program needs the right physicians available at the right times to ensure that care needs are met. Each patient on the unit must have an attending physician who should be the primary coordinator of the medical care.

Each attending physician must also ensure the availability of suitable alternates. Covering physicians may not be as familiar with this level of care. However, during that coverage period, an on-call physician assumes responsibilities comparable to those of the attending physician. The program medical director should create guidelines for the attending physicians to review with their covering physicians. For example, this could include an information sheet about the subacute program and physician roles and responsibilities.

Like the attending physicians, covering physicians must manage new-onset symptoms and condition changes consistent with the current care plan, including advance directives and other patient wishes. The nursing staff is responsible for conveying adequate, correct information to the covering physician. The covering physician should respond in a timely fashion to phone calls from the nursing staff, and should be willing to discuss clinical issues with staff, patients, and families as needed. For instance, covering physicians cannot simply order a mildly unstable patient transferred back to the hospital, place a patient on a psychoactive medication in response to an acute behavior or cognitive change, or order an expensive medication not ordinarily used in the program. They must consider the existing care plan and previous agreements with a managed care payer.

Oversight.   The program medical director is the principal individual to oversee the physician services. This person's functions would be comparable to the combined roles of officers (president, vice-president, secretary-treasurer), department chairmen, and the medical executive committee (quality of care review, privileges, and so on) in a hospital-based organization. Overall, medical staff structures can be flexible as long as essential physician functions are accomplished and key lines of authority and responsibility are defined and understood.

Nursing Service

An organized system is needed for delivering nursing care to subacute patients (Table 8–19, p. 246). The nursing service should be overseen by a qualified registered nurse (RN). Like the medical director, the program nursing director must distinguish clinical and administrative oversight functions. Clinical oversight functions relate to the care of individual patients and to issues related to the care of all patients, and administrative oversight covers such things as the operations of the unit, personnel issues, interdisciplinary relationships, and quality concerns. These functions may be handled by the same person or divided among several individuals.

Staffing.   Nurse staffing is a major challenge for subacute programs. Depending on the patient and the service, nursing staff hours for subacute care ordinarily range from 4 to 8 hours per patient per day, with a typical program average of 5 to 6 hours of care per patient per day. Typical nursing time for rehabilitation patients averages 5 to 6 hours per patient day. Subacute medical nursing hours occasionally run as high as 10 hours per patient day. This varies with the services offered and the complexity of the patient's needs.

However, nursing time includes more than just RN time. Different patients require various combinations of RNs, licensed practical nurses (LPNs), and nursing assistants (NAs) for the care. For instance, a patient who is being weaned from a ventilator may require a lot of RN time; a vegetative ventilator-dependent patient who is not progressing may require mostly LPN and NA time.

Each program is challenged to balance staffing needs with costs and availability. The staffing should be based on the scope and complexity of the care and services provided. For instance, on a 10-bed subacute ventilator unit, some tasks (medication administration, vital sign monitoring, and assessment of nutrition and hydration status) must be performed on all patients; and others (suctioning, turn and position, or ventilator weaning) will be relevant to only some. Chapter 10 presents evidence that relevant patient characteristics can be used to predict staffing prospectively for many patient categories.

The staffing process should also be linked to the quality management program. For example, inefficiencies in performing individual tasks that must be repeated for the care of each individual and throughout each shift can add up to substantial amounts of wasted time and staff frustration. In an efficient system, these time-consuming tasks that do not require a health care professional's expertise are streamlined, automated, or assumed by other, less expensive practitioners or staff.

Options for Organizing Nursing Care.   The changes in the health care system are inevitably affecting the way directors of nursing (DONs) in skilled nursing facilities (SNFs) and nursing facilities (NFs) hire and schedule staff. Patient classification systems are being used to categorize patients, such as by required treatments or physical dependency levels. In hospitals, a system was developed to help modify staffing to accommodate diagnosis-related group (DRG) classifications. For NF and SNF care, the resource utilization groups (RUGs) patient classification and case-mix payment system were developed. Based on the Minimum Data Set (MDS) database, the RUGs system classifies individuals with common characteristics into hierarchical groups, used to predict resource utilization. Each category is weighted according to resources, and the payment reflects the weighted value.

Nurse staffing and skill levels may vary depending on the scheme used to classify and place patients. For instance, in the NF-based rehabilitation RUGs categories, nursing assistants provide considerable hands-on care. Nurse staffing is more likely to be based on predetermined nurse staff time for various types of patients, based on these classifications. For subacute patients, the nurse staffing must be expanded or modified to include the numbers and skill levels needed to meet the care required by these various categories. Factors that may impact staffing include regulatory requirements, location, referring hospitals, facility design efficiency, internal operational efficiency, availability of nursing staff, and staff turnover (Harris, 1994).

There are several models for organizing delivery of nursing care to patients. Staff may be assigned by room, patient, function, program (ventilator, wound care, and so on), or some combination. One approach, primary team nursing, is based on the belief that care can be improved when it is given as consistently as possible by the same nursing personnel. In this approach, various licensed and nonlicensed direct care providers share functions within a team structure, rather than having each individual assigned to perform only certain functions. For instance, essential functions include communicating with other disciplines such as physicians and therapists, giving treatments and medications, and documenting assessments, treatments, and patient responses. The team leaders participate in the ITCs for patients for whom their teams provide care. The primary team leader ensures that the case manager or utilization review coordinator is aware of progress and condition changes that would affect length of stay and possible discharge.

In this model, the team leader may substitute for the clinical coordinator and report directly to the nursing director, or may report to a clinical coordinator who is responsible to the DON. Primary assignments for admissions may be divided by time of day of arrival; for example, all admissions before or after a certain time might be handled by the day or evening team. On average, each team is responsible for about 10 to 12 individuals. For units with less than 24 beds, swing beds can be located in middle rooms to allow for flexible staffing assignments based on bed location.

A day-shift RN team leader is responsible for seeing that these functions are completed consistently on a 24-hour basis. This role may also be divided between the day and evening shift team leaders. Primary team leaders are responsible for overseeing the care for all patients managed by their teams during their shifts. The team is permitted the flexibility to do its own scheduling and task coordination, as long as the necessary processes occur appropriately and consistently.

Communication of Patient-Related Information.   Effective communication within the nursing staff and with other disciplines is essential. General mechanisms to improve communications are discussed in Chapter 9. Change of shift reports—where vital information about current problems and processes are transmitted from one shift to another—are also valuable. Many programs have found it helpful to have walking rounds in conjunction with chart rounds so that the staff can point out issues concerning patients, procedures, equipment, and the like. Additionally, the medical director and DON should make rounds periodically—jointly, if possible—to get a first-hand view of the unit, its staff, and its patients.

Nursing Documentation.   There should be a systematic approach to nursing documentation. As with all the practitioners, documentation should be problem-oriented as much as possible because that is an important framework for viewing the needs and care of subacute patients. Documentation components may vary with the patient's condition, stability, and service needs. For instance, the information and discussion needed for a cancer patient who is receiving a preplanned treatment will be narrower than that for a medically complex or postoperative patient with some instability and multiple coexisting conditions that need monitoring.

A systematic approach to consolidating documentation and focusing on the essential items for each patient is important. Computerized charting of medication administration and of concise data such as vital signs can potentially help in this regard by allowing the same information to be used for multiple purposes without duplicate entry and by permitting transformation of textual data into graphic and flowchart form, making it easier to analyze information and detect trends. In the future, voice-activated dictation and direct recording of automated monitoring should help improve the scope and accuracy of documentation while also improving efficiency.

Oral Health Service

Intermediate-stay patients, such as those in subacute care programs, often have oral health needs (Table 8–20, p. 247). The oral health service does not necessarily need a dentist or other supervising individual on site, but it should be organized around the roles of relevant disciplines in defining and managing oral health problems. All programs should include enough oral health care to at least address basic needs including good oral hygiene, conditions affecting food intake, and monitoring for oral complications of other illnesses and treatments (for example, painful oral lesions in someone receiving chemotherapy or long-term antibiotics). Most oral health care can be delivered effectively by nursing assistants and other support personnel.

Dentist participation may be accomplished by contracting with outside dentists, by referral to a personal dentist or to other health care organizations that have dental services, or by using an on-site dental program. Unless the subacute program is in a larger organization that has a readily accessible supervising dentist, the program nurse manager or medical director may need to oversee the clinical aspects of this service.

Pharmaceutical Service

Subacute programs need ready access to a broad range of oral, parenteral, and specially administered medications and nutritional alternatives such as total parenteral nutrition (Table 8–21, p. 247). The program must be able to provide continuous or life-sustaining IV drug therapies (such as inotropic drips, continuous chemotherapy, and continuous pain management) without interruption.

Pharmaceutical services and information must always be available or readily accessible. Options for making drugs and biologicals available include a licensed pharmacy within the facility, an agreement with an outside licensed pharmacy, or some combination. Programs need clear policies for expected delivery times for medications ordered during normal business hours and on-call hours, and for STAT or emergency drugs.

The clinical pharmacy portion of the service should provide important consultative and support functions for medication-related aspects of the patient care. Examples of special problems that can benefit from a consultant pharmacist's input include monitoring and calculating of appropriate aminoglycoside doses, calculating safe cumulative doses of chemotherapy agents, calculating infusion rates of cardiac medications, determining appropriate concentrations of total parenteral nutrition (TPN) components, and determining and modifying a regimen of standing and PRN narcotics orders for pain control.

The pharmaceutical service should provide a systematic approach to organizing, distributing, dispensing, documenting, and monitoring all drugs and biologicals. Pharmaceutical policies should cover dispensing, administering, controlling, storing, and disposing of all drugs and biologicals, consistent with applicable law and regulation.

Drug Distribution System.   A unit dose system is desirable because the patients require frequent changes in drug, dose, or administration times. A few longer-term patients with fairly stable medication regimens may be able to use an alternative dispensing system.

Drug Ordering System.   Any system should be stable, consistent, and have error-prevention capabilities. It should be able to provide information regarding the drug (indications for use, appropriate dosing, drug–drug interactions, cost of therapy, special warnings such as use in renal impairment, and so on) and related patient data (diagnoses, allergies, drug profile). Computer-based on-line, real-time drug ordering systems are now technically feasible and should be used widely in the future.

Formulary Service.   A formulary service may be desirable to help keep quality controls on utilization, complications, and cost. The pharmacy provider should collaborate with the medical director, DON, administrator, and clinical pharmacist. Sometimes, lower short-term medication costs are offset by more costly longer-term relapses or problems. Any formulary system should be flexible enough to allow physicians to make clinically relevant exceptions that can be demonstrated to be of value to the patient.

Quality and Infection Control Programs.   Medications are a major potential source of morbidity in those with multiple concurrent problems or who take a lot of medications. The various disciplines, including clinical pharmacists, should collaborate to solve and prevent such problems. Physicians and nurses must be vigilant about medication risks and complications and should not just leave these responsibilities to the clinical pharmacist. Experience in managing and correcting medication-related problems is invaluable for physicians and nurses to learn to anticipate and prevent them, or recognize their occurrence.

The pharmacy's quality programs should relate both to its own services and to clinical medication-related issues. Based on a computerized medication ordering and dispensing system, the pharmacy should be able to analyze the data and provide a range of useful reports that medical directors and DONs can use to evaluate the performance and practices of physicians and nurses.

The pharmacy should work closely with the clinical pharmacist, infection control coordinator, and contract lab to develop bacteriologic patterns for the facility. The program should assess the appropriateness and complications of its antimicrobial use.

The clinical pharmacist should review the medication regimen at least once for each month of a subacute patient's stay. Reviews of other special needs such as TPN should be conducted more often (weekly if necessary). The pharmacist should help establish a mechanism for reporting possible or actual medication-related complications or major drug interactions, and review any such reports with the DON and medical director.

The clinical pharmacist and the pharmacy provider should report at least quarterly to the organization's pharmacy committee about relevant aspects of the pharmaceutical service and medication-related issues. In a facility with multiple levels of care, data for the subacute program should be separated from other levels of service (for example, acute or long-term patient care).

For the future, subacute programs should vigorously address medication-related issues and must use information resources more effectively. For example, error checking and information about medication dosages, costs, and drug regimen risks can be made part of a computerized ordering system. This can provide physicians and nurses with real-time feedback as a potential order is being entered. The clinical pharmacist's role is likely to shift as health care practitioners make increasing use of computer-based knowledge bases, ordering systems, drug-selection algorithms, and dosage calculation and monitoring support.

Oversight.   A supervising pharmacist, who may be independent or employed by the facility or the contract pharmacy, should be responsible for developing, coordinating, and monitoring pharmaceutical activities. Oversight of the organization's medication-related activities should include at least a clinical pharmacist, administrator, medical director, and director of nursing.

Rehabilitation Service

The rehabilitation service (the organization of therapists and related practitioners) should be distinguished from the therapeutic treatments and programs (Table 8–22, p. 248). The purpose of a rehabilitation service is to coordinate the individuals who provide various treatments and perform evaluations related to managing the functional and psychological consequences of illness and injury. The rehabilitation program may offer medical and other services in addition to rehabilitation treatments. The rehabilitation service is typically involved in both distinct rehabilitation programs and in conjunction with other care. Besides treatments delivered on-site, rehab personnel also play a major role in home evaluation for adaptive equipment needs, safety issues, and reintegration into the home environment.

Availability. Rehabilitation services can be provided internally or through a written agreement with outside resources, such as hospitals, rehabilitation centers, state or local health departments, or licensed specialists. Rehabilitation services are given at least 5 days per week, but many insurers expect subacute patients to receive treatments 6 or 7 days a week to shorten their lengths of stay. A comprehensive subacute rehabilitation program may require increased therapist staffing to provide continuity of care and availability for additional days of treatment.

Rehabilitative and restorative care does not have to be limited to that provided by licensed therapists. Therapy aides, nurses, nursing assistants, and others may offer related services, including ADL assistance, turning and positioning, active and passive range-of-motion exercises, skin care and skin monitoring, supervised mobility care, and bowel and bladder training. Whatever the arrangements, the rehabilitation service should be part of a coordinated service delivery process which includes therapists, physicians, nurses, aides, and others such as psychologists and prosthetists.

Staffing. A majority of both intensive rehabilitation providers and medical/rehabilitation subacute providers directly employ therapy staff. Other programs either completely or partially contract out therapy services. Trends in either direction will depend on how ancillary costs come to be handled under managed care and Medicare.

A typical 20-bed rehabilitation unit would have approximately 5 to 6 nursing hours per patient day, one full-time equivalency (FTE) physical therapist (PT) and one FTE occupational therapist (OT) for each five to ten treatments per patient per day; one PT aide for every two to three PT FTEs; one OT aide for every ten OT FTEs; one-half to one FTE social worker; one-half to one FTE therapeutic recreation; and one-half to one FTE registered dietitian. The nursing hours could be affected by the acuity levels of the patients. For instance, more unstable or medically complex patients may require more nursing and less therapist time, and more stable individuals may require more therapist and aide time and less nursing time.

In the future, as care delivery systems become more integrated, it may make sense to have common rehabilitation programs for those of several levels of acuity or of rehabilitation need. The cost of each patient's care on the same unit would vary depending on the problems, stability, and overall service needs, instead of having a more homogeneous unit where the reimbursement is similar for each case.

Oversight. The rehabilitation service has several levels of players, and therefore requires several kinds of oversight. A chief therapist or other individual should oversee the various therapists and the care they render. A nurse with special training in rehabilitative nursing may oversee the rehabilitation unit and the nursing personnel on that unit. A general medical physician, physiatrist, orthopedist, or neurologist may also oversee the medical aspects of the program. All of these individuals should coordinate their functions both within the rehabilitation service and with other disciplines or individuals involved in the subacute program. For example, a nurse in charge of a rehabilitation unit should be accountable to the director of nursing or the clinical nurse supervisor for the subacute program; the physician in charge of the rehabilitation medical aspects should be accountable to the subacute program medical director; and the individual in charge of the therapists should be accountable to the administrator in charge of the subacute program.

Respiratory Care Service

A respiratory service (Table 8–23, p. 249) is an organized group of technicians and practitioners who give direct patient respiratory treatments and support for others providing the care. Respiratory care services may be needed either for patients with primary respiratory needs or for patients with respiratory problems complicating the care of other primary and secondary conditions.

Respiratory treatments and monitoring should be available from appropriately qualified providers. The subacute program should clarify which aspects of the care are provided by nurses and which are the responsibility of the therapists. It should have access to pulmonary function testing and should be able to assess patient oxygenation status at least via pulse oximetry. Blood gas analysis capability should be accessible, but not necessarily directly on site.

Hospital-based programs typically use their existing respiratory therapy (RT) services for their subacute units. Because of a peculiarity in the Medicare regulations, NF- or SNF-based subacute programs must still (as of early 1996) contract with hospitals for RT services. Again, it is hoped that time will change these and similar requirements that may inhibit flexibility to provide services more cost-effectively.

Oversight.   Where RT is provided by an outside contract service, the respiratory therapists should be supervised by someone from the provider or by someone from within the organization of the subacute unit. Depending on the program's size (including number of ventilator beds), a chief therapist may be stationed on site, or may be present intermittently. This individual monitors performance, ensures appropriate technician staffing, and reviews and gives feedback about performance.

Social Services

Social services (Table 8–24, p. 250) should be organized to systematically identify and help meet individuals' psychosocial, functional, and personal needs. These needs may relate to emotional and cognitive function, behavior, personal and family issues, and options for obtaining and paying for current and future care and support (aides, equipment, supplies, follow-up nursing care, and so on). Social services also helps with discharge planning and placement. In some programs, a social worker assumes case management functions.

Social services personnel should advocate for patients' rights and help ensure that patients and families have some means for expressing their concerns and problems to facility staff and management. They should also help current and prospective patients, their families, and others find and use financial, legal, mental health, and other community resources, and help manage guardianship and conservatorship proceedings as needed.

Organized social services should be staffed full-time or part-time by one or more qualified social workers. A subacute program should have a qualified social worker performing assessments, participating in care planning and discharge planning, and delivering direct patient services.

Oversight. Oversight of the social services program should be provided by a licensed social worker, who will often be the principal social worker in the organization or the program. Again, the clinical and administrative functions must be distinguished, and anyone serving a dual role should be skilled at both, or receive additional training and oversight as needed.

Spiritual Services

The purpose of spiritual services (Table 8–25, p. 251) is to provide an organized approach to meeting the emotional and spiritual needs of subacute patients. Patients' spiritual needs can be addressed by religious services within the facility or access to those outside the facility, and by contact with members of the clergy. Members of the clergy are also often helpful in dealing with family issues, questions and concerns about unfavorable prognoses, and discussions of withholding or withdrawing treatment.

REFERENCES

Harris C. Nurse management 2000. *Provider*. 1994; 20(8):42,44.

Joint Commission on Accreditation of Healthcare Organizations. *Survey Protocol for Subacute Programs*. Chicago: JCAHO; 1995.

FOR FURTHER READING

Buchanan AE, Brock DW. *Deciding for Others: The Ethics of Surrogate Decision Making*. New York: Cambridge University Press; 1989.

Freedman M, Stuss DT, Gordon M. Assessment of competency: The role of neurobehavioral deficits. *Ann Intern Med*. 1991; 115:203–208.

Hastings Center. *Guidelines on the Termination of Life-Sustaining Treatment and the Care of the Dying*. Bloomington: Indiana University Press; 1987.

Hegland A. LTC Nurses go high tech. *Provider*. 1995; 21(4):50–54.

Hoffman DE, Boyle P, Levenson SA. *Handbook for Nursing Home Ethics Committees*. Washington, DC: American Association of Homes and Services for the Aged; 1995.

JCAHO says credentialing and privileging are critical. *Briefings Subacute Care*. 1995; 2(5):1.

LaPuma J, Orentlicher D, Moss RJ. Advance directives on admission: Clinical implications and analysis of the Patient Self-Determination Act of 1990. *JAMA*. 1991; 226:402–405.

Levenson SA. *Medical Direction in Long-Term Care: A Guidebook for the Future*. Durham: Carolina Academic Press; 1993.

Litchfield M. Nursing in the computer age. *NZ Nurs J*. 1990; 83(1):10–12.

Office of Technology Assessment. *Life-Sustaining Technologies and the Elderly*. Washington, DC: U.S. Government Printing Office; 1989.

President's Commission for the Study of Ethical Problems in Medicine and Biomedical and Behavioral Research. *Deciding to Forego Life-Sustaining Medical Treatment*. Washington, DC: U.S. Government Printing Office; 1983.

President's Commission for the Study of Ethical Problems in Medicine and Biomedical and Behavioral Research. *Making Health Care Decisions*. Washington, DC: U.S. Government Printing Office; 1982.

Ross JW, et al. *Handbook for Hospital Ethics Committees*. Chicago: American Hospital Publishing; 1986.

Vaczek D. Who's in charge?: DON's management skills are challenged when subacute units enter the picture. *Contemp Long-Term Care*. June 1994:75–76, 81.

Wanzer S, et al. The physician's responsibility toward hopelessly ill patients. *N Engl J Med*. 1988; 310:955–959.

TABLE 8–1   ESSENTIAL ELEMENTS OF A CARE MANAGEMENT SYSTEM

- Appropriate philosophies
- Detailed roles and responsibilities of all players, including patients, families, and other patient support systems
- A system for interdisciplinary assessment
- A mechanism for developing individual interdisciplinary care plans for each patient based on comprehensive assessments
- A system for the regular review and revision of each patient's care plan
- A mechanism for dealing with patient choices, including ethical issues and limits on medical treatment
- A systematic approach to providing various treatments and clinical services and to assessing care outcomes
- A mechanism for ensuring that essential support services, such as lab and radiology, are available
- A system for ensuring that practitioners and other care providers have the appropriate knowledge and skills
- A system for providing essential policies and procedures
- A system for ensuring effective performance and appropriate results

TABLE 8–2   A FORM FOR DOCUMENTATION OF FULFILLED RESPONSIBILITIES FOR THE ESSENTIAL PROCESSES OF SUBACUTE CARE[a]

Process	Objectives	Principal Responsibilities	Verification	Reference/Comments
Patient selection	• Verified that the individual needs the services. • Determined that our program can meet the patient's needs.	Nursing Physician Administration		
Postselection, preadmission	• Information required to be given to the patient/family has been given. • Appropriate individuals have been prepared to accept admission.	Admissions office Administration Nursing		
Assessment	• All information about the individual relevant to proper definition of their problems has been collected.	All disciplines		
Problem definition	• The individual's problems and needs have been fully and accurately defined.	All disciplines Patient/family		
Identifying care objectives	• The objectives of the care, and the criteria that will be used to determine when the objectives have been met, have been established.	Nursing Physician Social services Patient/family		
Care planning	• A plan to address the individual's problems, including the responsibilities of various individuals and disciplines, has been created.	All disciplines Patient/family		
Management of known problems	• A plan has been created to address the individual's known, active primary (main reason for admission) and secondary (coexisting) problems.	All disciplines Patient/family		
Management of new problems/complications	• Problems that arose as a result of existing conditions or that did not exist previously have been identified and managed.	All disciplines		
Prevention of nosocomial/iatrogenic problems	• High-risk and potential problems that may arise as a result of medications and treatments, or by being in a health care facility, have been identified, and measures have been instituted to try to prevent those problems and to recognize them if they arise despite precautions.	Nursing Physician Dietitian Clinical pharmacist		

Preparation for completion of treatment course	• The problems for which the individual was admitted have been treated sufficiently to allow for transfer to another site.	All disciplines
	• A plan for discharge and transfer has been implemented, including providing information to the transfer site, follow-up of problems, and communication of information to the patient and family.	Physical/ occupational therapist Patient/family
Follow-up	• The care during the stay was reviewed.	Administration All disciplines
	• The problems and concerns of the providers and recipients of care have been reviewed and addressed.	
	• The subsequent course of the patient has been followed up.	

TABLE 8–3   FUNCTIONS AND ITEMS FOR REVIEW BY AN INTERDISCIPLINARY TEAM CONFERENCE (ITC)

Functions

Patient-related

- Discuss various disciplines' assessment of the individual.
- Establish comprehensive care plan and adjust as indicated.
- Establish realistic care goals and objectives.
- Help determine roles of various disciplines and individuals in care of individual patients.
- Discuss changes in condition and new problems and symptoms.
- Review the course of acute illnesses, complications since last meeting.
- Review patient's condition and progress toward discharge.
- Discuss concerns, questions, problems from various disciplines or from the patient and family.
- Consider expectations of payer, perform relevant utilization review functions.
- Prepare for discharge.

Program-related

- Identify obstacles to achieving care objectives, including discharge.
- Review adequacy of staffing, support, supplies, equipment, and so on.
- Assign responsibility for various functions, including specific problem-solving activities.
- Assess input and conduct of various players.
- Discuss issues of concern to players.
- Apprise management of clinical issues.
- Refer quality and support problems for subsequent review and action.

Items to Review

- Current condition
- Progress toward care objectives
- Degree of stability
- Patient/family concerns
- Test results/pending tests
- Acute problems interrupting the treatment plan
- Any complications or risk situations
- Payer expectations for discharge

| TABLE 8–4 | POSSIBLE REASONS FOR INEFFECTIVE PARTICIPATION BY PATIENTS OR SUBSTITUTE DECISION MAKERS |

Decision Makers

- They think they understand, so they do not request more clarification.
- They have personal limitations in comprehending information generally.
- They do not want to make a decision.
- They are afraid they might do the wrong thing.
- They hold out until they hear what they want to hear.
- They misinterpret the information they receive.
- They do not admit that they do not understand.

Health Care Providers

- Providers fail to give decision makers all relevant facts about the condition, options, risks, prognosis, and the like.
- Providers give decision makers incorrect information.
- Providers erroneously interpret the facts for decision makers.
- Providers fail to respond adequately to a decision maker's request for additional explanation or information.
- Providers fail to clarify or to understand the rationale behind the decision maker's conclusions.

| TABLE 8–5 | APPROACHES TO ENHANCE PATIENT AND FAMILY INVOLVEMENT |

Area	Possible Approaches
Patient rights and responsibilities	• Written explanation of patient rights and responsibilities • Routine review with admissions officer prior to admission, social services after admission, and as needed
Description of subacute processes and players	• Written material to explain who will be involved in the care, and the various processes (assessment, care planning, etc.)
Mechanism for addressing concerns, problems	• Procedures for appropriate individuals to refer issues to (primary: first-line individual; secondary: in case initial efforts unsuccessful or results are unsatisfactory)
System for addressing ethical issues	• Policies on advance directives, life-sustaining technologies and withholding of resuscitation, and foregoing or withdrawal of life-sustaining treatment • Synopsis of relevant laws and regulations governing advanced directives and Do Not Resuscitate orders • Relevant laws and procedures regarding organ donation
Participation in aspects of care planning and care	• Means for patient/family participation in various areas of care (care planning, discharge planning, interdisciplinary team conferences, etc.)

TABLE 8–6	**POLICIES AND PROCEDURES FOR MANAGING ETHICAL ISSUES AND MEDICAL DECISION MAKING IN A SUBACUTE PROGRAM**

- **Determining existence of directives**

  Policy: Every incoming patient should be asked about any existing advance directives (ADs). Everyone should be encouraged to make one. If one exists, it should be obtained for the record.

  Procedure: Upon or prior to admission, the admissions office will ask the patient or family if an AD exists. If one exists, the patient or family will be asked to provide a copy for the medical record. Answers to these inquiries will be documented in the admission paper work and transmitted to the care site or unit of admission.

- **Determining patient's decision-making capacity**

  Policy: A patient with decision-making capacity (DMC) should be consulted as the decision maker (DM). A competent person may appoint someone else to make decisions, even if they are not incapacitated. Before a substitute decision maker is consulted, there must be a determination that the patient requests it or does not have health care DMC.

  Procedure: Upon admission, the nurses, social worker, and other appropriate interdisciplinary team members will evaluate a patient's DMC. This may require the use of various tests or consultations. If the DMC is unclear, the attending physician will help in the determination. If needed, the attending physician will request consultative assistance from another physician. If the patient is considered to lack DMC, the attending physician (and second physician, if needed) will certify that the patient lacks DMC.

- **Selecting the primary decision maker**

  Policy: A person who has DMC should be consulted as the decision maker. For individuals lacking DMC, if there is no surrogate decision maker or a guardian has not been appointed, then a prescribed order for selecting a surrogate decision maker should be followed.

  Procedure: The patient will be consulted as the DM unless previously adjudicated incompetent, or unless they are documented (as noted above) to lack DMC. Any court-appointed guardian will be consulted as the DM. If an AD exists and names a surrogate decision maker (SDM), that surrogate is the DM. In the absence of a specified SDM or guardian, other individuals will be consulted in the following order: spouse, adult child, parent, adult sibling, close friend. Before consulting a close friend as the surrogate, the staff will obtain from that person an affidavit certifying the basis for claiming knowledge of the individual and their health care preferences. If all surrogates in one class (siblings, children, parents, and so on) are unavailable, are incapable of making decisions, or choose not to make them, then the physician will consult someone in the next class. If surrogates of the same class cannot agree about withholding or withdrawing life-sustaining procedures, and the issue cannot be settled, then the case should be referred to the facility's Ethics Advisory Committee (EAC). If the attending physician believes that the SDM's instructions to withhold or withdraw treatment are inconsistent with generally accepted standards of patient care, then the physician will refer the case to the facility's EAC. The nurse or physician will enter the names and relevant relationships of individuals to be used as SDMs on the appropriate portion of the certification form.

- **Conclusions about medical ineffectiveness of treatment**

  Policy: Attending physicians do not have to order treatments that they consider medically ineffective, but must first follow a specific process.

  Procedure: If the SDM requests treatment that the attending physician feels is medically ineffective, then the attending physician may decline to order that treatment after certifying and having another physician also certify that the treatment is medically ineffective (that is, to a reasonable degree of medical certainty, the treatment will not prevent or reduce deterioration of an individual's health or prevent impending death). The attending physician will inform the patient or an individual acting on the patient's behalf of this conclusion. The patient or surrogate will be offered the right to seek transfer to another provider. If transfer is desired, and a situation arises in which failing to honor the request for treatment would likely result in the patient's death, then the request for the treatment will be honored pending the transfer.

- **Documenting certifications and orders**

  Policy: A designated form shall be used to record key ethics-related information in one place.

  Procedure: Based on their assessments, direct care staff with pertinent knowledge will check off appropriate conclusions or information on the Certifications: Advance Directives and Substitute Decision-Making Form. The attending physician and any consultants will initial any applicable items on the form. Each new column should be used only for certifications made on the same date. Changes to a previous certification (for example, a previously incapable patient regains DMC) should be made in a new column, and the earlier conclusion should be marked through. These will be initialed as appropriate on the form. Any specific elements of the care plan will be written or otherwise authorized by the physician as medical orders on the order sheet. The attending physician will discuss with the patient or appropriate SDM any specific care wishes, such as CPR, hospitalization, or tube feedings. This form will remain in the medical record at all times.

TABLE 8–7   CONSIDERATIONS IN MANAGING ETHICAL ISSUES IN SUBACUTE PROGRAMS

Issue	Approaches
Discussing ethical issues with patients and families	• The program should inform the patient and family of their rights and of relevant legislation and regulations that may affect ethical decision making. • Providers should initiate discussions early in the stay to try to avoid crisis-oriented decision making. • Providers should use a collaborative interdisciplinary approach to managing these issues. • Care providers should encourage patients and families to ask questions and clarify information about the care, prognosis, or treatment options. • Care providers should provide relevant information to facilitate decision making. • Care providers should recognize the psychosocial and cultural factors influencing ethical decision making.
Patient participation in decision making	• The patient's capacity for decision making should be assessed. • Discussions should elicit the patient's direct wishes unless their limited ability to participate is appropriately defined. • The patient should be involved as much as possible, even if decision-making capacity is limited. • The patient's pace of decision making should be respected and supported.
Substitute decision making	• Appropriate substitute decision makers (SDMs) should be identified based on applicable law and standards. • Care providers may have to guide SDMs as to their appropriate roles. • The family's pace of decision making should be respected and supported.
Implementation of decisions	• Decisions should be documented and also translated into appropriate medical orders. • Care providers should monitor and manage patients' pain and suffering, regardless of other decisions about treatment. • Providers should establish a mechanism for managing situations where ethical or legal constraints inhibit or prevent them from honoring patient or family requests. • Considerations of medical futility should be from the perspective of the patient's requests and condition. • Transfer to another care site may be indicated when subsequent treatment of a patient's condition is limited by request or by failure to respond to previous treatment.
Methods for resolving disagreements	• A committee or other mechanism is needed to help assess and resolve disputes that cannot be resolved on a patient/practitioner level. • A mechanism should exist to handle those few cases that may require judicial intervention.
Other influences on the decisions	• A mechanism must exist to recognize and balance the influence of outsiders such as insurers or managed care organizations on these decision-making processes. • Managed care may be reluctant to pay for continuing treatment of those with limitations on care. • The program should include information and training about managing ethical issues in its policies and training materials. • The program should help ensure appropriate confidentiality while still enabling necessary disclosure of relevant information.

TABLE 8–8	TACTICS TO IMPROVE PERFORMANCE OF OCCASIONAL STAFF

- Easily accessible, clear policies and procedures
- Closer supervision
- Detailed, pictorial and computer-based representation of procedures and tasks
- Explicit written expectations
- Have individual sign a statement of expectations
- Give the individual and contract agency performance-specific feedback soon after their shift or tour of duty

TABLE 8–9	CORE SERVICES FOR SUBACUTE CARE

- Activities
- Dietary/food service
- Laboratory and radiology
- Medical
- Nursing
- Oral health/dental
- Pharmacy
- Rehabilitation
- Respiratory therapy
- Social services
- Spiritual services

TABLE 8–10	ACTIVITIES SERVICE

Item	Components
Purpose of service	• To provide coordinated therapeutic and recreational activities to patients whose medical, functional, and psychological status may benefit
Coordination/oversight	• Individual trained and certified in therapeutic/recreational activities
Availability	• Ready accessibility as needed
Individuals/disciplines involved	• Primary: Activities therapist • Others: Music therapist, pet therapist
Primary functions/tasks	• Assess or review patient's level of physical and social function, compensatory and adaptive mechanisms, education and occupational background, leisure and recreation preferences, lifestyle, cognitive and emotional functioning, communications skills, social function • Monitor response to activities • Provide activities such as exercise classes, socialization, reading and educational activities, community activities, spiritual activities, creative activities, intellectual stimulation
Staff education and training/policies and procedures	• Basic understanding of the conditions, problems, and potential complications of the various subacute patients • Options for therapeutic activities in those with complex or multidimensional illness
Special needs, issues, concerns	• Ensure that activities staff can recognize onset of complications/problems related to conditions of various individuals that may arise during activities programs

TABLE 8–11   DIETARY SERVICE

Item	Components
Purpose of service	• To provide a coordinated approach to meeting the nutritional and hydration needs of patients
Coordination/oversight	• Dietetic services supervisor or consultant dietitian • Clinical dietitian
Availability	• May be provided within the organization or via services obtained through a written agreement or contract with another health care organization or an outside food service or food management company • Staff or consultant dietitians
Individuals/disciplines involved	• Food preparation and handling staff • Dietitians
Primary functions/tasks	• Assess nutritional status • Help assess factors supporting or inhibiting adequate nutritional intake • Recommend therapeutic diet interventions, modifications, and supplements • Monitor parameters of nutritional status such as lab values, weight gain or loss • Identify and report problems and risk factors such as drug/food interactions • Prepare and provide meals, nutritional supplements, and therapeutic diets • Educate patients, families, and staff regarding dietary issues • Follow up with patients and families as needed
Staff education and training/policies and procedures	• Current therapeutic diet manual • Nutritional aspects of various illnesses and conditions • Drug/food interactions
Special needs, issues, concerns	• Flexibility to accommodate frequent diet changes

TABLE 8–12   LABORATORY AND OTHER TESTING SERVICES

Item	Components
Purpose of service	• To provide appropriate, timely laboratory monitoring and testing for the patients
Coordination/oversight	• Administrator • Medical director
Availability	• Routine and STAT lab testing as needed • Routine and special radiologic, imaging, and other testing as needed
Individuals/disciplines involved	• Technicians • Physicians
Primary functions/tasks	• Provide monitoring and testing capabilities as needed
Staff education and training/policies and procedures	• Laboratory procedures • Recognition of significant abnormal test results • Recognition and prevention of problems with specimen collection, storage, and identification
Special needs, issues, concerns	• Means to oversee quality and consistency of lab services • Mechanism for communicating results promptly and ensuring appropriate follow-up

TABLE 8–13   MEDICAL SERVICE

Item	Components
Purpose of service	• To provide coordinated, appropriate, and timely primary and specialty medical care to the patients
Coordination/oversight	• Facility medical director • Program and service medical oversight
Availability	• Attending physicians with backup coverage always available • Specialists and consultants accessible as needed
Individuals/disciplines involved	• Family physicians, general internists, pediatricians • Medical specialists (nephrology, pulmonary, neurology, cardiology, gastroenterology, dermatology, oncology, hematology) • Surgical specialties (urology, orthopedics, neurosurgery, plastic surgery, general surgery) • Nurse practitioners • Physician assistants
Primary functions/tasks	• Assess and define medical condition and problems • Order and authorize medications and treatments • Monitor progress and response to treatments • Support other staff providing care • Educate staff, patients, and families
Staff education and training/policies and procedures	• Principles of subacute care • Illnesses, conditions, problems, complications of subacute patients • Managing patients with multiple comorbidities • Recognition and prevention of iatrogenic illness • Principles of primary, secondary, and tertiary prevention • Management of ethical issues • Physician role in interdisciplinary approach and processes of care • Capabilities and limitations of the specific subacute care program • Decision making regarding patient transfer, discharge
Special needs, issues, concerns	• Performing credentialing and granting privileges • Relationship of subacute practice to other aspects of physician's practice • Effective integration of physician services • Constructive participation of covering and occasional physicians • Physician participation in quality improvement processes

TABLE 8–14   HOW PHYSICIANS MAY HELP OR HINDER THE OUTCOMES OF SUBACUTE CARE

Help	Hinder
Diagnose new onset illnesses or complications correctly	Inadequate diagnosis of new onset illnesses or complications
Perform an appropriate assessment, correlated with that of other disciplines	Incomplete or inaccurate assessment
Select pertinent treatments based on consideration of clinical and other relevant factors	Choose the wrong treatments, fail to choose the correct treatments, or choose undesired or inappropriate ones
Perform cost-effective medical workup, where needed	Order unnecessarily expensive or irrelevant tests
Authorize orders that others need to provide care	Inadequate response to requests for orders that others need to carry out the plan of care
Recognize and address side effects and complications of medications and treatments	Fail to anticipate or to recognize side effects and complications; fail to act soon enough after these are recognized to prevent worse complications
Communicate needed information to staff, patients, and family	Inadequate provision to staff, patients, and families of information they need to make appropriate decisions
Perform procedures correctly	Perform procedures inappropriately, resulting in avoidable complications
Obtain appropriate consultative support in a timely fashion	Fail to recognize need for consultative assistance; fail to obtain consultation soon enough; fail to implement appropriate recommendations
Help staff, patients, and families make appropriate decisions to limit, withhold, or withdraw treatments	Fail to participate sufficiently in care discussions; fail to provide relevant information about medical condition and prognosis that would help others select care options; refuse to allow certain decisions to be made or implemented because of personal philosophies or discomforts
Ensure that rights of patients and/or families are respected	Fail to recognize or acknowledge certain rights; fail to advocate for patient where appropriate
Balance cost and care quality considerations	Overemphasize one or the other

TABLE 8–15   HELPFUL ITEMS FOR SUCCESSFUL PHYSICIAN PERFORMANCE IN SUBACUTE CARE

Item	Discussion
Basic expectations	• Policies and procedures; written performance and attitude expectations
Confirmation of essential knowledge and skills	• Credentialing process • Application for staff privileges • Privilege delineation
Coordination of physician roles with patient need	• Clarifying physician roles as primary attendings and consultants
Integration of medical with other care	• Medical director interactions with other key leadership and players to deal with concerns
Review of quality of physician performance and participation	• Indicator development and use • Medical director participation in broader quality program • Medical director rounds and reviews of care • Performance evaluation linked to privilege renewals
Feedback mechanisms	• Individual contact by medical director • Staff meetings

TABLE 8–16   CATEGORIES AND EXAMPLES OF PHYSICIAN CREDENTIALS

Credential	Possible Sources of Relevant Information
Knowledge	Evidence of education; publications; lectures and presentations; awards and other recognition; evidence of continuing education
Skills	Evidence of experience; results of quality reviews done internally or elsewhere
Training	Residency and fellowship; other special training or study (special courses, summer institutes, etc.)
Certification	Certificates by relevant agencies, associations, boards, etc.
Experience	Description of similar care given elsewhere
General performance	Results of quality evaluations at former or current practice sites; malpractice experience; current or previous actions against license
Miscellaneous	Specialty society membership/fellowship

| TABLE 8–17 | RELEVANT INFORMATION ON PHYSICIAN APPLICATIONS TO PROVIDE SUBACUTE CARE |

Personal Information
- Name
- Birth date
- Title
- Degree
- Health status

Education and Training
- Medical education
- Specialty and subspecialty residencies and fellowships

Practice Information
- Years in practice
- Practice experience in other states
- Registered practice specialties
- Practice experience in subacute or transitional care
- Current hospital, nursing facility, and other care site affiliations
- HMO, PPO, and other managed care affiliations
- Voluntary and involuntary changes in membership or privileges at other organizations

Licensure and Certification Information
- Verification of current state licensure
- Federal and state controlled drug and any other state prescribing licenses
- Current and past licensure in other states
- Specialty board certification
- History of any adverse actions against license(s)

Professional and Specialty Society and Other Memberships and Affiliations
- Current memberships and fellowships
- Academic appointments and affiliations
- Involuntary changes in membership or privileges

Liability Situation
- Current malpractice insurance carrier
- Previous malpractice insurance carrier(s)
- Policy expiration dates
- Policy limits
- History of malpractice judgments and settlements

TABLE 8–18   SUMMARY OF PROCESSES FOR PHYSICIAN CREDENTIALING AND PRIVILEGING IN SUBACUTE PROGRAMS

- Define categories of care provided in program.
- Define areas of competence for practitioners generally and for physicians specifically.
- Provide physicians with relevant definitions and privilege request categories.
- Collect and verify credentials (or copies).
- Grant category-specific privileges.
- Educate physicians about explicit criteria for performance expectations.
- Review physician performance as part of quality program.
- Give physician frequent, relevant feedback.
- Obtain comparable feedback from physicians.
- Review and renew or revise privileges periodically.

TABLE 8–19   NURSING SERVICE

Item	Components
Purpose of service	• To provide coordinated, appropriate, and timely skilled nursing and support nursing services and functions to patients • To serve a coordinating role in the overall care of patients and the processes of care
Coordination/oversight	• Facility director of nursing (DON) • Program nurse manager • Charge nurse
Availability	• 24-hour availability of nurses and nursing assistants • Access to clinical nurse specialists
Individuals/disciplines involved	• Registered nurses • Licensed practical nurses • Nursing assistants • Medicine aides
Primary functions/tasks	• Assess and document patient condition, care needs, problems • Help assess, define, and triage problems and condition changes • Develop and implement nursing care plans • Administer medications and treatments • Monitor and document responses to treatments and overall progress • Provide support for patients and families • Inform patients, families, and other staff about various conditions, treatments, and care plan • Help assess and prepare patients for postdischarge care
Staff education and training/ policies and procedures	• Principles and practices of care of complex medical and surgical conditions, and care of those with multidimensional problems • Nursing role in interdisciplinary team approach • Assessment of basic health-related signs and symptoms • Ability to identify and monitor illnesses and their complications
Special needs, issues, concerns	• Clarifying roles and relationships of nurses with other disciplines • Relieving nurses of tasks not requiring that level of training and skills

TABLE 8–20   ORAL HEALTH SERVICE

Item	Components
Purpose of service	• To support provision of appropriate oral health care
Coordination/oversight	• Program medical director or nurse manager • Supervising dentist
Availability	• Accessible as needed through on-site service or outside dentists
Individuals/disciplines involved	• Nursing assistants • Nurses • Physician • Dentist
Primary functions/tasks	• Assess oral health and dental status • Monitor complications and problems arising secondary to other medical conditions and treatments (intubation, paralysis, chemotherapy) • Provide appropriate basic and advanced oral health care • Educate staff, patients, and families about dental and oral health issues
Staff education and training/ policies and procedures	• Appropriate oral and dental assessment • Recognition of oral lesions representing medical complications • Techniques of oral hygiene
Special needs, issues, concerns	• Presence of appropriate equipment and supplies • Access to outside dentists

TABLE 8–21   PHARMACY SERVICE

Item	Components
Purpose of service	• To provide coordinated, appropriate, and timely service and support for the medications and intravenous and parenteral therapies administered to subacute patients
Coordination/oversight	• Registered pharmacist/pharmD
Availability	• 24-hour availability or access
Individuals/disciplines involved	• Pharmacist/technicians • Clinical pharmacist
Primary functions/tasks	• Assess medication and treatment regimen • Advise physicians and nurses about potential and actual risks, complications, and other medication-related problems • Recommend medication choices, doses, and dosage adjustments • Educate staff about therapeutic and undesirable effects of specific medications • Educate patients and families about appropriate use and preventive aspects of medications • Follow up results of treatments and complications
Staff education and training/ policies and procedures	• Special aspects of medications and treatments for subacute patients • Problems and complications of medication use in those with complex acute and chronic conditions
Special needs, issues, concerns	• Availability of medications and pharmacist support during off-hours

TABLE 8–22   REHABILITATION SERVICE

Item	Components
Purpose of service	• To coordinate rehabilitative and restorative care that maintains or improves function, assists recovery from illness and injury, and supports the provision of other medical and nursing services • To help individuals adapt to significant irreversible changes in physical and functional status
Coordination/oversight	• Rehab program coordinator • Rehab nurse • Physiatrist
Individuals/disciplines involved	• Primary: physical therapy, occupational therapy • Other specialized services: psychology, therapeutic recreation, vocational rehabilitation, orthotics, prosthetics, speech-language pathology • Physical and occupational therapy aides • Social services, nursing, dietitian, physician
Availability	• Physical and occupational therapy readily available • Speech therapy available as needed • Other specialized services accessible as needed • Services given at least 5 days a week, sometimes daily
Primary functions/tasks	• Assess functional and related health status • Provide therapies • Monitor and report signs and symptoms during therapy sessions • Define measurable rehabilitation goals and objectives • Determine relevant time frames for achieving the objectives • Identify factors that may help or inhibit reaching the goals • Identify and provide pertinent rehabilitation interventions • Assess patient response to therapies and overall progress • Educate patients and families regarding progress toward goals, self-care, coping with deficits • Follow up with patients and families
Staff education and training/ policies and procedures	• Knowledge of options for various therapies • Skill in delivering treatments appropriately • Physical and occupational therapists should have degrees from accredited programs • Rehab aides should have adequate training and supervision
Special needs, issues, concerns	• Coordination of formal rehabilitation program with other forms of rehabilitative and restorative care in the subacute program

TABLE 8–23   RESPIRATORY THERAPY SERVICE

Item	Components
Purpose of service	• To provide coordinated, appropriate, and timely respiratory care to patients with pulmonary and functional respiratory problems
Coordination/oversight	• Chief respiratory therapist
Availability	• Part-time or full-time presence or 24-hour access
Individuals/disciplines involved	• Respiratory therapists • Physicians • Nurses
Primary functions/tasks	• Help assess patient problems and service needs • Help manage equipment and supplies • Administer respiratory treatments • Monitor response to treatments and therapies • Support nurses and physicians in managing respiratory/ventilator care • Educate patients, families, physicians, nurses • Follow up on issues and problems related to the services and the equipment
Staff education and training/ policies and procedures	• Operation, maintenance, and repair of ventilators and other respiratory therapy equipment • Ability to recognize possible complications or condition changes related to respiratory conditions or treatments • Quality indicators for respiratory services
Special needs, issues, concerns	• Division of responsibilities between respiratory therapists and nurses must be clearly defined

TABLE 8–24   SOCIAL SERVICES

Item	Components
Purpose of service	• To provide coordinated, appropriate, and timely assessment, management, and support for psychosocial issues and case management
Coordination/oversight	• Principal social worker or department head
Availability	• At least part-time
Individuals/disciplines involved	• Social worker
Primary functions/tasks	• Assess psychosocial, functional, and financial status • Assess patient and family strengths and weaknesses in resources, coping, communications • Help ascertain patient preferences regarding extent of medical treatment • Participate in care planning and discharge planning • Educate and support patients and families for postdischarge care management
Staff education and training/ policies and procedures	• Knowledge of available internal and external programs and services • Appropriate recognition and definition of psychosocial problems • Understanding of reimbursement/utilization issues
Special needs, issues, concerns	• Role of social worker in case management and other possibly overlapping functions

TABLE 8–25   SPIRITUAL SERVICES

Item	Components
Purpose of service	• To provide psychosocial support and counseling to patients consistent with their philosophical and religious foundations
Coordination/oversight	• Principal clergy
Availability	• Accessibility as needed
Individuals/disciplines involved	• Clergy • Social services
Primary functions/tasks	• Assess spiritual/religious needs • Provide spiritual support to patients and families • Help other staff deal with psychosocial aspects of patients/families • Help resolve complex ethical issues • Educate patients, families, staff regarding ethical, spiritual issues
Staff education and training/ policies and procedures	• Recognizing situations where intervention may be helpful • Understanding of medical ethical principles and how to define ethical issues for specific patients
Special needs, issues, concerns	• Effective coordination of advice and information about ethical decision making with clinical situation and information provided by clinical practitioners

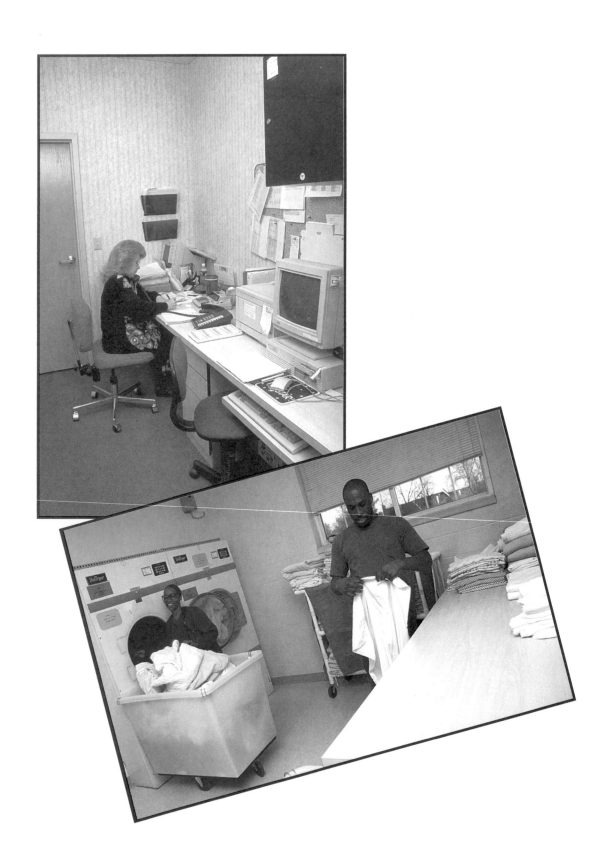

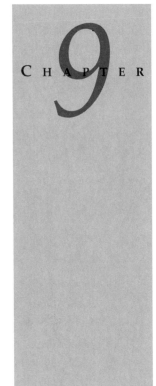

GENERAL SUPPORT SYSTEMS FOR SUBACUTE CARE

*H*ealth care is a service business. More so than in situations where the care is delivered one-on-one, complex care settings are strongly influenced by organizational and social psychological factors. A number of support systems are needed to evaluate and strengthen individual and collective performance.

In any setting, technical knowledge and skills alone do not ensure optimal performance. Care recipients and providers alike must understand that systems and processes must be optimized to achieve both effectiveness and efficiency in giving care. Processes cannot be ignored because they affect performance, which influences results. The trend toward total quality management (TQM) and process improvement is very relevant, and is not just a gimmick.

This chapter considers general support systems that influence those directly or indirectly involved in giving the care.

Many episodes of illness or injury are self-limited, requiring no professional intervention. Many others can be handled by a simple interaction between a practitioner and the individual needing help, with little or no involvement of other care providers or support staff. But still other situations—such as subacute care—require a systems approach to delivering the care.

In these last circumstances, the care involves substantial coordination of many individuals and processes operating within a broader framework. Health care practitioners and other disciplines (social workers, dietitians, physicians, nurses, and so on) provide the care with the help of clinical support staff (nursing assistants, technicians, and so on) within a facility, program, or organization that they generally do not organize or operate. Several categories of functions occur simultaneously: those involved in running the business (collecting revenues, maintaining buildings, paying bills, and so on) and those involved in providing the care (assessment, monitoring, problem definition, and the like). Anything that influences individual performance, which can be identified and appropriately reinforced or improved, can influence the outcomes (Table 9–1, p. 287).

Ultimately, any complex health care service requires a collection of support systems (Table 9–2, p. 288). Table 9–3, p. 289, illustrates the need for effective support systems, summarizing items from discussions so far in this book regarding subacute care and its patients. These are discussed at greater length below.

Characteristics of Subacute Patients.   Subacute patients have multiple complex problems. Their status and outcomes are affected by different combinations of past medical and personal history, coexisting conditions, psychosocial and functional factors, and their current treatment regimen. One individual may have ten or more problems, and may receive care from several physicians and others of many different disciplines who have different backgrounds, knowledge, skills, and ways of interpreting the same information. Each patient can have several different care objectives at the same time or at different times. Their care requires a unified plan, which must be achieved by reconciling these many variables.

Nature of Patient Risk.   Subacute patients tend to be at risk for complications, which could result from their conditions, treatments, or other aspects of their care. Any of the processes related to the care or the business could affect risk. Therefore, a mechanism is needed to anticipate and try to prevent such problems.

Variability in Desired and Achieved Care Outcomes.   Table 10–1, p. 337, lists the many different criteria for assessing health care outcomes and service quality. Some means are needed to anticipate and measure optimal results in individual cases. Several criteria may be relevant in a given case, and different criteria may apply to managing the same problem in different individuals. Often, the results of care can be anticipated, but sometimes they are unforeseen. Suboptimal results may occur despite effective performance or because of ineffective performance. Consistent processes are a prerequisite to effectively comparing outcomes among practitioners and care sites.

Influences on Decision Making.   Effective care requires complex decision making, which depends heavily on the interpretation of a sizable, multidimensional database and the available support of communications processes and information systems. Practitioners cannot rely only on their personal knowledge base. Often, those who need to use certain information are not necessarily responsible for collecting or documenting it. Significant information relevant to such decision making may be overlooked if it is not readily accessible or usable. Therefore, systems must support the information requirements of the care so that the appropriate information will be used correctly to make the most effective decisions possible.

QUALITY MANAGEMENT AND IMPROVEMENT SYSTEMS

A quality management and improvement system is dedicated to assessing and improving quality of care and services by doing several things:

- Establishing the proper *foundations* (attitudes, systems, processes) to enable effective operations and service delivery
- Employing quality *indicators* as a basis for comparing actual to desired or required performance
- Creating systems to *assess* actual performance and its precursors
- Developing a mechanism to *improve* quality based on these assessments
- Having methods to *anticipate* and *prevent* quality problems

An effective quality oversight and improvement program requires process quality, personal quality, and organizational quality (Figure 9–1). The result is continuous quality improvement (CQI). It includes facility-wide participation; effective coordination; support from leadership; cross-departmental expertise; an interdisciplinary approach to monitoring and assessment; appropriate collection, analysis, and reporting of data; and a system to implement various improvements and to monitor the impact of such changes on processes and outcomes (Ernst, 1994).

There are many potential obstacles to effective performance and outcomes in health care (Table 9–4, p. 290). Diverse individuals—however knowledgeable, skilled, well-intentioned, or credentialed—are not necessarily able to understand or accomplish the desired objectives of their performance or recognize the extent to which they are meeting the objectives without a system to organize, educate, and guide them. In health care organizations, considerable time is still spent dealing with dysfunctional interpersonal conflict and in investigating and reacting to performance failures.

Quality management and improvement systems should be the principal vehicle to optimize performance and improve care efficiency. The principles of total quality management (TQM) have been described and analyzed extensively during the past decade (Laffel & Blumenthal, 1989). However, there is still considerable misunderstanding of why this approach is important and of how to implement it properly. Some skeptics suggest that individuals should be able to work together effectively to accomplish their objectives without such "gimmicks."

The Vital Team Approach

Chapter 6 discussed the importance of the team approach to the care of subacute patients. The same principles apply to operating the support systems and the organization. Health care organizations are often still arranged primarily by

FIGURE 9–1   ACHIEVING A QUALITY ORGANIZATION: A SYSTEMS-WIDE APPROACH

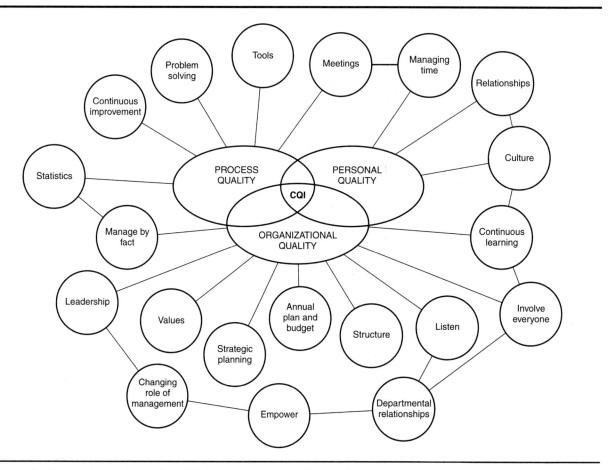

Reprinted with permission from Robert Myers, P.E., Asbury Services, Inc., Gaithersburg, MD.

functional areas or departments, which tends to create hierarchies within hierarchies. Whatever their structure, their operations should center on the functions that must be performed to provide the care and the roles of all individuals in achieving those functions.

There is evidence that an effective team approach can benefit organizations at several levels (Sherer, 1995): improving work processes, streamlining tasks, and improving overall organizational performance (Table 9–5, p. 290). The name (total quality management, continuous quality improvement, and the like) chosen for this approach is not as important as the key principles that must be followed to achieve the dual objectives of effectiveness and efficiency.

The Crucial Role of Organizational Leadership.

Organizational leadership (administrator, medical director, director of nursing, department heads, and so on) has several crucial roles in the success of the team approach and of the teams themselves. The leadership of an effective system must serve as coordinators, coaches, and referees. They must help elicit consistent performance from individuals and reinforce appropriate attitudes, and must help all players to recognize their common interests and identify and address their common obstacles. They must also embrace certain principles as a foundation for effective systems support in any health care setting, including subacute care (Table 9–6, pp. 291–294).

Leadership must help teams through their early stages when they are forming and then trying to overcome power struggles, old attitudes, unrealistic goals, diverse expectations, and concerns about excessive work. Once past these early stages, they establish new norms for team performance and turn more toward the tasks rather than toward dealing with each other. Ultimately, they transform themselves and thereby produce desired results for the organization.

But, unless the teams can advance past the critical early stages, they are unlikely to produce constructive change. Allowing dysfunctional teams to remain in place is harmful to staff, wasteful, and can adversely affect patient care. The enterprise bogs down in the focus on people trying to deal with each other rather than working jointly toward a common goal. This often happens when the leadership exhibits similarly dysfunctional qualities, which influence the performance of team members (Lumsdon, 1995).

These issues reinforce the important role of ownership and governance, especially in selecting the right kind of top executives and management and in setting the proper examples. The problems of executive teams may be more widespread than recognized. Certain personalities that tend to gravitate toward authority positions are ill suited for their roles and often have difficulty dealing with other people's anxiety, conflict, uncertainty, or confusion (Kagan, 1990). Many individuals reach executive status based more on their strong individualism than on their ability to work in teams. Some executives confuse the team building approach with undesirable "touchy-feely" exercises. They prefer to involve themselves in tasks and projects rather than improving performance (Sherer, 1995).

Whether trying to improve things or to correct urgent problems, boards and executives may compound the problems by bypassing their root causes. Many mistakenly bring in consultants who may present relevant generalities, but who do not uncover the specific reasons for performance problems in that particular organization. Sometimes, this happens because the very individuals who hire the consultants control the information that they are permitted to access or the conclusions they are allowed to reach.

Quality and Performance Improvement Methods

Every subacute program should familiarize itself with the various tools that are commonly used to analyze and improve performance in business and industry generally (Laffel & Blumenthal, 1989). These tools help discover opportunities for improvement, which the program leadership and care providers must then translate into changes in performance and practice.

These tools may be categorized as those used to collect and analyze data, to generate ideas, to determine the root cause of a problem, or to understand a process. Statistical tools—including line graphs/run charts, histograms, Pareto charts, scatter diagrams, control charts, check sheets, and decision matrices—are used to collect data, measure performance, display data, and investigate trends in outcomes and performance. Nonstatistical tools—such as brainstorming, flowcharts, and cause-and-effect diagrams—are used to focus on qualitative data, to describe and understand existing processes, and to decide on actions to be taken to improve performance (JCAHO, 1995a; Leebov & Ersoz, 1991).

COMMUNICATIONS SYSTEMS

It is generally accepted that effective communication is essential in any health care setting. Yet there is considerable variation in defining effective communication and determining when it has been achieved. Effective communications activities and systems have certain components.

Definition and Components

Information is a key component of effective subacute care decision making. Communication and information systems are related but not identical. Communication may be defined as the processes by which individuals try to provide, interpret, and act upon information in a meaningful way. Information systems are tools to assist communications and decision making. Thus, although communications can be helped by effective information systems, information systems alone cannot ensure effective communications. For example, installing a new phone system or purchasing a computer network and software are not equivalent to creating an information system, nor do they ensure better communications.

The three vital stages of communications are acknowledgement, understanding, and agreement. As senders, people are often satisfied that they have communicated successfully when they have delivered information in a format that they feel others should understand (for instance, they give a lecture or instruct an employee). They may assume that the recipients should be able to recognize and interpret their intended message correctly.

However, different people may have very different interpretations of the tone, intentions, and content of the same words. Recipients may not be able to understand a communication, may be capable of understanding but not understand it, may understand but not follow its intended message, or may understand and want to follow it but not be able to do so.

Communications that are offered for information only, which do not require action on another person's part (for example, the weather forecast), may be considered successful when they are sent. But health-care related communications usually are intended to trigger some action by a recipient (send supplies, take medications, perform a procedure differently, or the like).

Thus, a communication that is offered to try to influence performance may not be considered successful until one or more people have performed the desired actions. However, effective communication can occur and yet not have the desired effect on performance. Therefore, other systems must exist to help translate information into performance.

EXAMPLE

A nursing in-service presents appropriate information about how to deal with patient and family complaints and concerns. But some of the staff there do not agree with the information, some have difficulty correctly defining actual problems, and one nursing supervisor tells them to handle problems her way regardless of any proposed guidelines. Each of these factors will influence performance, despite the presentation of adequate, correct information.

Acknowledgement occurs when someone signals his or her effort to communicate, and the target acknowledges that an attempt is being made to convey information, permits the communication to occur, and pays attention (tunes in) to its content.

EXAMPLE

The administrator of a subacute program repeatedly sought information primarily to reaffirm his predetermined conclusions. For instance, in his preoccupation to fill beds, he would listen to any information about why a patient was appropriate, but routinely rejected concerns that the program was admitting patients it was not prepared to care for. When problems arose later, he claimed that no one had warned him.

This individual was a major obstacle to effective communications because he only selectively acknowledged attempts to communicate important information. Significant problems affecting patient care persisted because they could not even be presented effectively—much less debated—by the staff giving and overseeing the care.

Understanding occurs when the recipient comprehends the intentions and content of the attempted communication, regardless of agreement with the sender on either.

EXAMPLE

Upon admission to a busy subacute program, a physician and nurse discussed medical conditions, treatments, current condition, and discharge plans with a patient and family. The patient and family appeared to be listening, but later seemed vague about the care processes and why the condition was not improving as quickly as they expected. They took up a lot of staff time asking the same questions repeatedly.

In this case, information was provided and acknowledged, but there was little effort made to evaluate understanding. The patient and family may not have understood all that was said, or may have understood the words but not their implications, or may have understood but not agreed with the conclusions presented.

Agreement may occur when the sender and recipient both accept some or all of the conclusions, recommendations, or intentions of all or some part of the communication as correct.

EXAMPLE

A managed care payer contracted with a subacute program for the care of a patient for a 10-day period. A complication occurred on the seventh day. The physician felt that the patient needed to remain longer than 10 days, and provided the insurer with the supporting information. The insurer agreed that there had been a complication, but did not consider it serious enough to pay for an extended stay.

In this case, there may have been effective communication, but there was disagreement about its implications, resulting in two substantially different conclusions about subsequent action.

Enhancing Successful Communications

Both senders and recipients of information face some important tasks to achieve successful communications and desired performance. The scope and complexity of these tasks vary depending on who is involved, their knowledge and experience, and the ultimate purpose of the communication.

Table 9–7, pp. 295–296, lists the prerequisites for successful communication in a subacute care program, some examples of why it might fail wholly or partially, and some possible strategies for improving it. A few basic categories of causes may be identified as the source of most communications-related problems. Therefore, successful communication may be enhanced by addressing the issues that often inhibit it. It is surprising how often this simple principle is overlooked for various reasons, such as the rush of "more important things." But a prudent subacute program recognizes the extraordinary value of optimal communications as a problem-solving and risk-management tool. Such a program will periodically assess the strengths and weaknesses of all aspects of its communications processes.

Communications Tools.   Practitioners must be attentive to effective communications, but are also concerned about efficient communications (those that take the least possible time). When a communication effort is too complicated or time consuming, important information may not be conveyed. The recurrence of this problem can easily pose significant care quality and risk-management implications. Therefore, every subacute program should scrutinize the processes and tools that enable or inhibit efficient practitioner communications efforts.

For example, nurses spend much of their time handling telephone calls. Yet many calls are not urgent, and the intended target of the call is often not readily available. Therefore, a subacute program needs mechanisms to improve the efficiency of managing such calls. Nonurgent phone calls should be sent to voice mail or triaged by a unit secretary or clerk, and those needing prompt response forwarded or otherwise handled in a timely fashion. Computer networks should have electronic mail (E-mail), and faxes should be used to provide more complete information to physicians at their offices or to receive information from potential referral sources and labs.

Physicians also often react to receiving numerous phone calls, especially if they feel that those calls are not triaged properly or do not contain adequate information. This situation can be improved by more effective assessment, consistent and timely provision of appropriate information, using faxes to convey more detailed information (such as test results), using standing protocols to handle nonurgent patient problems (Table 7–12, pp. 200–201), and having all essential information available when calling a physician. In the off-hours (evenings and weekends), there should be a mechanism for efficiently handling phone calls (for example, a physician trying to return a nursing supervisor's call) and messages.

Some programs use a physician communications book or other alternative for non-emergency conditions, so that nursing staff can record important but not urgent information for subsequent review. Some also use a communications book to enable patients and families to record observations, comments, and questions that can be screened by the nursing team leader or social worker, and directed to appropriate individuals such as a physician.

INFORMATION SYSTEMS

All players in health care systems are information managers. The direct care providers collect, interpret, and document information about individual patients. The support staff and management provide information to the care providers and receive information from them, as well as other internal and external sources.

Effective information management is essential for consistently high-quality, cost-effective patient care—especially in an integrated delivery system where the emphasis is shifting from independently functioning service sites (such as hospital, nursing facility, or clinic) to coordinating services for a person with changing needs, delivered by different individuals at different sites over many months or years. Reliable, objective information can also help determine optimal treatments, effective practices and practitioners, and cost-effective programs. Inaccurate, incomplete, unavailable, or unusable clinical information handicaps decision making. Both the problems of past and current information and records management systems, and the potential for improvement, are widely recognized (Dick & Steen, 1991).

An information system is a coordinated approach to the systematic collection, storage, retrieval, transfer, analysis, and use of information concerning individuals, their personal and health-related conditions, and the associated needs and problems. An effective clinical information system must collect, organize, and distribute information coming from many different sources, such as the progress notes of various disciplines, test results, and other programs, facilities, and practitioners. Table 9–8, p. 297, indicates some potential benefits of a useful information system.

The Processes of Care.   The primary objective of a clinical information system should be to support each of the processes of care (assessment, monitoring, and so on) as fully as possible (Table 9–9, pp. 297–298). Two major components are the patient-related database and the knowledge base (the collection of facts about health and illness, and support for diagnostic processes and treatment choices). Just giving information to individuals (whether by written references, in-services, or continuing education) does not ensure either understanding or successful performance. Therefore, information systems should be linked to education, training, and other systems that facilitate its use. Effective performance—not just gaining knowledge or skill—is the desired endpoint.

The Subacute Patient Database

Table 9–10, pp. 298–299, lists the various categories and components of information in the subacute patient database. The information needs of subacute care are both complicated and simple. They are complicated because the complex care of these patients involves many different individuals, facts, and interpretations. However, because the same core issues, conditions, and problems tend to recur frequently, a relatively compact database can support most of the care delivery and decision making. A portion of the same database also supports important business functions such as billing and justifying reimbursement, and other clinical functions including monitoring responses to treatment, facilitating transfer and continuous care provision, and enabling care quality review.

The Subacute Medical Record.   The medical record (MR) is the organized collection of patient-related data based on, and used primarily for, providing and documenting the actual care. It has traditionally been—but does not need to be—paper-based and arranged in some kind of folder or binder. The medical record may not contain all of the patient database (for instance, preadmission information or financial eligibility data may be stored elsewhere). Its arrangement is less important than whether the documentation system enables the most efficient collection, storage, access, retrieval, and use of essential information. Table 9–11, p. 299, summarizes its several different uses, which are all directly or indirectly related to the care.

Ultimately, the medical record should be relevant throughout the various components of a health care system, protect privacy, be updated conveniently, and provide easily accessible, accurate, and complete information for care-related decision making. The composite information from the care of many different individuals should enable detailed understanding of the patients and analysis of the care processes and outcomes. Computerization can help streamline and enhance documentation systems and processes.

Components of the Patient Record.   The acute care record focuses on information related to managing a specific condition that necessitated the admission. The care involves a relatively few disciplines functioning within a brief time frame (a few days to several weeks). The long-term-care record emphasizes detailed assessment and management of functional status and multiple coexisting problems by many different disciplines over an extended period (months to years). As a hybrid of acute and long-term care, subacute care requires multi-disciplinary management of both acute conditions and the assessment and management of functional status and coexisting chronic problems, within an intermediate time frame (several weeks to several months).

Therefore, the subacute medical record must include information related to the important processes of care (assessment, problem identification, problem management, care objectives, patient response to care, and so on) pertinent to all these dimensions (Table 9–12, p. 300). Examples of relevant documentation might include confirmation that medications and treatments were given, descriptions of any complications or adverse reactions, evidence of the nursing care provided, and descriptions of the current status and condition changes.

Medical Records Policies and Services.   The medical records must be appropriately organized, stored, completed, and accessible. Each patient should have a personal medical record, which is maintained in accordance with accepted professional standards and applicable law, and which reflects the patient's total condition from admission to discharge.

Each physician visit should be documented with a progress note, and each nurse–physician interaction (for example, phone discussions) not resulting in a patient visit should be recorded. For subacute care, a physician should reevaluate and document a patient's progress at least weekly. Less frequent visits should be justified by the condition, and more frequent ones should be justified by the instability or complexity of the condition and/or the care. Subacute program medical directors must hold physicians accountable for their compliance with these policies. Other disciplines should document their routine and episodic evaluations, conclusions, and opinions.

Someone with adequate training in medical records management, who knows the pertinent standards and regulations, should coordinate this function. This individual is likely to be either a part-time employee or independent contractor for the subacute program, or someone who performs similar duties for other programs in the facility. In an automated future, this person should also help evaluate the formats and uses of computer databases and policies for record security and patient privacy, and the means for accurate, timely transmission of information.

Computers and Subacute Care Information Systems

Effective computerization can help achieve these desired goals of subacute care information systems, and thereby help achieve the care objectives. In the future, it is likely to be indispensable to providing cost-effective care, making the best possible use of valuable practitioner and staff time, and reducing the incidence of avoidable risks, including iatrogenic and nosocomial illness and other potentially preventable complications of the care or the setting.

Some forms of automation may help speed the collection and entry of patient-related data. But even more important is computerization's capability to allow many individuals to randomly and independently collect information for subsequent search, retrieval, rearrangement, analysis, and use for many diverse purposes. This can substantially reduce the time spent on internal and external planning, reimbursement, quality oversight, and regulatory compliance. Computerization also allows more ready access to a relevant knowledge base (for instance, medical references) and rules for decision making (for example, medical diagnostic support).

Computer Systems Acquisition and Implementation. Small personal-computer-based networks are now both reliable and cost-effective enough to be used in any subacute program. It is harder to find, choose, and use appropriate software. Planning and implementing an effective information system requires that all key participants understand the nature and processes of the care, the desired database, the potential outcomes of care, the possible influences on those outcomes, and the means to measure these things (see Chapter 10). Therefore, both clinical and business leadership must understand what they and their practitioners and staff need from the system (queries, reports, and the like) to ensure its proper design. Computer experts cannot design or adapt effective software without substantial input from the ultimate users. Although most individuals do not need computer expertise, everyone involved in documenting the care or in using a computer-based record should think in terms of their roles as information managers.

Flexible software should support the output needs of many disciplines and individuals, rather than of a few primary users. For several reasons, it is imprudent to choose software for the business or management aspects of the facility or program, and then try to graft clinical software onto it. The provision of care principally drives revenues and reimbursement, not vice-versa. The database needed for accounting purposes is only a small part of that needed to provide the care. Finally, the care providers and business staff need significantly different query and reporting capabilities out of the same database.

Support for Coordination and Integration of the Program and the Players.   An effective computer system can help coordinate the interactions and communications of participants at all programmatic levels (Integrated information management, 1994; Stead, 1991). It should also permit multiple forms of data integration and representation; for example, incorporating data analyses into reports or plotting vital signs or functional status graphically across time. Some valuable existing software may be seen as the prototype of such an approach. For example, some hospitals now allow physicians to view test results and place orders via modem from their home or offices (Hospitals attack a crippler, 1994). Other software—exemplified by Lotus Notes—permits effective integration of text, data, and graphics for a variety of clinical and business functions, across a network and even among various sites and practitioners. The use of digital phone transmission of data is now technically feasible and is increasing. Subacute programs should begin to investigate the possibilities for using such methods as direct data transmission of X-rays and EKGs to physicians' offices or other remote online consultation sites.

Support for Documentation Requirements.   Subacute programs should be able to use computers to document basic patient assessments (Margolis, 1993). Table 9–13, p. 301, describes desirable capabilities of such software. Effective software must be flexible enough to support the management and documentation of both acute medical conditions and coexisting or chronic conditions and problems. It must also allow users to expand or omit detail for different patients as needed. For instance, care of a patient receiving intensive rehabilitation will require a detailed database of their functional capabilities, which can be updated periodically. In contrast, the care of a comatose patient requires a less detailed collection of functional information, which is not likely to need much updating during the patient's stay.

Many subacute programs are located in facilities that already provide long-term care. Carefully selected software packages may be usable for both levels of care. Such software must be flexible enough to allow customization of key components such as care plan libraries and problem lists. It must also allow for both medical diagnoses and nursing problems as the basis for care planning, and must enable both periodic documentation of predictable, longer-term problems and frequent documentation of acute onset problems such as new infection or altered cardiovascular status. Because of the acute episodic and results-oriented nature of the acute care database, most acute care software is not likely to be as applicable to other care levels.

In the near future, as computerized records evolve, other components of an efficient, automated documentation system should become more prevalent. These include scanners, fax modems, large-capacity optical or magnetic storage drives, optical character recognition, and electronic document transfer and manipulation software.

Support for Clinical Decision Making.   Computer-based diagnostic support software can be indispensable in the care of subacute and similar patients, with their multiple coexisting conditions, often vague or nonspecific signs and symptoms, and unusual manifestations of common problems. Two prime examples of this software are Iliad and Quick Medical Reference (Barron, 1992; Bergeron, 1991; Buckner, 1991). Each of these programs allows physicians and others to enter combinations of signs, symptoms, and test results, and then guides them through differential diagnoses, suggests additional tests to order based on costs and patient risk, and enables them to look up characteristics of hundreds of diseases and conditions. Every subacute program should provide its practitioners with access to some such software (Bankowitz, 1991).

Additionally, an effective patient database provides a wealth of accumulated information that practitioners can use to evaluate and improve the care. There is strong evidence that physicians and other health care providers will obtain and use such clinical information if they are provided with appropriate tools (Safran et al, 1989).

Support for Searching Information Relevant to Patient Care. Computerized versions of many substantial medical and related references are now available. Two examples of useful general references relevant to the care of subacute patients are MAXX from Little, Brown and Scientific American Medicine (SAM). Such comprehensive electronic medical references allow users rapid access (generally within seconds) to multiple references to a given topic occurring through a variety of chapters or texts.

For example, if a patient came in with a rare disease or had the possible onset of a complication or a new illness, nurses and physicians could use MAXX (a CD-ROM based compilation of over 12,000 pages of text on several dozen medical areas such as gastroenterology and emergency medicine) to look up discussions of the pathophysiology, signs and symptoms, clinical course, complications, manifestations, workup, associated conditions, treatment, and prognosis of that condition. Several versions of software to access the National Library of Medicine's "MedLine" are also available (Horowitz & Bleich, 1981). These permit quick search over phone lines of comprehensive bibliographies of several decades' worth of articles on health and medical topics. A combination of CD-ROM-based references and on-line reference searching capabilities should enable efficient access to most vital information needed by most of those providing the care, at very little cost.

Support for Staff Education and Training. Besides the more sophisticated references such as those mentioned above, an increasing number of health-care-related journals and less sophisticated general health care references are available. All levels of staff should be able to access these databases so that they can improve their knowledge and skills in the process of caring for patients.

Additionally, business and industry are increasingly making use of computer- and CD-ROM-based software for real-time access to policies and instructions for performing procedures. Hardware is now available (for example, CD-ROM and optical disk recorders) for businesses to consolidate and index large internal databases. Interactive multimedia (computers, video, and audio) is also being used effectively in a number of educational and business settings to allow for more self-instruction, even as a service is actually being provided. Although effectively adapting these technologies takes some time and sophistication, they are likely to become commonplace within several years because of their potential enhancement of performance of a diverse work force and their efficient support for real-time instruction and performance oversight.

Support for Patient and Family Education. A substantial amount of computer-based health-related information for laymen is now available (Baig, 1993). For instance, inexpensive (under $100) CD-ROMs now contain entire health encyclopedias and drug reference manuals for laymen. In combination with the considerable amounts of written, audiovisual, and multimedia materials available for laymen, these could easily be used on a subacute unit to allow patients and families to teach themselves about various conditions, treatments, medications, and other relevant topics (Kahn, 1993; Sechrest, 1991). Such approaches can conserve valuable staff time, and help free up individual care providers to give some direct instruction and follow up additional patient and family questions.

Support for Program Quality Assessments.   Because quality assessments are ultimately based on the provision of care, a properly designed patient database and reporting system can be used for quality of care review purposes. For example, if medical orders for drugs and treatments include a data field for the reason or problem for which the medication or treatment is ordered, it is then possible to evaluate the composite information to see which patients with which problems receive various treatments, and then to assess the program's patient characteristics, treatments, and procedures, and to try to relate the medications and treatments to various outcomes, complications, or side effects. Compared to performing such functions manually, the time spent generating a report from existing computer-based data is small, especially when a single reporting format can be used repeatedly over time. This is an ideal example of the benefits of automation.

Support for Risk Management.   Although effective data analysis helps achieve useful quality improvement and risk management, it is cumbersome and time consuming if done by hand. Computer systems should help identify and flag high-risk situations, and help the analysis of incidents and accidents. Especially important is the capability to readily sort and group the results by various factors such as unit, time of day, patient, diagnosis, or principal physician. Some patient care and documentation software includes or can link to such capabilities, or it is possible to customize generic spreadsheet or database software. Again, doing this successfully requires first identifying desired output (reports, quality improvement objectives, etc.) so that the database and relevant reports can be set up properly.

Support for Effective Program Management.   Computers can also help in program management and reimbursement activities. A managed care environment demands intimate understanding of the costs of the care and the business. Cost accounting functions must be based upon understanding the care, as well as labor, supplies, and capital costs. Analyzing the actual services requires knowledge of the quantity, frequency, and cost of individual services actually delivered. Cost accounting makes much more sense when these are clarified first. A common mistake is to try to establish a cost accounting system without first having an intimate knowledge and analysis of the care and the services.

RISK MANAGEMENT AND SAFETY SYSTEMS

Many managers and practitioners conceive of risk management (RM) primarily as focusing on safety, liability control, and malpractice or other lawsuit claims loss. But a risk may be defined as any event or process that could ultimately cause a person, program, or organization to suffer economic losses or damage its reputation. Legal risks will arise primarily from patients, staff, or third parties (for example, insurers or government agencies).

Risks may be related to any of the patient care processes or to other aspects of operations that directly or indirectly affect the care or those giving or supporting it. In any program or facility, thousands of actions or encounters could potentially represent or lead to significant risk (Table 9–14, p. 302). Examples could include statements made by marketing staff during a family visit for possible admission, things that occur during the stay, or things not told to a patient or family at the time of discharge.

Although no program can manage all possible risks or prevent all potential problems, most major problems result from a relatively few predictable, preventable occurrences. An effective facility and programmatic risk-management program seeks and manages causes of risk, not just symptoms. Much of this book is about establishing systems with built-in risk-management features; that is, they are set up so that anticipating and preventing risk are part of routine care and support processes. When done this way, a risk-management program can be much more effective and efficient. Examples of tactics discussed in this book that represent built-in risk-management approaches to everyday operations include the following.

- Understand the nature, processes, and possible pitfalls of subacute care.
- Be aware of the capabilities and limitations of care providers involved in the program.
- Have an effective system of problem identification, resolution, and prevention.
- Use an effective information system to support those making decisions about the care.
- Provide regular, pertinent feedback to all parties involved in the care or the program.

A subacute care RM program should be part of the facility-wide RM program, involving all management, personnel, and departments in the facility. All of them represent potential sources of increased risk and potential contributors to reducing risk. The program should identify known and potential environmental problems in the physical building, the equipment used, and the activities performed. Additionally, it should address certain aspects of the direct care (Table 9–15, p. 303) that may present additional or special risk possibilities.

Table 9–16, p. 304, includes examples of some of the many things that subacute programs can do to anticipate and try to prevent these various risks. Table 9–17, p. 305, lists some tactics to try to minimize risks associated with treating managed care patients. In addition, a safety program should be used as the basis for managing the environment of care, including security, emergency preparedness, and hazardous materials and waste management. This safety program should include an orientation program covering fire plans, incident and/or hazard reporting systems, smoking policies, and general safety policies; safety-related information through continuing education programs; a system for reporting accidents, injuries, and safety hazards; and an organization-wide safety committee (JCAHO, 1995a, pp. 37–44).

EMERGENCY RESPONSE SYSTEMS

Every program needs a systematic approach to handling emergencies. Emergency preparedness also refers to knowing what to do if something happens to partially or completely disrupt the way an organization normally provides care. Disasters might include floods, hurricanes, fires, hazardous material incidents, or electrical power outages (JCAHO, 1995a, pp. 59–64).

Subacute programs should be able to identify clinical emergencies in a timely fashion, make a preliminary assessment of the nature and possible causes of the emergency, and institute basic CPR or other measures to at least try to stabilize a patient. Table 9–18, p. 306, lists some essential functions and support processes for clinical emergency management.

The emergency response system should include appropriate communications, policies and procedures, staff training, and equipment and supplies. Each program must determine and indicate the extent of its ability to manage emergencies on site. For instance, can it do basic or advanced CPR, and can it handle intubation and the administration of cardiotonic medications? There must be clear policies and procedures regarding management of emergency situations, including outside sites and referral sources (for example, local ambulance companies, transfer hospitals, and consultants).

The program should have arrangements with the community's Emergency Medical Services (EMS) and a local hospital for rapid transfers of emergency cases. A consistent process is also needed to ensure that advance directives and other patient wishes are communicated effectively and that EMS crews are aware of limits on resuscitation.

PHYSICAL PLANT, EQUIPMENT, UTILITIES MANAGEMENT, AND CENTRAL SUPPLY SYSTEMS

Plant management systems are essential to ensure that the physical plant is adequately maintained and that a system of preventive maintenance exists. Important clinically relevant physical plant issues include the ventilation, air conditioning, electrical system, and oxygen supply. Equipment management involves both the equipment itself and the staff who use, test, and monitor it. Examples of relevant equipment include scales, suctioning machines, special beds, and other electrical equipment used in patient care. The system must also ensure compliance with laws and regulations (for instance, the 1990 Safe Medical Devices Act) on reporting equipment and devices that may have harmed patients (JCAHO, 1995a, pp. 83–104).

Equipment management should be a joint effort between clinical and maintenance staff. The organization or facility should establish a vigorous preventive maintenance program. Given the scope of their direct care workload, clinical staff should collaborate with maintenance staff, but should not be primarily responsible for coordinating equipment maintenance or repairs. They should anticipate timely response to their identification of a physical plant or equipment issue, and should also be able to count on the support of an administrator or program manager in these matters.

Supplies should be maintained routinely, and also be accessible for special situations (for example, for a patient who arrives with problems and needs beyond those reported by the referring program or ascertained when the patient was accepted). Care providers should have to spend as little time as possible trying to obtain or replenish supplies. Designated nonclinical personnel should be responsible for delivering, ordering, and stocking supplies to save nursing staff time. In addition, adequate, properly maintained supplies should be available for procedures done by physicians, technicians, and others.

Optimally, with a computerized inventory system linked to the care system, the change in available stock could be reflected in Central Supply as supplies were used. When the inventory fell below a predetermined level, it would trigger reordering. This approach would also provide useful data for cost analysis, budgeting, and managed care contract pricing.

PROBLEM-SOLVING SYSTEMS

This book has emphasized the importance of the problem-oriented approach to subacute care. Only some causes of those problems can be found, only some causes respond to treatment, and some of those treatments may themselves cause problems. Additionally, problem resolution often depends on how issues are defined and on the established objectives.

In any complex situation such as subacute or long-term care—where a very diverse group of individuals tries to evaluate and resolve the problems of an equally diverse group of patients—successful results require the successful definition, identification, and solution of problems. Problem solving involves a series of identifiable steps: identify the symptoms or concerns, define the issues, collect data, determine causes, review and select options for addressing the issues, implement the selected approaches, follow up to see to what extent the issues are resolved, and modify the approaches as needed to improve the end result.

Problem-solving systems are approaches to recognizing, defining, preventing, and solving problems. All problems may be viewed as an actual or potential disruption of homeostasis; that is, they either disturb, or have the potential to disturb, an existing personal or systems balance. The perception that such situations are causing or threatening to cause such a disturbance is a source of individual anxiety representing a call to action. However, the response of various individuals to that call may take any of several markedly different forms, such as denial or avoidance, the rush to suppress the problem as quickly as possible, or the inclination to seek causes before taking definitive measures. How individuals respond to identifying and trying to solve problems typically reflects their customary approaches to dealing with things that make them anxious or afraid.

As discussed in Chapter 7, neither treating symptoms nor causes is necessarily the same as solving problems. Instead, the treatment or proposed solutions must be directed toward an objective so that something happens to improve or restore an individual or collective balance. An effective problem-solving system recognizes the need for a set of objective rules that compensate for inevitable differences in personal interpretation and response to the same situation. Otherwise, the approach to solving and preventing problems depends on personalities and whims, which is typically both ineffective and inefficient.

Reconciling different approaches to identifying and solving problems may be more of a problem than the challenge posed by correcting the problem itself. Failures of effective problem solving may not be due to a lack of possible solutions as much as to an unwillingness to admit a problem might exist, the failure to identify the specific cause, the failure to consider all feasible solutions, and the failure to tailor the solution to the specific problem and its causes.

This book has also stressed the problem-oriented approach to dealing with facility-wide, programmatic, and interpersonal issues. All of the steps mentioned apply equally to patient care and to the systems and process issues involved in giving and supporting care. Although the problems may differ, the underlying principles of effective problem management are identical. As with risk management, constructive problem solving should simply be built into everyday activities and should use the same tools and methods described earlier for quality improvement.

The Leadership Role.   The clinical and organizational leadership again play an essential role. Effective leadership must be able to recognize problems in their early stages so that they may lead others to make changes before problems become crises. Those who can do this well are invaluable participants; those who cannot do it well may put programs and organizations at higher risk of failure. This anticipatory intervention is also made harder by frequent pressures to reduce expenditures, and by control of budgets by individuals or departments who may not understand what is indispensable to effective care or recognize the value of preventive measures.

The processes of defining, identifying, analyzing, and anticipating problems and initiating subsequent actions must be personality-independent and cannot be allowed to become entangled in individual perspectives and ambitions. The problem-solving approaches of those who are being considered for management and supervisory positions should be assessed carefully. Those who are unable or unwilling to use a systematic, objective approach should receive appropriate training, guidance, and corrective feedback. They may not be good candidates for important management or supervisory positions because their limitations can have a broadly negative influence.

For example, effective problem solving cannot thrive when some possible solutions are excluded ahead of time, some individuals exempt themselves from consideration as needing change or improvement, or where people feel intimidated about giving feedback about situations or individuals that hinder their own performance. But many individuals have some difficulty in admitting that they may have caused or contributed to a problem. In positions of authority, these individuals may try to manipulate the process, the information, or the conclusions to serve their own purposes. The repeated occurrence of this undermines any quality improvement process. It establishes two incompatible sets of rules—one for those who evade responsibility and the other for everyone else.

EXAMPLE
A nursing director was hired at a facility with a subacute program. She had no experience in that aspect of care, and had a long history of undistinguished performance and poor interpersonal skills. She also used the political approach to problem solving; that is, those who she liked would be excluded from consideration as possible contributors to problems, and those who she did not like would be maneuvered into being blamed, even if they were actually the victims. She rarely tried to solve conflicts and problems within the nursing staff or between nursing and other departments, instead constantly trying to blame them on others, including the physicians. Despite her often disruptive be-

havior, she consistently refused to acknowledge any responsibility in causing problems for other staff. She even destroyed documentation that implicated her or her allies. However, the program administrator liked her because she was willing to help him make trouble for people who he disliked. The two of them joined forces to drive those who tried to address these flagrant problems out of the organization. The result was a cynical attitude among many of the staff, and a long series of uncorrected performance problems.

Physicians may also be a source of such root cause exclusion. For instance, some physicians have learned to evade accountability by invoking their authority as a physician, or by characterizing every attempt to influence their practices as interfering with the practice of medicine. But this, too, is an example of high-risk behavior. The solution to a medical problem may often be much less difficult than trying to get the physician to even admit that the treatment might be a cause. For example, it is easy to discontinue a medication that is determined to be causing, or possibly causing, a complication. But some physicians are reluctant to acknowledge that the medication may be a possible culprit because they equate the possibility with some attack on their abilities.

In summary, effective problem solving is a vital clinical and management tool and an integral component of any quality improvement program. Most care-related and systems problems can be identified, anticipated, and prevented or resolved effectively, even when there are no ideal solutions. The leadership of the program and organization must establish and reinforce appropriate rules and set an appropriate example.

POLICIES AND PROCEDURES SYSTEMS

Systematic Approach to Policies and Procedures

Organizations have goals and objectives. Goals are the general approaches that support meeting their broad objectives. For example, a facility might agree on an objective of establishing a subacute program. Its goals would be to provide a level of high-quality service, to be financially viable, and to offer those services that meet patient needs.

Achieving desirable objectives requires a collection of effective individual efforts to apply knowledge and skills at the right time in the right way to achieve desired objectives. Both subacute care provision and the business operations include many processes. Most processes (giving medications, assessing condition changes, communicating among care providers, and so on) are recurrent. Processes involve several individuals (nurses, nursing assistants, physicians, dietitians, and the like), and most individuals are involved in many different processes. To provide effective patient care, these individuals must combine their skills and perspectives to perform many functions and tasks consistently and effectively.

Policies are more specific statements of the means to obtain goals. Processes are systematic collections of activities that help achieve these goals. For example, a facility policy would be to admit those individuals who need a level of service provided in a subacute program, and whose needs can be met by the program. A related policy would be for each prospective admission to receive a preadmission assessment to determine if they need the service and if the program can meet their needs safely and effectively. The assessment process involves physicians, nurses, and others with designated roles.

Subacute programs need procedures to cover all care processes such as assessment, care planning, and medication administration and monitoring. These procedures consist of specific functions and tasks such as performing an examination, preparing a piece of equipment, checking blood pressure, or documenting a finding. Determining the functions and tasks needed to make these processes effective helps define appropriate participant roles. A procedure prioritizes responsibilities such as various roles in the assessment process, where and how the information should be recorded and used, who should use which information to help define an individual's problems, and so on. For example, an admission procedure would include the steps (contact referral source, ask certain questions, record the answers, and so on) and disciplines involved in obtaining referrals and evaluating whether the patient needed the care and the program could care for the patient.

Policies and procedures also relate to staff selection and performance evaluations. Individual job descriptions represent the collection of functions and tasks needed to accomplish the various processes involving each individual. A properly designed job description can thus serve as the basis for individual performance evaluations (comparing actual to expected performance), including the individual's skill in performing those functions and tasks and his or her contribution to accomplishing the organization's goals and objectives.

Policies and procedures are also a basis for quality improvement and risk-management programs. Because individual performance is influenced by the systems in which people function, quality improvement programs should analyze specific processes as well as outcomes, including individuals' roles in those processes. Successful RM programs analyze and adjust systems and processes to try to reduce the frequency and severity of undesirable occurrences.

Policies and procedures thus serve several important purposes for subacute programs. They provide the ground rules for the effective interaction of people of diverse backgrounds, knowledge, skills, and motivations. They coordinate responsibilities for managing care processes, addressing problematic and high-risk areas of care, and preventing and solving problems (risk management). They help support performance assessment, identify potential obstacles to performance, and promote process improvement efforts.

Effective policies and procedures must promote rather than inhibit desired performance. They reflect, or should change successfully, the realities of the system for which they are created, and should be linked to efforts to enable effective performance. They may change systems by changing or influencing the responsibilities of individuals, the expectations for their performance, the processes by which they interact, the resources allocated for enabling performance, the consequences for inadequate performance, or the rewards for appropriate performance.

Specific Policies and Protocols.   Many subacute units use specific protocols for managing various conditions and situations; for example, caring for joint replacement patients, weaning patients from a ventilator, or treating wounds. These protocols are often referred to as "critical pathways," which are specific treatment regimens that specify the component processes or activities, time frames, laboratory tests, documentation, discharge planning, and other aspects of the care (Graham et al, 1995). These pathways can help staff recognize patient condition changes by comparing observations to expectations, and may help both patients and providers anticipate and understand the course of treatment.

These pathways should be developed or adapted by a group of key individuals, including the nurse manager, medical director, and key clinical staff. Other individuals may need to be consulted, depending on the item. For example, an orthopedist would be helpful in developing a critical pathway for joint replacement patients, and a wound care nurse for pathways concerning wound management. Figure 9–2 represents an abbreviated critical pathway for a post-joint replacement subacute patient.

Critical pathways work best for individuals with limited active problems or prominent diagnoses uncomplicated by associated medical conditions or frequent acute episodes of illness. However, many individuals have multiple underlying problems and intermittent acute clinical events that may complicate the stay. For them, the critical pathways may need to be modified or to be more problem-oriented, rather than focusing on the specific reason for admission to the unit. For example, Table 7–9, pp. 190–198, represents the tasks involved in managing various problems common in subacute patients, which could be adapted as a critical pathway to manage those conditions.

Critical pathways should be adjusted if review finds that a substantial number of the patients do not follow a predicted clinical course. Or, if the prescribed course is appropriate, then the care may need to be reviewed to ascertain the reasons for frequent deviations.

Other Protocols.   Other policies and protocols for managing various conditions, and for performing procedures and tasks, should address common high-risk or problematic circumstances, or any situation that can benefit from greater consistency or standardization. These can help reduce individual performance variation, take advantage of new knowledge in the field, and help improve the reliability of outcomes measurements.

These patient care policies and protocols should be developed by appropriate disciplines or interdisciplinary teams, in consultation with the medical director and medical and nursing staffs, and approved by the administrator or governing body. Some protocols from other settings can be used unchanged, but many will need some program- or patient-specific modification. For example, parts of the protocols developed by the Agency for Health Care Policy and Research (AHCPR) for various conditions (depression, heart failure, pressure ulcers, and so on) are valid without changes, and others need some modification and supplementation to be most useful in a transitional or long-term care setting.

Examples of topics for relevant subacute care policies and protocols include, but are not limited to, managing complex medical patients; tracheostomy care; hemodialysis; renal diets; discharge planning; family education; management of disruptive patients; infusion therapies (that is, administration of blood products, chemotherapy, IV antibiotics, IV pain management, dobutamine, dopamine, IV push medications, and so on via peripheral IVs, long lines, and PICC lines); insertion and management of infusion catheters (Broviac/Hickman catheters, implantable ports, PICC lines, heparin locks, epidural catheters, subcutaneous

FIGURE 9–2   CRITICAL PATHWAY (ABBREVIATED) FOR A POST-JOINT REPLACEMENT PATIENT

Time	Assessment	Laboratory Tests	Documentation	Expected Outcomes
Day 1	• Pain symptoms • Mobility • Range of motion • Wound site	• Check prothrombin time results if anticoagulated	• Pain symptoms • Wound site condition • Mood and affect	• Progression of activities of daily living toward independence
Days 2 to 3	• Condition of wound incision while changing dressing • Surgical site for evidence of infection	• Check prothrombin time results if anti-coagulation needs adjustment	• Surgical site condition • Mobility • Ability to participate in therapies	• Progress in therapy participation • Wound site healing • Decrease in pain
Day 4	—	— —	—	• Suture removal
Day 14	• Condition of surgical site • Strength and mobility of joint area	—	• Any pain complaints • Condition of surgical site • Patient's level of function	• Discharge to community

infusions, central venous or arterial lines); cardiac monitoring (that is, telemetry, EKG monitoring, Holter monitors); monitoring pacemakers; electrocardiover- sion; organ donation; blood drawing/venipuncture; cardiopulmonary arrest re- sponses; hospice care; acute pain management; rehabilitation care; home visits; transfer and gait training; care of casts and external fixation devices; seizure management; ostomy care; whirlpool/sterile debridement; total hip replacement protocols; total knee replacement protocols; shoulder replacement protocols; manual joint manipulation; dysphagia protocols; provision of respiratory thera- pies; maintenance of ventilators and respiratory equipment; obtaining arterial blood gases; pulse oximetry; handling accidental extubation; postural drainage; nebulizer treatments; use of oxygen; procurement of cylinders; and tra- cheostomy weaning (JCAHO, 1995b).

For example, a common concern in both subacute and long-term settings is physician notification of acute condition changes and abnormal lab results. Some triage is essential because there are so many condition fluctuations and lab abnormalities and because the patients cannot just be sent to the hospital for evaluation. On the other hand, the significant condition changes and abnormal- ities must be addressed appropriately and in a timely fashion. Therefore, every subacute program should have a protocol for this situation. Figures 9–3 to 9–5 give examples of a policy for managing abnormal lab test results, a fax cover memo to convey adequate information, and a letter to physicians explaining their roles in all of this. Table 7–12, pp. 200–201, offers examples of guidelines for triaging such condition changes.

HUMAN RESOURCE SYSTEMS

As a service business, subacute care depends heavily on those providing direct patient service and those supporting them. The skills, attitudes, personal char- acteristics, and knowledge that are essential to effective performance in sub- acute settings have been discussed above and in other chapters. Human resource (HR) systems are essential to adequately attract, train, retain, ensure adequate qualifications, and improve the performance of those at all levels of the program and facility. In addition to other standard personnel functions, two components of HR systems that are particularly relevant to subacute programs are performance evaluation and education and training.

Performance Evaluation and Improvement

Any living being requires feedback to maintain proper balance (homeostasis). For example, the body maintains a constant temperature range by being able to sense both the external temperature and the internal body temperature, and making adjustments accordingly. Similarly, all humans need some feedback to perform properly and to change their behavior. Such feedback compares actual versus expected performance, both from within themselves (internal feedback) and from other people and the environment (external feedback).

All players in a subacute program need some feedback to optimize their participation. Desired performance must be defined in relation to the needs of patients, colleagues, co-workers, and the individual performer. External feed- back is important so that individuals do not just use their own standards and self-assessment to evaluate how their performance impacts outcomes or others'

FIGURE 9–3   POLICY ON INTERDISCIPLINARY APPROACH TO MANAGING TEST RESULTS

Rationale

Many tests are obtained on the facility patients, either during routine screening or as a result of a condition change or new-onset illness. Only some of these results represent clinically significant situations, requiring some significant change in the care plan or treatment orders. There is no requirement to do something about every abnormality, or to render treatment when it is not indicated. When results represent clinically significant situations, there may or may not be an effective treatment. Or, if something can be done, there may be a reason (for example, advance directives) not to do anything. However, the results must be compared to previous ones and correlated with the individual's clinical status, in order to determine whether action is needed and the urgency of that action. It is just as important to explain decisions not to do anything about a potentially clinically significant result as it is to explain reasons for making a particular choice.

Policy

Handling of test results shall be a cooperative effort between the nursing staff and the physicians. All lab test results shall be related to the potential or actual urgency of the individual's clinical situation. All potentially significant abnormal test results, or all results that may relate to an individual's current status or condition change, shall be commented upon by a nurse, physician, or both, to clarify the thinking about any decisions about taking or not taking further action.

Procedure

1. Test results will be reported to the nursing station or facility by the laboratory, radiology service, or other source.
2. The test results will be communicated to the attending physician, with the urgency of doing so depending on the seriousness of the abnormality and the patient's current condition.
3. The nursing staff will refer to available guidelines in making these decisions about urgency of notification. If necessary, a staff nurse will have a nursing unit manager or supervisor review the results and the patient's condition to help decide on the urgency of notification.
4. Test results may be faxed to the physician. They should be accompanied by a cover memo explaining the current situation, which includes clinically relevant information that the physician may need to understand the significance of the results, any specific questions that the physician needs to answer, and the urgency of the response needed.
5. Test results will be called to the physician when they represent clinical situations requiring urgent intervention, where the patient's life and safety may be in immediate jeopardy, or when requested by the physician.
6. The nursing staff will follow appropriate procedures to decide whether to hold off on giving a scheduled medication or treatment while awaiting a response from the physician.
7. When physicians respond to notification, they may decide either to do something about the abnormality (more tests, a treatment, a new or changed order, or the like) or not to do anything at present (further observation, no further observation, no treatment). If they decide that nothing needs to be done, the physician will provide (or the nurse will request) enough information to be able to document the reason why no further action is needed.
8. If a physician or physician extender is on site later to assess an individual with a significant condition change or other problem, this individual should clarify or supplement any existing documentation about the reasons for the medical decisions to do or not to do anything about the abnormality.

Examples of Appropriate Documentation

1. *Digoxin level 0.5*: "Patient is stable, has no dyspnea, rhythm is only rarely irregular. Therefore, current digoxin dose is considered adequate despite low blood level."
2. *BUN 37, creatinine 0.7*: "BUN is increased from before, but patient shows no clinical signs of dehydration, is alert and taking food and fluids OK. Still needs diuretics because of history of congestive heart failure. Will recheck and may consider adjustment if BUN continues to rise."
3. *Hematocrit 32*: "Hematocrit is somewhat lower than usual (34–36). No evidence of GI bleeding. Not on any medications that could be causing blood loss. Has no symptoms that might be related to anemia. Iron levels normal. Problem probably due to chronic illness. Will recheck."

FIGURE 9–4   PATIENT INFORMATION FAX COVER MEMO

Dear Dr. _____ :

　　Information about _____ , one of your patients at the facility, is being faxed to you.

I. **IS A RESPONSE NEEDED, AND WHEN?**

　☐ No response is needed.

　☐ Please contact (☐ any nurse on unit _____   ☐ the unit coordinator   ☐ the house supervisor) at

　　telephone # _____ to discuss this information or the patient's clinical status:

　　　☐ AS SOON AS POSSIBLE
　　　☐ Sometime before the end of the day
　　　☐ At your next regularly scheduled visit or phone call

II. **PLEASE NOTE THE FOLLOWING INFORMATION**

　☐ We are faxing to you laboratory or test results that we have received.

　☐ Please advise about what to do about the following lab or test result:

　☐ Please advise about what to do about the following patient problem(s):

　　　　　　　　　　Thank you for your cooperation.

Dear Physician:

　　As you know, subacute patients often have abnormal lab test results and condition changes that should be reported to a physician. However, not all abnormalities require a physician action. Also, what is to be done about any abnormal result depends on the context. For example, a BUN of 61 is a problem if the last BUN was 32, and an improvement if the last BUN was 73. A dilantin level of 9 is very important if a patient has seizure activity, and not very important if the condition is stable and the last dilantin level was 11.

　　As part of our efforts to streamline and improve physician–nurse communications at this facility, we propose to change the way in which laboratory and test results are communicated to you. A phone call or fax will be accompanied by:

- A description of the clinical context or any symptoms or signs that were the reason for the lab work or test being ordered
- Specific requests as to what (if any) response and action is desired.

　　During the day, the unit nurse coordinator or another nurse on the unit will provide this information. During the evenings and nights, and on weekends, the house supervisor will review the information first, and decide on its urgency and its clinical context. As much information as possible will be kept until the following regular working day, and then transmitted routinely.

　　In return, I request that you do the following:

- Collaborate with the nurse making the call to determine the significance of the information, and whether it requires any action by a physician.
- Accept the information courteously, even if you do not think it needed to be called in at that time.
- Ask for any additional information you need to decide if there is a problem, what the problem is, and what should be done about it.
- Provide me with feedback about how the system is working, so that I can work with the nursing department to give feedback to individual nurses, and thereby improve the triage of these situations.

　　I believe this systematic approach can help improve the care, accommodate your requests for more effective management of information and phone calls, and help the nurses meet their responsibilities to report abnormalities in a timely fashion. Thank you for your cooperation.

Sincerely,

Medical Director

performance. Using the wrong criteria to assess performance can reinforce undesirable behavior. For example, desirable behaviors relevant to problem solving and risk reduction should be supported and undesirable ones should be discouraged. Reinforcing the right behavior often enough is likely to produce more of it, and repeated feedback or various consequences are usually necessary to reduce undesirable behavior.

People need both specific examples and generalities to change their behavior. Feedback must be frequent and specific enough so that the recipient can connect it to certain aspects of performance. For instance, to try to reduce medication-related complications by improving physician ordering practices, it is often more effective to give feedback about a specific order when it is being written than to give general feedback about medication usage weeks or months later. It also is important to explain the rationale for the feedback (why is the medication less desirable?) and to offer an acceptable alternative (what medications or other actions might be more appropriate?).

Performance evaluations are a form of cumulative feedback. They provide an overall picture, but may not be specific or frequent enough to influence behaviors related to defined areas. For example, a performance evaluation may tell someone overall if they have done an acceptable job and may suggest general areas for improvement, but can rarely tell them specifically which tasks could have been performed better, or how it was determined that certain aspects of that performance could stand improvement. Performance evaluations should be based on job descriptions and on standards of practice and performance (including technical skills, attitudes, and interpersonal relationships). Management and staff should know what each other ought to be doing (job descriptions) so that they can hold each other more accountable for actual performance.

In health care settings, individuals have multidimensional relationships. They are accountable to someone else in the organization (for example, supervisor, department chairman); others are accountable to them (for example, attending physicians are accountable to a medical director); and they also should be accountable to others who depend on their performance (nurses serve patients and also perform tasks that influence the performance of physicians, other nurses, and other individuals such as therapists and social workers). Each of these relationships differs based on the varying roles. Therefore, a cross-section of feedback is needed to obtain the different perspectives and avoid overlooking potentially significant problems. Individuals are less likely to respond appropriately to those whose feedback does not influence something they desire (a good evaluation, a promotion, a bonus, and so on). A fair performance evaluation must be multidirectional, including those who hold the individual accountable, those who are accountable to the individual, and those who the individual is supposed to serve most directly.

Thus, for example, a medical director should be evaluated by the administrator, other department heads, the physicians, and the nurse unit managers. Similarly, an administrator or CEO should be evaluated by a board, by the top management, and by the staff and practitioners whom the CEO or administrator should be supporting.

EXAMPLE

The administrator of a facility including a subacute program considered his major priority to be satisfying the board. He convinced the board that balancing the budget and getting good accreditation results would prove that he was doing his job. He balanced the budget by shortchanging his own staff, ridiculed them for any licensure or accreditation deficiencies, demanded that the beds be filled, suppressed efforts to discuss honestly the program's quality problems, carefully controlled all information going to the board, and refused to acknowledge his own behaviors as causing high staff and management turnover and his demands as ultimately harming patients. Because the board had no other realistic perspective from which to judge his actual conduct, they refused to believe the evidence even when major crises and staff departures made the problems plain. The more they praised and rewarded him, the worse and more frequent these behaviors became.

This individual's performance criteria should have been developed with the input of the management staff and others in the facility, and his performance evaluation should have been based on feedback from the facility practitioners, patients, and management staff whose performance he influenced. The board reinforced all the wrong behaviors by rewarding the results without recognizing that most positive results occurred despite, rather than because of, this individual.

Use of Quality Assessment Findings in Performance Evaluations. Relevant findings from quality assessment and improvement activities should be part of the basis for an overall performance assessment. Figure 9–6 is an example of a physician performance evaluation summary instrument that the medical director or another supervising physician could use. The assessments themselves should be based on feedback from a physician's patients and families, and from nurses and physician colleagues who have worked with the physician enough to be familiar with his or her practice and performance. This feedback should be received and provided regularly, and the cumulative results can then be used at the time of privilege renewals. Some similar and some different items could be used for evaluating line staff, support staff, management, and owners and governing bodies (Figure 9–7).

Education and Training Systems

When care outcomes and cost-effectiveness were not emphasized much, optimizing individual performances was less important. It was typically assumed that someone's background, training, experience, and licensure or certification sufficiently reflected their knowledge and skills, and that only the individual professions should evaluate or correct the performance of their peers. But these assumptions are often untrue.

The objectives of education and training programs are to assess the knowledge and skills of those at all levels of the program and to ensure that knowledge and information are used consistently to provide appropriate, efficient service. Those to be educated and trained include patients and families, practitioners, and other direct care staff, support staff, owners and governing body, and management.

Health care programs and organization should vigorously support such initiatives. The time and money spent on effective education and training activities are vital supports for care quality improvement and risk management, even though they do not contribute directly to revenues. For example, when ordered to make additional budget cuts by the administration, a hospital-based subacute

FIGURE 9–6   EXAMPLE OF A PHYSICIAN PERFORMANCE EVALUATION BASED ON DESIRABLE
                    CHARACTERISTICS IN THE CARE OF SUBACUTE PATIENTS

PHYSICIAN PERFORMANCE ASSESSMENT SUMMARY

Indicator	Optimal Performance	Minimal Performance	Individual's Score
Outcome of his or her patients	An optimal outcome is achieved in almost every case.	The optimal anticipated outcome is almost never achieved.	Minimal Optimal 0 1 2 3 4 5 6 7 8 9 10
Support for overall care management of individual patients	Practitioner is consistently helpful and cooperative, helps create a pertinent care plan, and supports the goals and objectives of the care.	Practitioner is rarely helpful and cooperative, does not usually help create an appropriate care plan, and often does not support the goals and objectives of the care.	Minimal Optimal 0 1 2 3 4 5 6 7 8 9 10
Quality screens	Practitioner's care is consistently compatible with quality standards, as evaluated by peers.	Practitioner's care is rarely compatible with quality standards evaluated by peers.	Minimal Optimal 0 1 2 3 4 5 6 7 8 9 10
Rate of possibly preventable complications	Few of practitioner's patients have significant complications related to the treatment or unrelated to the illnesses or conditions.	Almost all of practitioner's patients have significant complications related to the treatment or unrelated to the illnesses or conditions.	Minimal Optimal 0 1 2 3 4 5 6 7 8 9 10
Technical skills	Practitioner consistently demonstrates substantial skill in patient assessment and management.	Practitioner's skills in assessment, treatment selection, and managing cases are inconsistent or questionable.	Minimal Optimal 0 1 2 3 4 5 6 7 8 9 10
Process support	Practitioner responds in a timely fashion when contacted about problems, and consistently helps other staff deal with documentation and other process requirements.	Practitioner rarely helps (or actively resists helping) with process, documentation, and other requirements.	Minimal Optimal 0 1 2 3 4 5 6 7 8 9 10
Patient/family satisfaction	Patients and families are almost always satisfied with the quality of the physician's care and his or her support in providing information and helping them make vital decisions.	Patients and families are almost never satisfied with the quality of the physician's care and his or her support in providing information and helping them make vital decisions.	Minimal Optimal 0 1 2 3 4 5 6 7 8 9 10
Legal and regulatory status	Practitioner continues to fully meet relevant general and specialty licensure criteria, based on overall practice.	Practitioner's ability to remain licensed in the state is in jeopardy.	Minimal Optimal 0 1 2 3 4 5 6 7 8 9 10
Improvement of knowledge and skills	Practitioner maintains and tries to improve current knowledge and skills relevant to care of the program's patients.	Practitioner does not make any effort to try to improve current knowledge and skills.	Minimal Optimal 0 1 2 3 4 5 6 7 8 9 10
Overall interest and concern	Practitioner consistently exhibits substantial interest in the patients' well-being and in the success of the facility's programs and services.	Practitioner is rarely interested or openly indifferent to the patients, care, and facility.	Minimal Optimal 0 1 2 3 4 5 6 7 8 9 10

*Reviewed by*_____, M.D.   *Date*_____

FIGURE 9–7   EXAMPLE OF OTHER ITEMS THAT MIGHT BE INCLUDED IN PERFORMANCE EVALUATIONS

Indicator	Optimal Performance	Minimal Performance	Individual's Score
Reliability	Highly reliable and consistent in performance, with rare exceptions. Can be depended upon to carry work and problem solving to completion without having to be closely monitored or frequently reminded about responsibilities.	Inconsistent, unpredictable, not reliable. Typically does only part of a task. Does not carry work and problem solving to completion. Must be closely monitored and frequently reminded to follow through.	Minimal Optimal 0 1 2 3 4 5 6 7 8 9 10
Fairness	Shows sense of balance and fair play when mediating among those with contrasting perspectives. Usually balances self-interest with interests of others or with common interest.	Plays politics to the extreme. Shows favoritism without regard to objective information. Emphasizes personal interests and preferences.	Minimal Optimal 0 1 2 3 4 5 6 7 8 9 10
Communications (from)	Presents information so others can understand. Makes effort to see if others understand. Goes out of way to clarify communications.	Does not generally present information so others can understand. Does not try to see if others understand the message. Tends to fault others for failure to understand communications.	Minimal Optimal 0 1 2 3 4 5 6 7 8 9 10
Communications (to)	Is receptive to communication from others. Goes out of way to ensure that messages are being interpreted correctly. Is able to accurately restate in own words what others are trying to say.	Makes it clear that communication from others is undesirable. Does not try to ensure that messages are being interpreted correctly. Often misrepresents what others are trying to say.	Minimal Optimal 0 1 2 3 4 5 6 7 8 9 10
Ability to carry out functions and tasks	Can consistently carry out tasks exactly as needed or directed. Almost always follows policies and procedures correctly. Does right thing in right way consistently. When given feedback, does not repeat same mistake twice.	Often does the wrong thing, or right thing in the wrong way, or the wrong thing in the right way. Actively resists conformity to agreed on procedures. Does not correct performance when given appropriate feedback.	Minimal Optimal 0 1 2 3 4 5 6 7 8 9 10
Problem solving	Consistently demonstrates ability to define situations accurately, evaluate causes, and recommend appropriate solutions. Follows up on problems to ensure adequate resolution.	Often addresses symptoms, not causes. Rarely searches beyond limited personal knowledge of reasons or causes. Does not suggest helpful solutions. Causes problems by how he or she addresses problems.	Minimal Optimal 0 1 2 3 4 5 6 7 8 9 10
Technical proficiency	Knows his or her job/profession and does it as well as anyone possibly could. Consistently shows high level of technical skill, consistently does the right thing in right way, and knows limits of knowledge and when and where to get help.	Employee does not perform his or her job very well technically, does not ask for assistance, and often does the wrong thing or only partially the right thing, or the right thing in the wrong way.	Minimal Optimal 0 1 2 3 4 5 6 7 8 9 10
Knowledge base	Keeps informed about knowledge in his or her own	Does not keep up with information in own profession or	Minimal Optimal 0 1 2 3 4 5 6 7 8 9 10

(continued)

FIGURE 9–7   EXAMPLE OF OTHER ITEMS THAT MIGHT BE INCLUDED IN PERFORMANCE EVALUATIONS (CONTINUED)

Indicator	Optimal Performance	Minimal Performance	Individual's Score
	area; understands how job fits into the bigger picture; also understands how his or her work affects the work of others and relates to the care and services given in the facility.	work area. Does not know or understand much about his or her work or context in which it is given; does not understand how his or her work affects the work of others and relates to the care and services given in the facility.	
Peer relationships	Has excellent working relationships with colleagues and other employees. Treats peers and subordinates with respect. Tries to be supportive and helpful. Considers others' interests as well as own.	Has poor working relationships with others. Does not treat peers and subordinates with respect. Is not supportive and helpful. Routinely emphasizes own interests over those of others.	Minimal Optimal 0 1 2 3 4 5 6 7 8 9 10
Use of authority	Uses authority rationally to help others get things done. Does not make decisions that create obstacles. Sets a good example by helping remove obstacles, and by not creating them for others through power moves.	Uses authority to coerce and control. Does not use it to help others do what needs to be done. Does not help remove obstacles. Often uses authority to get his or her own way. Actions tend to create obstacles for others.	Minimal Optimal 0 1 2 3 4 5 6 7 8 9 10
Acceptance of responsibility	Has a fair, balanced attitude towards personal responsibility. Rarely makes excuses or passes responsibility to others. Tries to act responsibly even when circumstances make it difficult to do so.	Rarely accepts personal responsibility. Frequently makes excuses or passes responsibility to others. Often uses "circumstances beyond control" as an excuse to justify not having done something, or having done something other that what was supposed to have been done, or having done something incorrectly.	Minimal Optimal 0 1 2 3 4 5 6 7 8 9 10
Feedback (from)	Generally offers constructive, comprehensible feedback to others based on accurate information and observations.	Offers no feedback, or offers feedback that is unclear, unfair, not supported by objective information, or often intimidating or demeaning.	Minimal Optimal 0 1 2 3 4 5 6 7 8 9 10
Feedback (to)	Acknowledges feedback, and tries to understand it even if not agreeing fully with it.	Rejects most feedback, even when given constructively. Cannot evaluate self from the viewpoint of others.	Minimal Optimal 0 1 2 3 4 5 6 7 8 9 10
Overall service attitude	Conveys an attitude that service is the primary objective of work responsibility, whether directly to patients or indirectly via those caring for them. Goes out of way to try to help.	Views other staff as nuisances or obstacles to accomplishing work tasks. Frequently gets annoyed with other staff for calling or trying to get help. Conveys direct or hidden message of being "too busy to be bothered." Does not go out of way to ask what can be done to help.	Minimal Optimal 0 1 2 3 4 5 6 7 8 9 10

FIGURE 9–7 EXAMPLE OF OTHER ITEMS THAT MIGHT BE INCLUDED IN PERFORMANCE EVALUATIONS (CONTINUED)

Indicator	Optimal Performance	Minimal Performance	Individual's Score
Dedication to improvement	Strives for improvement; seeks ways to do things better. Can acknowledge potential benefits of new approaches. Is willing to change habits when there is some demonstrated benefit in doing so.	Very resistant to new suggestions. Immediately rejects new approaches without trying to understand them. Conveys attitude of "this is the way we've always done it; why change?" Actively resists new approaches and tries to undermine new procedures.	Minimal Optimal 0 1 2 3 4 5 6 7 8 9 10

program administrator decided to eliminate most staff instruction about how to perform procedures correctly. Upon further inquiry, the program medical director learned that there was no cognizance of the possible risk-management implications of such a move.

Components.   Chapter 6 reviewed the different kinds and levels of knowledge and skills for the various players. Table 9–19, p. 307, lists some essential areas for education and training for subacute staff, management, and practitioners, including conceptual understanding, factual knowledge base, performance skills, and general rules and expectations. Each of these also has general, program-specific, and patient-specific aspects.

Knowledge.   Knowledge, which may be general or function-specific, reflects the possession of factual and conceptual understanding. General knowledge may include a basic understanding of the principles, processes, and objectives of subacute care; the principles of the care environment (for example, managed care); and the relationship of the care of individual patients to the goals of the overall system.

Function-specific knowledge includes understanding specific roles and responsibilities, appreciating the relationship between performance and outcomes, knowing how to perform required functions and tasks correctly, and appreciating how people can identify what they do not know, when they have done something correctly or incorrectly, and how and when to obtain help. Patient care-specific knowledge covers understanding of how to identify, manage, and monitor the various illnesses and conditions that affect subacute patients.

Skills.   Skills represent the potential to do something consistently and correctly. For example, assessment skills include the ability to identify and define patient findings and characteristics (for example, physical abnormalities and functional deficits). Problem-solving skills involve the ability to identify and define existing and potential patient problems. Patient management skills include the ability to select and initiate appropriate treatments and other relevant interventions (for example, to try to prevent complications).

Program- or service-specific skills include an understanding of various programs such as pulmonary care, dialysis, or wound management. Procedural skills include performing procedures correctly and safely, and identifying any associated complications. Educational skills include the ability to explain information or to train patients, families, or other staff. Interpersonal skills include the abilities to relate to, and communicate with, other individuals effectively, and to participate in problem-solving, quality improvement, and risk-management activities.

Although didactic instruction (lectures, continuing medical education, and the like) is useful to provide knowledge, actual performance is the best reflection of the caliber and relevance of an individual's skills. This may be observed, measured, or inferred from outcomes. Often, people know intellectually how to perform a task but may be less adept at actually doing it, or at doing it in a particular way to fit a specific situation. Some individuals know how to do a procedure but may not be as adept at explaining to others how to do it. Managers and supervisors must be able to not only evaluate staff performance but also to ascertain the causes of any performance-related problems and to show individuals how to adjust their performance appropriately.

Methods.   Education and training processes should be both subject-oriented (to enhance knowledge) and case-related (to evaluate and improve skills). They should be an integral part of everyday operations (the concept of the "learning organization"), so that people learn as they work or while they are receiving care.

For example, orientation and in-service programs are common in health care settings, but must be followed up to see if they result in effective performance. The postinstruction period is a desirable time to observe and adjust performance through feedback. It is generally easier to correct performance early before bad habits become ingrained.

Consistent with overall program objectives of both effectiveness and efficiency, education and training processes should be efficient for both the teachers and the learners. As much as possible, subacute programs should use available technologies including video and computer-based multimedia, and emphasize self-learning supported by trainers and skilled practitioners. On-line, real-time information and databases have enormous potential to teach and train individuals as they work. All subacute programs should seriously investigate these options, which should eventually become integral parts of health care organizations.

REFERENCES

Baig E. Patient, heal thyself—via PC. *Business Week*. July 12, 1993:157.

Bankowitz RA, McNeil MA, Challinor SM, et al. A computer-assisted medical diagnostic consultation service. *Ann Intern Med*. 1989; 110:824–832.

Barron D. The Iliad. *Phys Comput*. February, 1992:28–31.

Bergeron B. Iliad: A diagnostic consultant and patient simulator. *MD Comput*. 1991; 8(1):46–53.

Buckner JA. Help with tough diagnoses. *Phys Comp*. December 1991:36–38.

Dick RS, Steen EB, eds. *The Computer-Based Patient Record: An Essential Technology for Health Care*. Washington, DC: National Academy Press;1991

Ernst DF. Total quality management in the hospital setting. *J Nurs Care Qual*. 1994; 8(2):1–8.

Graham MJ, Pettus T, Klava S. Critical pathways link services to outcomes. *Provider*. September 21, 1995:31–32.

Horowitz GL, Bleich HL. Paperchase: A computer program to search the medical literature. *N Engl J Med*. 1981; 305:924–930.

Hospitals attack a crippler: Paper. *Business Week*. February 21, 1994:104–106.

Integrated information management paves the way to better decision making on patient care. *Hosp Health Netw*. January 5, 1994:56.

Joint Commission on Accreditation of Healthcare Organizations. *Plant Technology and Safety Management Handbook: Managing the Environment of Care*. Chicago: JCAHO; 1995a.

Joint Commission on Accreditation of Healthcare Organizations. *Survey Protocol for Subacute Programs*. Chicago: JCAHO; 1995b.

Kagan D. Unmasking incompetent managers. *Insight*. May 21, 1990:42–44.

Kahn G. Computer-based patient education: A progress report. *MD Comput*. 1993; 10:93–99.

Laffel G, Blumenthal D. The case for using industrial quality management science in health care organizations. *JAMA*. 1989; 262:2869–2873.

Leebov W, Ersoz CJ. *The Health Care Manager's Guide to Continuous Quality Improvement*. Chicago: American Hospital Publishing; 1991.

Lumsdon K. Why executive teams fail, and what to do. *Hosp Health Netw*. 1995; 69(15):24–31.

Margolis N. Life-saving data sharing. *ComputerWorld*. July 26,1993:28.

Safran C, Porter D, Lightfoot J, et al. ClinQuery: A system for online searching of data in a teaching hospital. *Ann Intern Med*. 1989; 111:751–756.

Sechrest RC. Educating your patient with multimedia. *Phys Comput*. October, 1991:18–26.

Sherer J. Tapping into teams. *Hosp Health Netw*. July 5, 1995:32–35.

Stead WW. Systems for the year 2000: The case for an integrated database. *MD Comput*. 1991; 8(2):103–110.

FOR FURTHER READING

Abdulla AM. Teachers aide. *Phys Comput*. December 1993:12–17.

Berwick, D.M. Sounding board: Continuous improvement as an ideal in health care. *N Engl J Med*. 1989; 320:53–56.

Blum B. *Clinical Information Systems*. New York: Springer-Verlag;1986.

Computer, heal thyself. *Multimedia World*. December 1993:80–82.

Dewey J. Living quality. *Provider*. October 1994:38–48,77–78.

Fournies FF. *Why Employees Don't Do What They're Supposed To Do; and What To Do About It*. Blue Ridge Summit, PA: Liberty Hall Press;1988.

Hegland A. Computers empower nurses. *Contemp Long-Term Care*. August 1993:58,60.

Kritchevsky SB, Simmons BP. Continuous quality improvement: Concepts and applications for physician care. *JAMA*. 1991; 266:1817–1823.

McDonald CJ. Computer-stored medical records: Their time is nigh. *MD Comput*. 1987; 4(1):7–8.

Minard B. Growth and change through information management. *Hosp Health Serv Admin*. August 1987:307–318.

Pozgar GD. *Long-Term Care and the Law: A Legal Guide for Health Care Professionals*. Gaithersburg, MD: Aspen;1992.

Stahl DA. Critical pathways in subacute care. *Nurs Manage*. 1995; 26(9):16–18.

Taft C. Managing the cardiac arrest in the long-term care and subacute medical facility. *Geriatr Nurs*. 1995; 16(2):84–88.

TQM/CQI: The CEO experience. *Hospitals*. 1992; 66(11):24–36.

TABLE 9–1   REINFORCING DESIRED OR UNDESIRED PERFORMANCE

Increase the Behavior	Decrease the Behavior
Positive Reinforcement	**Negative Consequences**
Desired performance may be increased by the following:	*Desired performance* may be decreased by the following:
• Make it faster and easier to do something in the desired way. • Repeat specific performance feedback periodically. • Clarify overall goals and objectives. • Help individuals understand why they should do something; especially, how it relates to achieving goals and objectives.	• Provide negative feedback for appropriate performance.
	Undesired performance may be decreased by the following:
Undesired performance may be increased by the following:	• Provide corrective feedback for suboptimal performance. • Provide corrective feedback to those who obstruct desired performance by others.
• Make it faster and easier to do a less desired thing or to do the right thing suboptimally. • Reward achieving objectives regardless of the means used to do so.	
Remove negative consequences	**Remove positive reinforcement**
Desired performance may be increased by the following:	*Desired performance* may be decreased by the following:
• Remove or prevent placement of obstacles to doing things in the desired way. • Eliminate unpleasant consequences for doing the desired thing. • Provide an effective strategy for circumventing obstacles.	• Withhold pertinent positive feedback for appropriate performance. • Fail to repeat specific performance feedback periodically
	Undesired performance may be decreased by the following:
	• Do not reward inappropriate performance.

Adapted with permission from Levenson SA. Implementing policies and procedures. *Clin Ger Med.* 1995; 11:449–465.

TABLE 9–2   ESSENTIAL GENERAL SUPPORT SYSTEMS FOR SUBACUTE CARE

System	Description
Quality oversight and improvement	Systems that help establish guidelines for effective performance and desirable outcome, that monitor compatibility of performance with those guidelines, and that try to adjust and improve performance
Communications and information	Processes and tools (e.g., databases, decisional support, data collection and input) by which individuals effectively obtain and provide information needed to make decisions and perform essential functions
Risk management and safety	Systems that can identify high-risk areas of care and business operations, and anticipate and prevent problems
Emergency response	Systems that enable effective handling of serious unanticipated or life-threatening occurrences
Physical plant, equipment, and utilities management	Systems to manage the physical plant and environment, and to solve and prevent related problems
Central supply	Systems to ensure that adequate supplies are available in a timely fashion
Problem solving	Systems that facilitate the identification, management, and prevention of care-related and operational and management problems
Policies and procedures	Systems that help create and implement effective policies and procedures that enable consistent performance and processes, and help solve and prevent problems
Education and training	Systems that assess and try to improve the knowledge and skills of individuals to help them make the best possible decisions and provide consistently high-quality results through appropriate performance
Human resources	Systems to identify, hire, train, support, and retain the best possible individuals to provide direct care and support services Systems to offer feedback about individual performance related to expectations, to allow for appropriate performance adjustment and improvement

TABLE 9–3   WHY SUBACUTE CARE AND ITS PATIENTS NEED EFFECTIVE SUPPORT SYSTEMS

Factor	Reasons for Its Impact
Characteristics of subacute patients	• Multiple complex problems • Multiple influences on patient status • Impact of both medical and nonmedical factors on care outcomes • Different treatment objectives at different times for the same patient, or for the same problem in different individuals • Practitioners with different knowledge, training, perspectives, and ways of interpreting the same information • Need for a single care plan for each patient • Systematic approach needed to reconcile all these variables
Nature of patient risks	• Patients tend to have multiple risk factors • Complications may result from conditions, treatments, or care site • Mechanism needed to anticipate and try to prevent such problems, and to identify them when they occur
Variability in desired and achieved care outcomes	• Many different criteria for service quality • Same criteria not always applicable to the same degree in different cases • Variable expectations and interpretations by different providers and recipients of care • Some means needed to assess optimal results in individual cases
Influences on decision making	• Effective care depends heavily on complex decision making • Complex decision making heavily influenced by availability and accuracy of information • Multiple internal and external parties influence the care, reimbursement, and quality considerations • Considerable differences of opinion about which information is relevant, and how it should be coded and organized
Performance influences on outcome	• Ultimately, care outcomes depend on collective individual performances • Many influences on individual performance may impact outcomes • Things that promote or inhibit effective individual performance can be identified and appropriately reinforced or improved • Practitioner variance in attitudes, knowledge, and understanding • Technical knowledge and skills do not ensure correct performance • Systems must appropriately influence and adjust individual performance

TABLE 9–4   EXAMPLES OF OBSTACLES TO EFFECTIVE PERFORMANCE IN SUBACUTE CARE

Obstacle	Examples
Inappropriate regulatory requirements/penalties	• Requirements that inhibit essential flexibility • Regulations that mandate processes and performance requirements unlikely to positively impact the care
Territoriality/power and control	• Individuals or disciplines who may not participate in an interdisciplinary process • Decision-making processes that are dominated by personal ambitions and perspectives
Irrational authority	• Owner, CEO, administrator, or department heads who make decisions without understanding the impact on care providers
Inadequate resources	• Reimbursement that does not allow adequate treatment duration • Insufficient or inadequately trained staff
Denial of responsibility	• One or more individuals or departments who do not agree with their roles or acknowledge their responsibilities
Inappropriate problem management	• Tendency to react to symptoms instead of seeking and addressing causes of problems
Root-cause exclusion	• Individuals who use their authority to excuse themselves from consideration as potential causes of problems or source of solutions
Inadequate knowledge base	• Individuals who do not know how to manage various problems or handle complex equipment correctly
Inadequate information systems support	• Inadequate references or resources for ready access to relevant clinical information
Multidisciplinary rather than interdisciplinary approach	• Individuals from all disciplines may be present but not coordinating or synchronizing their performance
Excessive common variation disguised as special variation	• Inconsistency from shift to shift, or from person to person, which is excused as being clinically valid variation
Inadequate or insufficient guidelines, standards, policies, procedures	• Harmful or potentially risky performance failures or inconsistencies among practitioners in handling the same problem • Lack of standards for performance/mutual expectations
Unclear roles, responsibilities	• Conflict among various disciplines over roles and task responsibilities

TABLE 9–5   CATEGORIES OF TEAMS TO PERFORM VARIOUS FUNCTIONS IN HEALTH CARE ORGANIZATIONS

Category	Principal Functions
Work teams	• Transform organization operations and functions. • Evaluate, improve, manage, or change work processes.
Integrating teams	• Consolidate tasks organization-wide (e.g., streamline purchasing processes across several locations).
Management teams	• Ensure that organization's design helps rather than hinders it from accomplishing its mission.
Improvement teams	• Suggest processes that will improve operations.

TABLE 9–6	ESSENTIAL PRINCIPLES FOR A SYSTEM THAT EFFECTIVELY SUPPORTS SUBACUTE CARE PROVISION	
	Principle	**Management and Leadership Objectives**
Governance and management role	• Management's job is to see that collective performance achieves desired goals and objectives. To do this, it must enable the work force. To do that, it must try to remove obstacles to effective performance, and must not deliberately or inadvertently place such obstacles. • To serve the patients well, the staff must be well served. • Governance and management must set a good example. Most people cannot be fooled for long by recurrent discrepancies between what they are told to do and what is done by those who tell them to do it. • The role of leadership is not just planning and oversight, but strong support for creating systems that help those giving direct care.	• We will try to remove the obstacles that hinder performance and provide the resources that enable it. • We will try not to place obstacles in others' paths, and will always try to remove obstacles that we or others may have placed in their way. • We will use our authority to referee disagreements as objectively as possible. • We will provide staff with necessary training and support to perform well, and with ongoing feedback to help improve their performance. • We will allow the staff to have a voice in adjusting systems so that they meet their needs better. • We will support the credibility of our value systems and goals by practicing what we preach. We will point out when performance, behaviors, attitudes, or actions are not compatible with our goals, no matter who is out of line.
Attributing responsibility	• The conclusion that performance failure is due to personal inadequacies is a diagnosis of exclusion. Of all the reasons for failed performance, only a few relate to personal limits such as motivation and intelligence, while many concern some aspect of the system in which individuals must function. • Anyone, from governance and top management to front-line staff, may share some responsibility for causing or preventing a problem. • All of the leadership are accountable for the system in which the care providers must function because they establish it and make key decisions about policies and priorities. • Attributing responsibility appropriately requires the collective perspectives, both favorable and unfavorable, of different individuals affected by a situation or by other people. • Many people resist being held responsible because they fear being blamed, and blame typically is accompanied by some punishment. • To be responsible for their actions, people must understand clearly what	• We will not permit people to deny personal responsibility by trying to blame it on the system, but we will consider other causes of performance failure before deciding that an individual is the cause of the problem. • We will evaluate individual responsibility without having predetermined conclusions about who wishes to be excused from such considerations. • We will include those of various relevant perspectives in these discussions. • We will solicit staff input regarding appropriate means of attributing and enforcing responsibility. • We will encourage the staff to help hold one another accountable and to point out failures of accountability when they occur. • We will not automatically assume that those with authority are correct and those working under them are wrong until proven otherwise. • We will distinguish responsibility from blame. Any disciplinary actions will be consistent with the severity of the performance problem.

(continued)

TABLE 9–6   ESSENTIAL PRINCIPLES FOR A SYSTEM THAT EFFECTIVELY SUPPORTS SUBACUTE
                   CARE PROVISION (CONTINUED)

	Principle	Management and Leadership Objectives
	they are responsible for, and how to do it correctly.	• We will ensure that staff and management understand the general goals and objectives of the care and of this facility, and their own place in the overall scheme. • We will strive for policies, procedures, and job descriptions that clarify individual and collective responsibilities, and an information system that makes it easy for people to find what they need in a timely fashion.
Giving performance feedback	• Feedback does not equal criticism. No one likes criticism, but everyone needs feedback to change their behavior for the better. Feedback should both be given and received appropriately. Bad feedback, and entrenched resistance to receiving it, are major causes of failures of communication and performance. • No one should be immune from receiving feedback. Everyone has the right to challenge the feedback they receive, but no one should be able to ignore it. • Feedback from one source is not enough to form a fair picture of how someone is doing. It should be multi-directional. • People tend to deliver or to discern a lot of hidden messages and motives when giving or receiving feedback. • Many people's lives are strongly influenced by demeaning messages from others in authority. Through long, unpleasant experiences, they may equate feedback about their performance with a general attack on their personal adequacy. • Feedback cannot always be positive, but it can be accurate, clear, and pertinent. • A manager must not only say that something is wrong or could be done better, but must also explain why and be able to show how to adjust performance appropriately. • Feedback must be timely, task-specific, and include relevant instructions or demonstrations of the correct approach. • Giving feedback properly is a learned skill. As part of their per-	• We will give accurate performance-based feedback. It will include information to help individuals change performance in the appropriate direction. We will try to ensure that people have what they need to be able to change appropriately. We will encourage an active dialogue about the details of such feedback and the specific changes desired. Once these expectations are clarified, we will expect them to be willing, active participants. • Feedback will be offered upward, downward, and laterally. Everyone will receive feedback from a cross-section of their peers, bosses, and subordinates, and of those they are supposed to serve, and they will be expected to pay attention. • We will explain clearly to all staff why they are being given feedback, and will help them clarify the messages that are being delivered. • We will be responsible for knowing the staff's responsibilities and functions, and how these should be done correctly, so we may offer appropriate, specific advice about how they may do better. • We will use and provide appropriate references and resources to ensure that the staff are being told the right thing to do and how to do it correctly. • We agree to receive feedback from others about how well we give feedback so we can adjust our own performance accordingly. • We support a system in which job- and pay-related rewards are based in part on how well we support and participate in the TQM process. These conclusions should be based in part on feedback and evaluations from others whose performance and outcomes depend on the program.

TABLE 9–6	ESSENTIAL PRINCIPLES FOR A SYSTEM THAT EFFECTIVELY SUPPORTS SUBACUTE CARE PROVISION (CONTINUED)	
	Principle	**Management and Leadership Objectives**
	formance evaluation, everyone should receive appropriate feedback about how well they offer and receive feedback. • Individual performance in relation to quality improvement principles should be included among the criteria used to judge eligibility for bonuses and other rewards.	
Exercise of authority	• In exercising authority generally, a position somewhere between the extremes of authoritarianism and the total hands-off approach is desirable. • Some forms of power may seem more expedient than others, but in the end give less desirable results.	• Although some authority-based hierarchy will still exist, its primary purpose will be to ensure that the system and its individuals function well and strive for improvement. • We will use coercive power as a last resort, and instead use power based on information, reward, expertise, and leadership by example, as much as possible.
Problem solving	• Any problem-solving effort must begin with appropriate problem definition. Failing this, the proposed solutions may not be pertinent or may make the problem worse. • Defining a problem and determining its causes requires perspectives largely unhindered by preconceptions and hidden agendas. • In effective problem-solving processes, lines of authority are largely irrelevant to correctly identifying and defining problems. • An accurate picture of reality requires a merging of viewpoints that transcends the needs or desires of any one individual or group. • Typically, front-line staff may be too close to the action and the management and ownership too far removed from it. Therefore, defining a problem may require merging these perspectives. • A vital leadership role is to identify potential problems before they are fully apparent, and to know when and to what extent to intervene prospectively.	• We will include all relevant disciplines and individuals in efforts to define problems and identify their causes. • In trying to establish the facts, we will focus on a person's hands-on experience, direct observation, and relevant understanding and insight regardless of their position or authority in the organization. • To resolve differences in opinion about the facts in any situation, we will establish and use an objective system of data collection and analysis that does not favor any one individual, discipline, or department. • We will try to define problems properly and determine their causes before choosing solutions. If short-term solutions are chosen of necessity, we will be willing to reassess and change them as appropriate. • We will support a prospective risk-management approach that tries to anticipate and prevent problems, rather than waiting and reacting to problems after the damage has been done.
Communications	• There are many prerequisites for successful communications, and	• We will try to verify the extent to which other people accurately and completely

(continued)

TABLE 9–6	ESSENTIAL PRINCIPLES FOR A SYSTEM THAT EFFECTIVELY SUPPORTS SUBACUTE CARE PROVISION (CONTINUED)	

	Principle	Management and Leadership Objectives
	numerous reasons why communications fail. • There are ways to test for the success of communications, and ways to adjust communications approaches to increase the likelihood of such success. • Often, communications fail because of the lack of easy access to complete, accurate, timely information by those who depend on it for making decisions.	understand the information we try to give them. • We will try to identify specific reasons for communications successes and failures. • We will try to modify attitudes and preconceptions that may obstruct effective communications. • We will create a mechanism to give individuals feedback about their communications skills. • We will try to develop more efficient and effective documentation and information management systems. • We will try to create more effective and efficient education and training methods, and a means to assess effective performance.
Overall political climate	• Some amount of politics is inescapable, but its impact may range from usually constructive to very destructive. • Traditional hierarchy-based, power politics is not supportive of efficient, high-quality performance.	• We will strive to emphasize common interests and objectives. • We support the creation of a constructive political arena that balances various interests and does not allow any one interest to overpower the rest. • We will set the appropriate tone for one another and for the staff, patients, and families by providing business and clinical leadership by example.

TABLE 9–7 PREREQUISITES, WEAKNESSES, AND POSSIBLE SOLUTIONS FOR SUCCESSFUL COMMUNICATION

Attribute	Need	Examples of Causes of Problems	Possible Approaches to Improvement
Comprehensible message	The sender must deliver a comprehensible message to the receiver.	A practitioner may not speak loudly enough to be heard by a hearing-impaired patient, may speak too fast, may not write legibly, or may use terms without defining them.	• Ask recipient to rephrase messages as they understand them. • Use computer-generated documentation and information. • Establish policies requiring clarification of illegible information.
Level of receptivity	Both sender and receiver must be alert and able to pay attention.	A patient may be sleepy, sedated by medications, have a short attention span, be preoccupied by something else, or be so uncomfortable with the information or the message that he or she tunes it out.	• Monitor effects of medications on cognitive status. • Carefully assess attention span and cognition. • Ask recipients to explain their understanding of a message in their own words.
Potential for understanding	The recipient must be able to comprehend the information.	A patient may be cognitively impaired, or cognitively intact but not have the background or ability to understand the information presented.	• Assess patient sensory, cognitive function. • Tailor information presentation to try to accommodate patient limitations.
Basis for interpreting message	There must be a common ground of understanding.	A physician may be trying to explain technical details about a medical problem although the staffperson, patient, or family member lacks the training or information base to evaluate either the facts or the conclusions.	• Use or explain appropriate terminology. • Anticipate, encourage, and respond to questions and requests for clarification. • Carefully establish the factual basis for communications, and distinguish the facts from any opinions or conclusions based on those facts.
Clarification process	The receiver must recognize the need for further clarification and must request clarification as needed.	A nurse may not understand what a supervisor said to do, but may not be comfortable admitting lack of understanding A patient or family member may want to ask questions about a medical condition or a decision they are asked to make, but not know the appropriate questions to ask.	• Create a system that helps all players to feel comfortable in asking questions and requesting clarifications. • Anticipate, encourage, and respond to questions and requests for clarification.

(continued)

TABLE 9–7   PREREQUISITES, WEAKNESSES, AND POSSIBLE SOLUTIONS FOR SUCCESSFUL COMMUNICATION (CONTINUED)

Attribute	Need	Examples of Causes of Problems	Possible Approaches to Improvement
Receptivity to requests for further communication	The sender must be receptive to the receiver's need for clarification or additional information.	A nurse may ask for clarification of an order, or a patient may ask for additional information about a procedure, but the physician may claim to be too busy to to take the time.	• Establish guidelines for communications-related responsibilities of all players. • Provide consistent, frequent feedback regarding individual performance in communicating. • Include questions in patient, family, and staff surveys regarding the quality of communications efforts.
Ability and motivation to use the information appropriately	The receiver must want to, and be able to, process the message.	A physician may tell a family member that further aggressive medical treatments are unlikely to have any substantial benefit, but the family member may not want to hear that conclusion.	• Use various mechanisms such as interdisciplinary team conferences and the ethics committee to resolve disputes. • Extensive use of written materials to reinforce verbal information.

TABLE 9–8   BENEFITS OF AN EFFECTIVE INFORMATION SYSTEM

Area	Benefits
General	• Allows the same information to be used for multiple purposes (e.g., a single list of diagnoses can be used in different formats for a problem list, insurance form, patient education, discharge summary, and quality of care review).
Provision of care	• Provides factual information about illnesses and conditions and their management. • Provides easily accessible decision support. • Facilitates communication of results of decisions to others who need to know. • Speeds documentation time. • Reduces risk by providing information and indicating potential problems. • Provides protocol-based reminders and guidelines. • Facilitates providing information and instruction to patients and families.
Financial/business	• Facilitates timely translation of service into billing. • Optimizes revenue collection. • Enables better analysis and understanding of resource need and use. • Provides more relevant detail for planning and budgeting.

TABLE 9–9   HOW CLINICAL INFORMATION SYSTEMS SHOULD SUPPORT SUBACUTE CARE
                                    CLINICAL PROCESSES

Process	Objectives
Patient selection	• Provide complete, timely information about the current status and needs of prospective admissions. • Enable rapid determination of whether the program can meet a prospective patient's needs by matching their problems and service needs with the program's capabilities.
Postselection/preadmission	• Facilitate provision of relevant and required information to the patient/family. • Enable quick, consistent transmittal of essential information about the individual to prepare appropriate staff to accept the admission.
Assessment	• Centralize database of relevant patient information. • Reduce duplication of data entry by allowing the same data elements to be used repeatedly for multiple reports and other purposes.
Problem definition	• Facilitate correct, complete definition of the individual's problems (diagnoses, conditions). • Track progress of problems to ensure appropriate follow-through.
Identifying care objectives	• Help staff relate the services and orders to the care objectives, and help them recognize when those objectives have been met.
Care planning	• Facilitate creation of a care plan to address the individual's problems, and the responsibilities of various individuals and disciplines (e.g., staffing, work assignments).
Management of known problems	• Facilitate identification of relevant problems, and make available information about appropriate treatment alternatives. • Help select the most pertinent treatments with the lowest risk.
Management of new problems/complications	• Help identify and respond in a timely fashion to condition changes and complications • Facilitate consistent, timely reporting of potential and actual complications to ensure appropriate follow-through.

(continued)

TABLE 9–9	HOW CLINICAL INFORMATION SYSTEMS SHOULD SUPPORT SUBACUTE CARE CLINICAL PROCESSES (CONTINUED)
Prevention of nosocomial/ iatrogenic problems	• Help staff identify areas of high risk and potential problems that may arise as a result of medications and treatments, or by being in a health care facility, and institute measures to try to prevent those problems and to recognize them if they arise despite precautions. • Warn of potential risk-management problems such as drug interactions.
Preparation for completion of treatment course	• Help staff plan for discharge and transfer, and efficiently provide required information on discharge to patient, family, finance office, payers, and those who will be providing continuing care. • Help match patient needs to available resources by providing access to a database of such options.
Follow-up	• Enable more timely collection of reimbursement. • Facilitate review of care outcomes for individual patients and for the program collectively. • Enable communication of information regarding problems and concerns of the care providers and recipients. • Facilitate follow-up to ensure problem resolution. • Help analyze care patterns, resource utilization, and service needs.

TABLE 9–10	CATEGORIES AND COMPONENTS OF A SUBACUTE PATIENT DATABASE

Personal Information
Name/Nickname or preferred name/Patient ID number/Current or last known address/Date of birth/Social security #/Sex/Race/Marital status/Religion/Birthplace/Primary language

Significant Others
Name/Relationship/Address/Phone numbers

Admission-Specific Information
Date admission approved/Admission date/Transfer source/Reason for admission/Anticipated length of stay/Current discharge plans

Care Providers
Provider name/Role (consultant, specialist, community social worker, etc.)/Address/Phone numbers

Supplementary Social and Personal Information
Current living situation/Current support systems/Work history/Education/ Driving/Smoking history/Alcohol use/Advance directive and treatment code status

Functional Status and Other Assessments
Individual's overall perception of health

Activities of daily living (ADLs): Eating/Ambulation/Dressing/Personal hygiene/Bathing/Toilet use/Bladder control/Bowel control

Instrumental activities of daily living (IADLs): Shopping/Cooking/Financial management/Cleaning/Laundry/Telephone use

Appetite/Dentition/Communications capability/Vision/Hearing/Behavior/Mood/ Short-term memory/Remote memory/Following directions/Sleep pattern/

TABLE 9–10	CATEGORIES AND COMPONENTS OF A SUBACUTE PATIENT DATABASE (CONTINUED)

Level of energy, fatigue/Decision-making capacity/Dietary restrictions, preferences

Tests of cognition, mood, and behavior/Level of consciousness

Medical History

Previous acute hospitalizations (reasons and dates)/Previous inpatient or outpatient psychiatric treatment/Previous surgical procedures (reasons and dates)/Family history/Allergies/Immunizations/Diet/Current symptoms or conditions

Physical Status

General/Height/Weight/Nutritional and hydration status/Skin condition/Level of consciousness
Vital signs

Body systems: Skin/HEENT/Mouth/Teeth and gums/Pharynx/Neck/Chest/Lungs/Heart/Peripheral vascular/Breasts/Abdomen/Rectal/Genitalia/Extremities/Musculoskeletal/Neurological

Studies and Test Results

Study or test/Problem or reason why done/Date done/Result/Need for follow-up

Medications and Treatments

Medication: Name/Dosage/Frequency/Reason/Duration

Treatments: Description/Frequency/Duration

Problems and Diagnoses

Problems: Description /Onset date/Severity/Resolution date/Present on admission?/Present on discharge?

Medical diagnoses: Description/ICDA code/Onset date/Severity/Resolution date/Present on admission?/Present on discharge?

Risk Assessments

Coma score/Depression score/Fall risk score/Nutrition risk score

TABLE 9–11	POSSIBLE FUNCTIONS OF THE SUBACUTE PATIENT RECORD

- Communication among care providers
- Information source for follow-up
- Legal record
- Basis for payment
- Source of data for quality improvement activities
- Resource for research

TABLE 9–12   COMPONENTS OF THE SUBACUTE MEDICAL RECORD AS THEY RELATE
TO CARE PROCESSES

Care Process	Relevant Medical Record Component
Patient selection	• Preadmission assessment forms • Contact information for practitioners, sites providing care prior to admission
Assessment	• Assessment instruments (activities of daily living scales, depression scales, cognitive function evaluation, etc.) • Minimum Data Set assessment where required
Problem definition	• Medical problem list (diagnoses) • Nonmedical problem list (health-related, functional, psychosocial, and other problems)
Identifying care objectives	• Interdisciplinary care plan • Data and discussions to support selection of specific objectives • Advance directives and other evidence of patient wishes
Care planning	• Initial interdisciplinary care plan and evidence of periodic review and revisions as indicated, covering acute, chronic, and other relevant problems
Management of known problems/new problems and complications	• Physician orders • Problem-oriented medical, nursing, and other progress notes • Lab, X-ray, and other test results • Evidence of problem resolution
Prevention of nosocomial/ iatrogenic problems	• Risk assessment scales (e.g., skin breakdown potential, fall potential) • Documentation of actions taken to prevent and manage problems
Preparation for completion of treatment course	• Progress notes indicating movement toward discharge • Assessments of home or other discharge setting • Contacts made with other organizations, support systems • Documentation of patient/family education and instruction
Follow-up (separate from clinical record)	• Closed record review • Quality improvement minutes, notes

TABLE 9–13   DESIRABLE FEATURES OF COMPUTER SOFTWARE TO SUPPORT SUBACUTE
CARE PROCESSES

Process	Objectives[a]
Patient selection	• Should permit preadmission data collection on prospective patients, which can then either be archived or transferred to their active file if they are admitted • [Should help compare patient's needs and characteristics to program services and capabilities to flag patients who may have special requirements or needs in excess of the program's capabilities]
Postselection/preadmission	• Should enable automatic notification of relevant departments and individuals about a prospective admission, including important information (admission date, diet, precautions, etc.)
Assessment	• Should permit both a standardized and user-defined assessment • The data collected in the assessment should be usable in various combinations for multiple reporting purposes • Users should be able to initiate queries on any data item or combination of items
Problem definition	• Should allow for a standardized and user-defined problem library, which is used to create problem lists on each patient • Should allow for defined problems to become the basis of a care plan • Should enable comparison of admission and discharge problems as part of program quality outcome measurements
Identifying care objectives	• Should allow for user-defined care objectives library, and permit use of such information in program quality outcome measurements
Care planning	• Should be able to create a care plan to address the individual's problems, using both standardized and customized care plan libraries • [Should be able to use the care plan to produce lists of the functions and responsibilities of various individuals and disciplines, such as nursing aides]
Management of known and new problems/complications	• Should allow for problem-specific medication and treatment orders • Should allow for documentation of progress in resolving both existing problems and those that arise during the stay • [Should provide physicians and other practitioners with knowledge-based assistance in diagnosing causes of problems]
Prevention of nosocomial/ iatrogenic problems	• [Should help identify and flag areas of high risk and potential problems that may arise as a result of medications and treatments, or by being in a health care facility, and recommend measures to try to prevent those problems] • [Should allow incident/accident analysis]
Preparation for completion of treatment course	• [Should allow user-defined libraries of internal and external referral sources and discharge options to facilitate transfer and discharge planning] • Should allow for rapid generation of most portions of discharge and transfer summaries, incorporating essential components (e.g., problem list, medication list)
Follow-up	• [Should allow program to analyze impact of various aspects of its care on eventual outcomes] • [Should allow for follow-up of concerns of providers and recipients of the care, as basis for program quality analyses]

[a]Items in square brackets are secondary capabilities that may require separate software or customizing existing patient care software. Nonbracketed items should be part of a single program, and should be capabilities of basic systems.

TABLE 9-14   EXAMPLES OF AREAS OF POTENTIAL RISK EXPOSURE IN A SUBACUTE PROGRAM

Area	Risk Situation
Administrative/governance	• Decisions based on too little or erroneous information • Insufficient attention to accident and incident reporting and follow-up • Preoccupation with coping rather than preventing crises • Cutting corners in service delivery and staffing to improve net revenues • Unwillingness or inability to address problems and enforce responsibilities • Creation of a highly political environment that leads to denial of responsibility and the passing of blame • Inappropriate criteria for patient selection • Pressure to admit patients who cannot be safely cared for in the program
Managerial	• Medical director failure to monitor quality of health care being given by physicians and other staff • Interpersonal and interdepartmental conflicts that result in buck-passing and failure to assume responsibility • Incomplete or outdated policies and procedures • Failure to monitor proper performance of procedures and delivery of care and to correct inadequate performance • Failure to ensure that all persons who need professional licenses are currently licensed and remain licensed • Failure to ensure that facility personnel become and remain trained in state-of-the-art knowledge and skills
Service delivery	• Program inability to consistently care for the patients admitted • Physician unavailability in the event of emergencies • Failure to comply with federal and state regulations for care and documentation • Policies and procedures that are not used consistently by staff • Failure to obtain and document informed consent for procedures • Failure to manage and document ethical decision making effectively • Occurrence of possibly preventable complications without evidence of efforts to identify and anticipate them • Use of inappropriate or unsupervised personnel (e.g., therapist is unavailable to oversee an aide who is giving a therapy session) • Failure to follow up on significant abnormal test results in a timely fashion • Failure to identify the right patient for medications and other treatments • Failure to keep patient records up-to-date and properly documented • Failure to carry out physician orders completely, correctly, and in a timely fashion • Failure to recognize, act on, and document changes in patient condition • Recording care not actually given, or altering medical records to try to hide something • Failure to identify problems or needs (e.g., suicide attempts where staff did not detect or respond to recurrent signs of suicidal behavior) • Providing the wrong drug, dosage, directions, expiration date • Failure to recognize predictable drug interactions • Failure to take precautions (e.g., to isolate when needed) • Inaccurate representations of program capabilities by marketing staff • Failure to give patient and family all necessary instructions at the time of discharge
Support staff	• Inadequate support of practitioners and direct care staff by support departments • Inadequate response to need for equipment repairs, supplies • Failure to practice preventive maintenance or to have emergency plans (e.g., loss of primary electrical power in a program that admits ventilator patients)
General	• Preventable employee on-the-job injuries • Inadequate or inaccurate information systems

TABLE 9–15   COMMON AREAS OF RISK INVOLVING MEDICAL AND NURSING CARE

Category	Examples
Follow-up of test abnormalities	Patient with slightly abnormal lab values, or whose lab values shift slowly with time; physician does not follow up or does not document reason for considering results clinically insignificant.
Treating conditions without sufficient reassessment	Physician orders medication dosage change by phone; patient does not improve significantly after several days, but physician tells nurse to continue treatment as ordered without examining the patient directly.
Deciding not to treat certain conditions without appropriately documented justification	Physician decides that patient's Do Not Resuscitate order justifies not working up new-onset bleeding, without clarifying expectations.
Failing to take action regarding an observed problem	Medical director does not follow up with a physician who is not reassessing patients when requested or who does not adequately communicate with patients or families.
Saying too little or too much	Weekend nurse fails to explain to family what has been done about patient's complication, or does not find out desired information or direct family's questions to appropriate practitioner.
Treating symptoms, not causes	Patient keeps falling and is confused; physician orders bed rest and sedation; later found to have hypotension from GI blood loss.
Failing to recognize obvious complications and side effects	Patient recently had orthopedic surgery; develops painful, swollen leg; treated symptomatically; later found to have venous thrombosis.
Damaging comments or high-risk actions by other providers, including hospitals	Patient treated conservatively for apparently minor infection suddenly gets septic; hospital emergency room staff (or outside consultant asked in on case) tells family that patient could have been helped more if the program had transferred the patient sooner.

TABLE 9–16   EXAMPLES OF RISK AVOIDANCE MEASURES IN SUBACUTE CARE PROGRAMS

- Explain the care to be provided and the potential limits and unavoidable complications.
- Clarify expected performance for all players.
- Respond in a timely fashion to concerns of staff, patients, and families.
- Consistently use specific patient selection criteria that are applied consistently.
- Do not overpromise and be unable to deliver.
- Clarify and document limitations on treatment and ensure that these are consistent with patient wishes and applicable state law and regulations.
- Explain and document decisions to withhold and withdraw treatment based on clinical appropriateness and compatibility with patient wishes.
- Explain to each patient his or her right to make decisions regarding care, including the right to refuse treatment.
- Ensure that limits on treatment (for example, Do Not Resuscitate) are well defined and are not overinterpreted (the patient may still desire testing, hospital transfer, or aggressive medical interventions).
- Clarify and advise patients of any policies about facility limits on honoring advance directive requests.
- Ensure adequate mechanisms to resolve disagreements among patients, families, and staff regarding treatment decisions or care plan, but ensure that they are not openly debated in the medical record.
- Perform and document detailed assessments of patients on arrival, including any active problems (pressure ulcers, confusion, fever) accompanying them on admission.
- Ensure appropriate understanding of OBRA '87 nursing facility regulations, where applicable.
- Investigate complaints carefully and report findings appropriately to concerned parties.
- Use an effective problem-solving system that does not permit any root-cause exclusion.
- Ensure appropriate consent for treatments and procedures.
- Ensure that medical orders are clear, or that they are clarified as needed before implementation.
- Adapt established, pertinent clinical practice guidelines and protocols where standardized procedures are important.
- Ensure that significant deviations from practice guidelines and established standards are well documented to justify variation.
- Have effective quality review mechanisms in place that assess performance, detect significant deviations from norms, and ensure appropriate supporting documentation.
- Ensure that policies and procedures are current and consistent with standards.
- Ensure that all staff know and use policies and procedures; for example, universal precautions, techniques for safe lifting, reporting condition changes to physicians.
- Ensure appropriate, regular performance-related review and feedback to all players.
- Have some mechanism for physician credentialing and privileging.
- Ensure that all staff, including physicians, understand appropriate attitudes and perspectives toward the care.

TABLE 9–17   RISK AVOIDANCE IN CARING FOR MANAGED CARE PATIENTS

Issue	Risk Avoidance Measures
Facility is concerned that managed care organization (MCO) may terminate a contract or not make referrals if too many patients are rejected.	• Facility should not admit a patient to an inappropriate bed, even for a short time. • Facility should be very familiar with its own strengths and limitations. • Facility should specify right to reject or discharge a patient who represents an unmanageable danger to safety or health of self or others.
MCO may have different policies or protocols for treating patients.	• Program should have a core of policies and consistent processes for delivering care to all patients, with exceptions made only after medical and nursing review for clinical appropriateness. • Program should have a policy that prospective admissions must meet certain criteria and admission must follow established procedures, including physicians' orders. • Skilled nursing facility-based program should ensure that MCO practices, protocols, and admission and transfer decisions are compatible with provisions of OBRA '87 regulations for SNF-based care.
MCO may put pressure on for rapid admission decisions.	• Program needs systematic preadmission assessments. • Program should be part of community-wide agreement on standards of information provision and support across care sites.
Facility and MCO may be liable for premature discharge, even though MCO decides continued stay is no longer necessary.	• Program and patient should clarify coverage with MCO upon admission. • Program should not permit retrospective reviews and denials. • Program should negotiate realistic "concurrent" review schedule, tied to progress toward achieving care objectives and problem resolution. • Program should establish mechanism for appeal of disputes over MCO determinations of length of stay. • Program should have MCO inform in writing when coverage limits are approaching. • Program should ensure that utilization reviews are performed by qualified personnel. • Facility has duty to give reasonable discharge notice. • Program should be prepared to provide continuing care if discharge may present risk of patient harm. • Program should ensure adequate and timely documentation of patient progress to support assertions that continued stay may be needed.
MCO may expect some or all of care to be given by its own staff and providers. .	• Facility should clarify any obligation to provide facilities, supplies, and support to outside staff (e.g., therapists, nurses, or physicians) employed or retained by the MCO. • Facility should clarify its rights to subcontract certain services, such as therapists. • Facility should clarify responsibility to review and give feedback about care given by all providers. • Facility should clarify rights of MCO to access its utilization review and quality review records.
MCOs may try to get facility to indemnify it against legal consequences.	• Facility should review MCO's financial and liability history. • Facility must carefully review any proposed MCO contract provisions. • Facility must balance its assumption of legal or financial risk. • Facility should consult with its own insurance carrier before agreeing to assume legal or financial liabilities, to ensure it is not violating its own insurance policy.

TABLE 9–18   ESSENTIAL COMPONENTS OF A SUBACUTE CLINICAL EMERGENCY MANAGEMENT SYSTEM

Function	Essential Components
Communications	• An accurate, updated list of essential services for emergencies, and their contact phone numbers • An accurate, continuously updated list of primary and consultant physicians caring for each patient • A telephone and paging system that enables incoming calls and messages to reach appropriate individuals in a timely fashion
Policies and procedures	• Readily available, current, detailed procedures for all processes associated with providing emergency services
Education and training	• Training and periodic retraining in CPR and the management of emergency equipment • Switchboard and phone handlers who fully understand how to handle incoming calls when there is an urgent situation • A pertinent assessment of the knowledge and skills of nurses, technicians, physicians, and others who may participate in managing emergencies • Periodic disaster drills involving clinical staff
Equipment and supplies	• Emergency drug box, with periodic review of contents and procedures • Equipment compatible with the level of emergency response offered in the program (e.g., defibrillator, EKG machine) • A program for periodic preventive maintenance and testing of all equipment, including emergency equipment

TABLE 9–19   VITAL COMPONENTS OF EDUCATION AND TRAINING FOR ALL PLAYERS

Category	Examples
Conceptual	
General	• Definition and scope of subacute care • Place of subacute care in the health care continuum • Forces influencing the care
Program	• Organization's mission, vision, philosophy, and goals • Program's goals and objectives • Services offered in program • Program organization • General roles and functions of various disciplines • Principles by which the program operates • Principles of interaction and relationships among disciplines
Patient	• Patient rights and responsibilities • Approach to formulating care goals and objectives for patients • Identifying high risks for each patient • Problem-specific and patient-specific measures to reduce risk • Care planning processes • Principles of effective documentation • Principles of effective communication with other staff, patients, families • Principles of patient and medical record confidentiality
Knowledge	
General	• Organization's personnel policies and procedures • Relevant health care law and regulation • Relevant practice standards and guidelines • Fire prevention and safety procedures
Program	• Program's actual services, staffing, and structure • Roles of various disciplines and individuals in each phase and process of the program • Actual policies and procedures • Responsibilities of the individual's position • Procedures for accident prevention and incident management
Patient	• System for assessing and defining patients' problems and prognosis • Relevance of specific findings in individual patients • Defining condition and prognosis • High-risk, problem-prone areas for the patient • Care plan for individual patients • Tactics to reduce complications in high-risk patients • Handling advance directives, surrogate decision makers, and other ethical issues
Skills	
General	• How to define, solve, and prevent problems • Tactics for effective communication • Useful ways to offer and evaluate feedback
Program	• Total quality management-related principles and practices
Patient	• How to perform specific procedures correctly • How to identify potential problems or actual onset of new problems • What to say and what not to say to patients and families

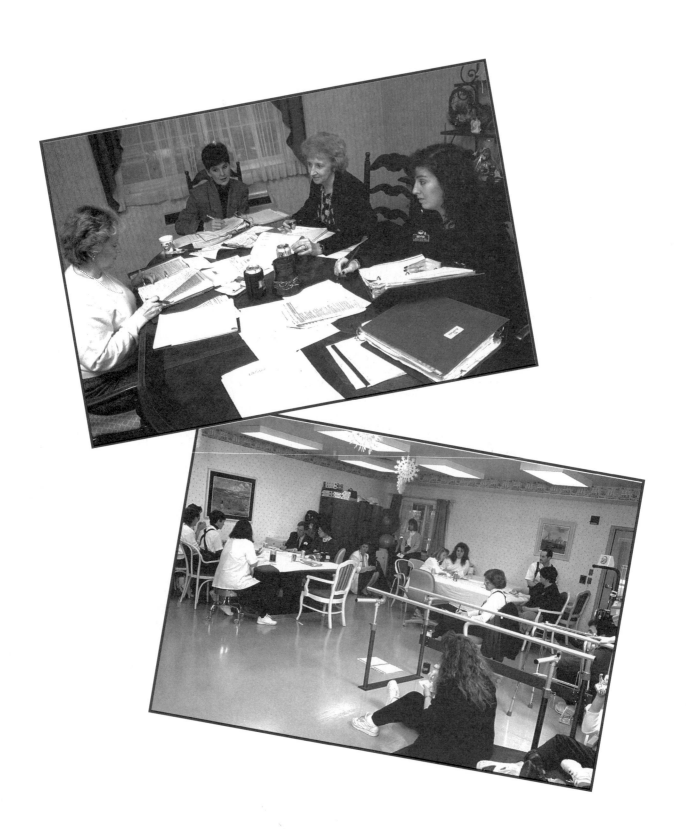

ASSESSING AND IMPROVING PATIENT OUTCOMES AND SERVICE QUALITY

*F*or various reasons, many individuals and organizations are interested in health care outcome measurements, including those for subacute care. Many relevant factors must be considered, including individual versus aggregate results, time frames for results, risk adjustment, and care objectives. Few studies have been done specifically in subacute sites, but patient-related factors that can predict risk and outcomes have been identified in other settings for similar patient populations.

Quality indicators are an important basis for providing and improving the care. Subacute programs should use certain steps in creating their quality indicators and quality management programs. Programs should create indicators for care-related processes and for outcomes.

Quality-related findings should be used to improve the direct care and the processes related to providing and supporting the care. An effective quality program should be considered a valuable investment.

Subacute programs are also seeking accreditation as a way to demonstrate compliance with pertinent standards. Accreditation has positive aspects but also some limitations. Compliance with standards must be combined with an effective quality program and the development and use of industry-wide protocols and guidelines.

The purpose of this chapter is to review the many issues related to measuring and improving quality in subacute programs, and to propose how practitioners and other staff can develop and use their quality indicators to improve outcomes and evaluate risks.

Many individuals and organizations—including payers, utilization management organizations, regulatory agencies, certifying and accrediting bodies, public health authorities, researchers, and health policy makers—are interested in care outcome measurements. They may want to improve their ability to understand the efficacy and risks of alternative procedures for the same condition; to choose appropriate care options; to predict likely outcomes of care; to define the impact of specific practitioners, processes, or interventions on the outcomes; to assess and improve performance; to compare the performance of different providers and provider organizations; to receive rational reimbursement of relevant treatments and procedures; to optimize lengths of stay; and to identify provider organizations and practitioners who require focused review as part of the licensing, certification, or accreditation process.

Meaningful efforts to develop health care quality indicators and to study patient outcomes are a fairly recent development. The move to managed care has accelerated these efforts. Insurers seek the least expensive services and treatments that will achieve desirable care objectives, especially those that can help reduce the subsequent use of costly health care services. They also want to know that the care was essential; that is, that it helped achieve the outcome, or at least that a comparable or better outcome could not likely have been achieved without the care. Additionally, it is important to know if care achieves optimal results, that is, the best that anyone could reasonably have done under the circumstances.

The subacute care industry has claimed to be able to provide effective care that is less costly than alternatives such as hospitalization. For that and other reasons, many individuals and organizations are interested in measuring patient outcomes and the performance and results of subacute practitioners and programs. However, they must understand the factors impacting these assessments, and the subsequent interpretations of the data.

CHALLENGES IN MEASURING QUALITY IN SUBACUTE CARE

All health care providers render care processes (assessment, testing, treatment, and so on) to patients with certain problems and needs (case mix, severity of illness), which are reflected in identifiable results (functional status, quality of life, and so on). Table 10–1, p. 337, lists the various criteria for health care quality. Health care quality measurements either assess outcomes or the appropriateness of processes known or believed to produce those outcomes.

Subacute care provides various programs (Table 5–1, p. 92) and treatments (Table 5–2, pp. 92–93), via a series of identifiable processes (Table 7–1, p. 181). To guide performance, standards (expectations for minimum, optimum, or acceptable range of performance) are needed for both the processes and the results. Quality indicators then provide specific measurements for various aspects of these processes and results. These evaluations must also consider relevant patient characteristics such as case mix and severity of illness.

For example, a quality standard for subacute care might relate to the appropriate selection and admission of patients to a subacute unit. A related quality indicator might be that no more than 5% of patients should be transferred back to an acute hospital within 3 days of admission. Or, a quality standard related to the care of ventilator patients could be linked to a quality indicator that at least 60% of ventilator patients admitted for postacute care should be weaned from the ventilator.

Presently, quality standards and indicators for subacute care are still being developed and refined. One purpose of this chapter is to explore the factors that should be considered in developing them.

Although patients and outsiders (researchers, regulatory agencies, policy-makers, and so on) are primarily interested in outcomes, providers must be equally attentive to processes. As discussed throughout this book, the means to the end are just as important as the results, especially when both effectiveness and efficiency are desirable. As discussed later in this chapter, this should include both the clinical and the general support systems and processes.

Considerations in Measuring Outcomes

Results of episodes of illness and injury may be measured relative to individuals or to groups of individuals (Table 10–2, p. 337). Practitioners and programs are primarily interested in individual results, and outsiders focus more often on aggregated and comparative results. Overall, both are important.

Assessing Individual and Collective Results.   Like other health care settings, subacute programs typically try to demonstrate their efficiency and effectiveness by comparing their outcomes with other subacute programs or other care settings treating similar individuals (for example, lengths of stay for cardiac patients, percentage of wound care patients whose wounds are healed, and percentage of complications or home discharges among ventilator patients).

However, many issues affect the validity of such comparisons. As in any health care setting, the information gathered about various patients must be reliable. Data elements must be defined and coded appropriately. For example, various practitioners at the same and different sites must use roughly the same criteria to make a diagnosis of depression or pneumonia, and the diagnoses must be recorded and coded correctly and completely. Clinicians must be able to recognize new onset of complications or condition changes, including potential nosocomial or iatrogenic illness. They must be available to do assessments in a timely fashion so that similar conditions are assessed at a corresponding point in their natural history. As long as such processes vary significantly among individual practitioners and across care sites, they will affect the validity of outcomes comparisons. This is another compelling reason for greater process standardization, including the further development and use of protocols and practice guidelines. Also, collecting data over time (either for many individuals or the same individual at various intervals) requires adjustments for any changes in the factors that affect the outcomes, for instance, if the standard of practice for managing a condition changes, or the patients age significantly.

Additionally, many other things are relevant to developing quality indicators and standards (Table 10–3, p. 338). Most subacute patients have different combinations of problems and begin their subacute care at different points in their illness even though they may be receiving the same core service (ventilator care, rehabilitation therapies, and so on). Many of these patients improve only partially, and only some of their conditions benefit from continuing or aggressive medical intervention. It is often difficult to specify the exact relationship between the outcomes of a patient's condition, the outcomes of the care, and the performance of a provider organization or clinician.

Relevance of Care Objectives.   It is simpler to relate processes to outcomes when a specific treatment can be linked to eventual full recovery from a single discrete condition in an otherwise well individual. However, subacute patients may have any one or several of the objectives listed in Table 10–4, p. 339. Only some patients can realistically expect full reversal of their underlying conditions during their stay. The case mix of individuals with these diverse objectives varies among different subacute programs and even among patients in the same program with similar illnesses or receiving comparable services or treatments. Many patients have a single care objective during their stay; for others, the objectives vary at different points. For example, full recovery may be anticipated early in a comatose patient's stay, but the prevention of complications or further decline may be a more realistic objective if the patient later fails to emerge from the coma. In addition, patients are often just as interested in outcomes related to their quality of life (such as psychological and social functioning) as they are in their physiological improvement or their long-term survival.

Thus, evaluating outcomes for subacute patients requires comparing each person's achieved to predicted or desired objectives. Each subacute program should be able to accurately establish care objectives for most of its patients. Eventually, it should be possible to establish benchmarks for an appropriate percentage of admissions who achieve predicted objectives. Programs would want to assess reasons for consistently achieving more or less than predicted results. Reasons for overachievement may include high-quality care, limited patient selection (for example, only lower-acuity cases), or failure to establish accurate objectives. Reasons for underachievement may include quality problems, inadequate initial assessments, or unrealistic objectives.

Outcome measurements must also consider any patient- or family-directed limitations on medical interventions. They must also weigh the important difference between achieving specific treatment goals and accomplishing overall care objectives. A successful treatment does not necessarily achieve a desired outcome. For example, a patient may undergo successful surgery but not regain much function, may be resuscitated but remain comatose, or may have a cancer spread despite successfully administered chemotherapy.

Care objectives are also important in comparing outcomes across care sites. For instance, it is possible to compare subacute care in hospitals to that in free-standing skilled nursing facilities, but comparing subacute care outcomes to those of high-acuity care in hospitals requires that individuals be in similar stages of their illness with comparable goals.

Time Frames.   Outcomes must also be related to a time frame (Table 10–5, p. 339). "The closer a measured outcome is in time to the activities of the provider organization or clinician whose performance is being evaluated, the more likely that the level of performance has at least partly contributed to the outcome; the longer the elapsed time between the treatment and the measurement of the outcome, the more likely that other patient-related factors, community-related factors, or even factors related to other provider organizations or clinicians will have affected the outcome . . . . Intermediate outcomes (e.g., degree of freedom from pain at discharge after a total hip replacement) generally can be more reliably measured than long-term outcomes (e.g., functional mobility 2 years after hip replacement) because of the difficulties in following ambulatory patients over time" (Schyve, 1995, pp. 29–30).

Based on these definitions, the immediate effects of specific procedures or treatments may be considered a short-term outcome, and patient status at the end of a subacute stay should ordinarily be considered an intermediate outcome. But a broader assessment of the value of health care requires longer-term measurement such as performance following discharge. Although subacute programs cannot be directly responsible for postdischarge services or outcomes, the value of paying for subacute care must be related in part to its ultimate impact on longer-term outcomes. Care that does not have a positive longer-term impact may not be worthwhile despite some shorter-term improvement. Eventually, integrated health care systems must address these and other patient-related issues that transcend specific care sites.

FACTORS THAT INFLUENCE SUBACUTE PATIENT OUTCOMES

To assess subacute outcomes, and the impact of the care on those outcomes, it is important to recognize the things that influence the course of illness and the rate of individual recovery, including the relative roles of acute illness, underlying or coexisting conditions (comorbidities), and the different care components.

Table 10–6, pp. 340–342, summarizes factors that are often considered in evaluating patient risk and outcomes of episodes of illness and injury. Although few studies have been done specifically in subacute settings, Table 10–7, p. 343, lists factors that have been found to be relevant to the risks and outcomes of individuals with the illnesses and overall status typical of subacute patients. The following sections summarize the major issues.

Patient-Related Characteristics

Diagnoses.   One possible way to assess subacute patient outcomes would be based on their diagnoses; for example, group those with hip fractures, those with left-sided strokes, or those with uncomplicated myocardial infarction. Efforts have been made to extend the hospital-based diagnosis-related groups (DRGs) to the subacute setting.

But subacute patients often fall in between several diagnostic categories. Patients with the same diagnosis can have significantly different levels of severity because of different coexisting conditions, factors not readily discernible on admission, and different levels of overall systems failure based on past history and age.

Furthermore, those in the same DRG categories often do not consume comparable health care resources (Soeken & Prescott, 1991), and available systems to further subcategorize DRGs offer relatively little useful gain. DRGs are based on anticipated resource consumption and modified by complications and comorbidities, which were defined as significant if their presence was likely to increase the length of stay by one day in 75% of the cases (Rosko, 1988). But these criteria are much less relevant to the subacute than to the high-acuity patient because subacute care is usually more broadly focused on managing a spectrum of problems than on aggressively treating a discrete diagnosis.

For those whose treatment is initiated in a hospital, the principal illness should have been diagnosed and enough treatment begun to stabilize them prior to transfer to a subacute program. Therefore, they are usually in another phase of their illness and the original DRG may not apply. For example, a patient admitted to the hospital with an acute myocardial infarction no longer has that problem when discharged to the subacute program, but will still be burdened by some consequences such as limited self-care, arrhythmias, or reduced cardiac output.

Thus, medical diagnoses or DRG categories alone cannot adequately differentiate subacute patients or predict their outcomes, resource use, or lengths of stay. They do not weigh sufficiently the multiple factors that may cause similar problems in different patients.

However, the number of medical diagnoses may help predict the likelihood of complications or eventual functional status. The number of concurrent conditions, compiled as the Index of Coexistent Disease (ICED) score, was found to predict complications and functional status one year postoperatively for total hip replacement patients (Greenfield et al, 1993). But the number of secondary medical diagnoses does not predict other resource needs such as the intensity of nursing care (Prescott, 1991).

Severity of Illness.   Severity of illness (SOI) measurements try to group patients to predict similar outcomes and resource use based on their levels of impairment from their medical conditions. For example, a typical SOI scale might have four groups, with those in the highest-severity group being considered to be severely affected and at the highest risk for complications or death. To date, most SOI scales have been based on physiological measurements and tend to focus on predicting the short-term risk of dying. For example, the Computerized Severity Index (CSI) is based upon the principles that severity is disease-specific, severity levels within diseases are not necessarily comparable across diseases, different diagnoses should receive different weights in rating overall patient severity, and overall severity should relate to the number of organ systems involved (Iezzoni & Daley, 1992).

However, those with similar physiologically oriented SOI scores on admission can have significantly different outcomes (Thomas & Ashcraft, 1991). Also, short-term mortality-oriented, physiologically based SOI scales are less relevant to subacute patients because relatively few subacute patients are highly unstable. Instead, they are more likely to have multidimensional problems (limited mobility, undernutrition, volume deficit, clinical instability, and so on) of diverse origin. Their outcomes—including the risk of dying—and their care needs are more likely to be influenced by the combination of their coexisting conditions and the frequency of acute complications and condition changes (Bernardini et al, 1995). Therefore, a SOI scale for subacute patients should accommodate these factors.

Table 10–8, p. 343, illustrates a way to group the risk levels of subacute patients based on the combined impact of acute and chronic conditions. The acuity categories range from those suffering little impact from acute illness to those with significant impact. The "coexisting impairments" categories range from none to severe global impairment. As Table 10–9, p. 344, illustrates, those in group 1 (minor or moderate acuity, no or low comorbidity) are more likely to recover to or beyond their premorbid state, are less likely to suffer complications of their current illnesses or treatments, and their lengths of stay and resource use are likely to be lower. Group 2 patients have an intermediate chance of all the above, and group 3 are the least likely to recover fully and the most likely to have complications, and are likely to consume the most care resources.

Thus, a chronically ill individual with a mild myocardial infarction (MI) may have the same overall risks and care needs as an otherwise fully functional person with a more severe MI. Those with a relatively minor acute illness and multiple underlying conditions often have the same level of risks, mortality, and service needs as those with a more serious acute condition but fewer comorbidities. For example, a combination of anemia, arrhythmias, and the side effects of medications used to try to control congestive heart failure may lead to volume deficit, confusion, and general deconditioning in a patient who has recently had pneumonia. Without those coexisting conditions, the patient may not have needed hospitalization initially or might have improved enough during hospitalization to not require so much postacute care.

Therefore, to assess risk and measure and compare outcomes, subacute programs must use severity of illness (acuity) measurements that consider each individual's stability and their overall burden of disease. An example of this approach is the Nursing Severity Index, which is problem-oriented rather than disease-oriented. It is comparable to, and simpler than, other SOI scales, and has also been found to predict both short-term mortality and length and costs of acute episodes of care (Rosenthal et al, 1992, 1995).

Functional Status.   Several studies (Cohen et al, 1992; Incalzi & Daley, 1992; Lichtenstein et al, 1985; Narain et al, 1988) have confirmed that activities of daily living (ADL) status is a useful predictor of outcomes and subsequent placement in the hospitalized elderly. These findings should be relevant to subacute settings because their patients often have comparable limitations, regardless of age. For example, in geriatric patients discharged from an acute hospital, a low ADL score—that is, greater dependency—at hospital discharge and the presence of neoplastic or cardiovascular diseases all predicted increased mortality and increasing physical dependency (Incalzi & Daley, 1992). Another study found that the inability to walk unassisted was a significant predictor of the risk of suffering iatrogenic complications in high-risk, long-stay, elderly medicine service inpatients (Lefevre et al, 1992).

"Ability in the areas relating to instrumental activities of daily living (IADL) that require increased interaction with the environment, whether household or community, appears to be a prerequisite for independent living in the community" (Chong, 1995). Therefore, measurements of an individual's ability to perform IADLs can help predict the likely discharge destination and required postdischarge support. Currently, several IADL measurement instruments exist, but none of them is considered a standard.

Level of Neurological Functioning.   An individual's level of consciousness reflects central nervous and circulatory system functioning plus general endocrine and metabolic status. The Glasgow Coma Score is a composite of three indicators of central nervous system function: motor responses, verbal responses, and eye opening (Teasdale & Jennett, 1974). As a reflection of altered levels of consciousness, it appears to be a useful independent predictor of mortality (Niskanen, 1991), and is one of the few independent predictors of increased risk of iatrogenic illness. In other words, those with more impaired levels of consciousness should be considered at higher risk of dying and of having complications related to their medications or treatments.

Other Factors.   A patient's total number of medications can predict the risk of iatrogenic complications (Lefevre et al, 1992) and mortality (Incalzi & Daley, 1992). Nutritional status is also very relevant to predicting outcomes. Involuntary weight loss greater than 4% of body weight appears to predict increased mortality (Wallace et al, 1995). Protein–energy undernutrition is a risk factor for 1-year post-hospital-discharge mortality, and serum albumin levels appear to relate to medical complication rate and functional outcome in geriatric stroke patients (Aptaker et al, 1994).

Based on the preceding, Table 10–10, p. 344, summarizes the core patient-related data that should be collected for all patients in all programs. This information is relevant both to providing care and to assessing care outcomes.

Resource Use and Site Characteristics

Efficiency (resource use and cost of care) is another important measure of quality. Related issues include the appropriate cost and duration of the care, and where it should be given.

Sites for Care Provision.   As discussed in Chapter 1, several different sites offer subacute care, at different licensure levels (hospital, SNF, NF). Anecdotal evidence suggests that a properly prepared program in any of these settings may potentially deliver effective subacute care. Although the quality of care undoubtedly varies among subacute programs, arguments about innate quality or outcome differences among the various sites remain unsubstantiated. Any significance of other variations in site characteristics (Table 10–11, p. 344) also remains unproven.

Cost and Duration of Care.   The appropriate amount and duration of any health care depends heavily on the care objectives. As discussed in Chapter 3, appropriate subacute care should achieve defined objectives that cannot be readily provided less expensively, or at the same cost but with other distinct advantages, elsewhere. Currently, there are some benchmarks for appropriate lengths of stay for uncomplicated procedures or problem management in otherwise stable individuals (for example, postoperative knee replacement surgery), but very few for more complicated problems or situations.

However, there is some evidence that the level of resources that various patients are likely to require can be predicted in advance based on measurable characteristics. A relevant area is the ability to anticipate the scope and intensity of nursing care. Traditional measures of nursing intensity have focused on dependency and have not usually included SOI measures. One study (Soeken & Prescott, 1991) determined factors related to acute care nursing intensity to include severity of illness, patient nursing needs (dependency), and complexity of care. Severity included both global severity and physiological status. Patient nursing needs included ADL needs, mobility, safety, and emotional need. Complexity included the complexity of nursing tasks and procedures and the complexity of decision making associated with the nursing process and level of provider needed according to a standardized scale.

However, although all three factors (severity, dependency, and complexity) relate to hours of nursing care, severity only does so to a point. In the aforementioned study, as severity increased, resource use increased at a decreasing rate, then plateaued, and finally declined. For example, a stable comatose patient may require a large amount of low-complexity care that could be provided by non-RN staff, but a newly diagnosed and unstable juvenile diabetic with multiple family and school problems may require fewer hours of care but need the skills of an advanced clinical specialist. Using hours of care alone to calculate the costs of providing care to these two patients would underestimate the costs of providing care to the latter individual (Soeken & Prescott, 1991).

In other words, those requiring more hours of nursing care have greater severity of illness and greater dependency needs and need treatments requiring a higher degree of judgment and skill. But sicker patients may not consume skilled nursing time as much as the time of other staff such as nursing assistants. Nursing resource utilization appears to depend more on the skill level of the care than on the quantity of care. Therefore, the availability of a mix of those with appropriate skill levels may be more relevant to the care of subacute patients than just considering staffing hours.

This is consistent with other evidence, discussed above, about the factors that are most relevant to assessing subacute patient risk and outcomes. It is also compatible with the findings of the Health Care Financing Administration (HCFA) case-mix project. The data collected by HCFA as the basis for its case-mix payment system for skilled nursing facilities (SNFs) and nursing facilities (NFs) suggest that service needs can be predicted by a combination of factors, including ADL dependency levels, and the presence of certain specific conditions including depression, neurological disorders, second- or third-degree burns, open wound or skin lesions, explicit terminal prognosis, hemiplegia or quadriplegia, and septicemia. More investigation of the impact of comorbidity and acuity on the cost and duration of care in subacute patients is desirable.

Availability and Frequency of Treatments and Services.   Much debate about subacute care and care sites has related to the nature and frequency of the treatments and therapies (for example, respiratory, physical, occupational, or speech therapy) that patients receive. However, although any treatments must be given by appropriately skilled individuals, both their optimal frequency or intensity and who should do them is still often unsubstantiated. Currently, who does procedures, and how often treatments are given, may depend on the availability of reimbursement or specific staff as much as or more than on actual patient need. Additionally, more frequent or complex treatment is not necessarily associated with better care or outcome. For example, a simple once-daily ventilator weaning program appears to be more effective than either intermittent mandatory ventilation or pressure-support ventilation, both of which are more complicated and time consuming for staff (Esteban et al, 1995).

Availability and Characteristics of Other Practitioners.   Principal areas of physician involvement with subacute patients are assessment of progress and response to treatment, help in properly defining patient problems and identifying their causes, recognition and management of causes of complications, prevention of nosocomial and iatrogenic illness, and provision of information and support for patient, family, and staff decision making.

All subacute patients do not need the same degree of physician intervention, which could range from several times daily to only occasionally. For instance, a patient with frequent predictable infections may be treated using protocols with little physician reassessment, but someone with fluctuations in condition or new onset of complications may need more frequent or intensive physician evaluation and intervention. The quantity of physician services that patients receive may or may not have much to do with their outcomes.

Subacute programs use several different models of physician coverage, which may also include nurse practitioners, physician assistants, or nurses to perform some traditional physician functions such as assessment, documentation, and monitoring. Regular physician availability is important for adequate management of actively unstable patients. However, there is no evidence that any one of these models is more effective than others, to relate the frequency of physician visits to outcomes for the subacute patient, or to support an optimal number of physician visits for any episode of illness.

AN APPROACH TO A SUBACUTE QUALITY ASSESSMENT PROGRAM

Currently, subacute care—like long-term NF-based care—is handicapped by the scarcity of comparative data and appropriate benchmarks. Although many of the factors affecting patient outcomes are being identified, their relative contributions need further clarification.

Efficient Data Usage.   Fortunately, many of the same data needed to assess quality are relevant to providing care. Therefore, a properly designed, appropriately computerized database for each patient and for related programmatic processes can support both the care and quality assessments. For instance, Table 10–12, p. 345, shows how clinically relevant data can be used to help improve the care. This information can be used to anticipate patient service needs, to prepare to deliver care (for example, staffing requirements), to anticipate possible patient risks, to try to prevent certain complications, and to assess the eventual outcomes.

For the foreseeable future, subacute programs will therefore be in the position of collecting data both for their own purposes and to help establish appropriate benchmarks. The time spent will be more worthwhile if some common approaches to data collection and outcomes measurement can be determined.

The next sections suggest steps for creating a clinically relevant, comparatively efficient quality assessment process (Table 10–13, p. 346).

Identify Care and Support Processes

First, each subacute program should recognize its overall purpose and understand vital processes of care and support needed to accomplish its overall objectives. The mutual impact of those processes and of individual performance should be assessed. Many process-related quality indicators may be drawn directly from clear policies, procedures, practice guidelines, and job descriptions. For instance, guidelines for wound care or pain management include processes such as assessment and treatment, which should influence policies and procedures (who should do what, and in what manner). The actual performance can then be compared to desired performance, providing the basis for quality indicators.

Define the Patient Database

Secondly, subacute programs should define their clinical patient database to include information that is relevant to delivering care and to assessing outcomes. They should ensure that the data are measured and coded reliably and consistently.

Subacute patient status and outcomes may be evaluated by objective anatomic and physiological measurements, functional measurement, and measuring overall patient function or performance including severity of illness (acuity) levels.

Assessing Physical Status and Improvement. Anatomic and physiological variables (such as blood pressure and range of motion of a joint) are generally easier to measure than functional levels (for example, ability to perform physical work and social functioning; Schyve, 1995). As much as possible, practitioners should use standardized, coded, objective physical measurements of both specific bodily functions (such as heart rate and rhythm, blood gases, and renal function tests) and general physical status (such as level of consciousness). For instance, patients who are admitted for pain management should have fairly detailed documentation of the number, frequency, duration, and intensity of their pain episodes, in addition to qualitative descriptions of their pain. Pain intensity should be coded on some objective scale that can be used by multiple observers (for example, ranging from 0 for no pain to 4+ for severe pain).

Assessing Functional Status and Improvement. Because functional status strongly influences various outcomes, subacute programs should measure functional status for all their patients, including those admitted with primarily medical needs—just as all patients who are admitted principally for rehabilitation therapies should have some physiological measurements.

There are several scales for measuring functional status. Common ones include the Functional Independence Measure (FIM), Barthel Index, Katz ADL Scale, and portions of the Minimum Data Set (MDS) for SNFs and NFs providing both long-term and subacute care.

For instance, the FIM, which is increasingly common among rehabilitation programs, contains 18 items covering areas of self-care, sphincter control, mobility, communication, and cognition. Each item has scores ranging from a maximum of 7 (complete independence) to a minimum of 1 (total assistance) based on actual performance rather than capacity. Thus, the total scores range from 18 to 126. Admission data should be collected within 72 hours of admission, and discharge data within 72 hours prior to discharge. The clinician observing the patient assesses function directly. When differences in function occur at different sites or different times of day, the lowest score is used.

Most SNFs and NFs must use a federally mandated resident assessment instrument for their long-term patients. It consists of two elements, the MDS and the Resident Assessment Protocols (RAPs; Chapter 9). The MDS is a collection of information regarding an individual's functional status, psychosocial status, medical conditions, cognitive patterns, communication and hearing patterns, physical functioning and structural problems, continence, diagnoses, skin condition, health conditions, and special treatments and procedures. The data are to be collected within 14 days of admission and periodically thereafter, depending on condition changes.

There is debate over which functional measurement scale is most appropriate. Investigations to date have reached different conclusions about the inherent value and relative merits of various scales (Kidd et al, 1995). However, measuring functional independence must be combined with other health-related assessments such as acuity to accurately evaluate outcomes. Therefore, it may be more important for outcomes measurements to determine an overall level or range of functional impairment (for example, none, minimal, moderate, total) than to be overly concerned about which scale is used. As long as comparable ranges can be developed for various instruments measuring function, any one of them may serve the purpose.

Assessing Overall Status and Improvement.   Important measurements of overall status include psychosocial status (return to work, patient well-being) and general medical status (primarily, the level of overall stability and comorbidities). These are relevant to all patients, not just those admitted for medical reasons. Although most reports on rehabilitation try to demonstrate the effectiveness of rehabilitation treatment by comparing the patient's previous functional levels with the final results, it appears that both medical stability and comorbidities must be taken into account. Comorbidities and adverse clinical events (any acute or subacute change in health status—indicated by specific signs, symptoms, and/or laboratory findings—suggesting the appearance of acute or subacute illness) both influence functional recovery (Bernardini, 1995). Again, a problem-oriented SOI scale such as the Nursing Severity Index (Rosenthal et al, 1992, 1995) deserves more investigation as a relevant tool for subacute care because it takes these factors into account, is simple to use, is clinically relevant, and also has the advantage of representing both comorbidities and severity of illness in a single instrument (see Chapter 7).

Collect the Data

Every subacute program should thus assess its patients in several dimensions, including indicators of physical, functional, and overall status and improvement. It should measure severity of illness, the overall burden of coexisting diseases, and the intermittent occurrence of acute clinical events. It should record such information on admission and on discharge, and periodically during the patient's stay—especially if the stay is prolonged or when there is a significant condition change. Discharge data should be compared with assessments performed prior to or at the time of admission. It should determine and document care objectives and note the occurrence of other relevant factors, such as the onset of probable nosocomial or iatrogenic illnesses. It should also be part of a broader approach that considers longer-term results.

Analyze Individual and Aggregate Data

It is important to evaluate individual patient outcomes. Because of the great variety and scope of service needs of these patients, it is useful to subgroup them by common characteristics and to aggregate the outcomes of many subacute patients, adjusted statistically to control for the differences caused by the other factors known to affect those outcomes (such as severity of illness and comorbidities; Table 10–14, p. 346).

But subacute outcome and quality assessments must recognize the difference between grouping results and average results. "Average" results do not reflect the variations among individual cases, or the variable case mix among programs. For example, it is not enough to say that 72% of a program's ventilator patients are weaned, or that 84% of stroke patients are discharged home. Such conclusions do not reveal the factors that facilitated weaning in some or prevented it in others, or about whether patients in either group had comparable severity of illness or levels of risk when they began their stay.

Thus, subacute programs should adjust individual patient outcomes for various risk factors, and then aggregate the risk-adjusted data appropriately to evaluate patient outcomes and care quality. Data from previous patients should be used to establish internal benchmarks, which can be compared to other sites and used to improve the care of subsequent patients.

Problem-Specific Measures.   Some outcome measurement tools for specific programs or treatment areas (such as back injury, trauma, or joint replacement) have been based on various combinations of physical, functional, and overall assessment instruments. For example, trauma patient outcomes could be assessed using an ADL functional rating scale, dependency scale, and work disability scale. However, each of these problem- or condition-specific approaches must still factor in severity of illness and comorbidity adjustments. Table 10–15, p. 347, is an example of some databases developed by a consortium of participants in the subacute industry to assess the outcomes of pain management and wound care patients.

Assessing the Quality of Subacute Processes

Care outcomes must be achieved both by doing positive things (for example, monitoring progress, delivering treatments) or by preventing negative occurrences such as iatrogenic or nosocomial illnesses. Outcomes assessments primarily help measure the effectiveness, efficiency, and supportiveness of care. But alone they are insufficient to evaluate all aspects of quality (Table 10–1, p. 337).

Process is important because it influences and reflects performance, which can affect the effectiveness and appropriateness of the care. Process-related indicators may also reflect other quality-related attributes including the timeliness, continuity, privacy, confidentiality, efficiency, patient and family participation, and safety of the care. Less than full recovery, the occurrence of complications, or a prolonged recovery period should be due to the unavoidable impact of disease processes, not to something about the care, care site, or practitioners. Consistent processes are also essential to improve outcomes comparison because excessive process variation among practitioners or care sites undermines such efforts.

Table 10–16, p. 347, describes the several kinds of processes in subacute programs. It is useful to differentiate these for the purposes of quality oversight.

Appropriate Patient Selection

Each program should have a process for patient selection and preadmission evaluation to ensure that it can care for the patients it accepts. Trying to prevent inappropriate admissions and premature transfers is an important risk-management function. It is unsafe and inefficient for patients to be admitted without adequate preparation by the receiving facility, or to have to be transferred out soon after admission because they are too sick.

Currently, there is no benchmark for an acceptable percentage of patients who have to be transferred out unexpectedly soon after admission. However, allowing for occasional changes in condition between the time of discharge and arrival at the facility, such transfers should occur very infrequently. A process that selects patients appropriately and rarely leads to premature discharge should be considered adequate.

Each subacute program should address the causes of admissions-related problems, including the circumstances surrounding each patient who must be transferred soon after admission. The results of those reviews should be considered within the quality program.

Other than referrals coming from within their own programs or network, a program's ability to make such decisions—for example, receiving timely, accurate information from the referral source—may not be readily within its control. Referral sources should be providing ample information for appropriate decision making. The subacute program should give referring programs feedback about how well they provide sufficient accurate information and support continuity of care for their referrals. A subacute program's reluctance to do this out of fear of not getting referrals may be a systems issue that needs to be addressed at a higher (community- or organization-based) level. Each program should also assess discrepancies between its own preadmission and postadmission assessment data. For example, it is important to know if a particular referring program consistently underreports the various secondary problems of its transfers, which in turn delays effective problem management by the subacute program. The failure of various components of the health care system to address such process issues cannot continue to be condoned.

EXAMPLE

Because of administrative pressure to fill beds, a subacute program almost never turns down referrals. As the lengths of stay in local hospitals have shortened, more patients have been transferred from those hospitals with inadequate information, or who are so unstable on arrival that they must be transferred back within 1 to 3 days. The administrator has refused to discuss this with the hospitals and has not permitted his admissions staff to address the problems or to turn down patients, telling the staff that a patient in a bed for even 2 days is better than an empty bed. He always blames the problem on the referral sources, and will not admit that the subacute program is not careful enough in its selection process. The staff physicians are aware of this problem but the administrator will not permit them or the medical director to address it at higher levels.

This disregard for dealing with a problem that jeopardizes patient safety should be considered a quality problem at both the referring and the receiving sites. It should affect each program's licensure and accreditation results. Unless all these players take it seriously, it will not soon be corrected.

Data Sources.   In reviewing issues related to admissions processes, the direct care staff and patient records are important sources of information. The reasons for discharge from the program should be coded (Table 10–17, p. 348). The warning signs or common characteristics of the premature discharges should be sought to allow the program to better anticipate and address the issues. For example, a program should focus more carefully during patient selection processes on referrals who have combinations of problems similar to those of former patients who had to be discharged soon after admission. The program should also review reasons for rejecting various prospective admissions to help it understand the characteristics of those patients and how they might better accommodate a broader patient spectrum. The program administration should help address any problems.

Postselection, Preadmission Preparation

Once patients are accepted for admission, the staff should be prepared to accept and manage them. Generally, the greatest workload for care providers is at the beginning and end of a patient's stay. Many tasks must be performed, including extensive assessment, documentation, and preparation either for the admission or for transfer.

Every program should assess the consistency, supportiveness, and efficiency of this process. Examples of relevant processes include the ease of obtaining equipment and supplies, the dependability of the admissions office in providing adequate notification and documentation regarding impending admissions, and the consistency with which the program adjusts to unanticipated patient needs. It is important to evaluate whether any delays or other process problems in preparation for admission might have contributed to premature discharge or other significant problems identified early in a patient's stay.

Data Sources.   The nursing staff and other disciplines involved in patient care, as well as support departments such as housekeeping and dietary services, are important sources of information about the consistency of the processes and the availability of essential supplies and equipment.

Assessments

Every patient needs a multidimensional assessment as a prelude to defining problems and identifying and addressing their causes. Standards for participation should avoid excessive structural indicators that mandate specific formats (in contrast to content) for the assessment or specific disciplines to do them, unless there are compelling reasons to do so. As computerization replaces discipline-specific paper forms with more flexible unified databases, traditional role divisions for performing and documenting assessments should also adapt.

Each program should ensure that the assessments contain appropriate items. Some items (for example, cardiovascular status, decision-making capacity, and nutritional status) should be assessed in every individual. Others (for example, details of extremity range of motion) may depend on the patient's problems and the reasons for the care.

Data Sources.   The assessments should be reviewed for content, completeness, and timeliness. The completeness and timeliness of medical and nonmedical problem identification, reflected in problem lists and other related documentation, are important indicators of the quality of the assessment process. Gaps in assessment should not contribute to delays in problem identification and management.

Problem Definition

The overall objective of the care of patients with complex illnesses is to manage all the problems necessary to accomplish the desired result. Review of the problem-definition process should ensure that it defines each patient's significant problems and diagnoses fully and correctly, so that they can be managed effectively.

It might be argued that effective problem management will demonstrate an effective problem definition process. If the patient improves completely and rapidly, the results might be used to assume the correct process; that is, that all relevant problems were addressed. But a prolonged stay or a less than full recovery cannot automatically be attributed to the illness without considering the process. Even if all identified problems were managed appropriately, it is still possible that some important problems could have been missed.

Review of the problem definition process should ensure that it includes all relevant disciplines, and that responsibility for problem identification and definition are coordinated with the responsibility for problem management. In addition to ensuring that these functions are done, there should be flexibility in specifying who should do them.

Data Sources.   The scope and severity of problems on admission should be compared to those upon discharge. Again, use of a problem-oriented approach to care can help streamline the process.

Care Planning

The management of diverse problems requires coordination of the performances of many individuals. A systematic care planning process should provide that framework. The care plan must also be flexible enough to ensure adequate response to condition changes and problems in achieving care objectives.

A review of the care planning process should ensure that a written care plan outlines a systematic approach to meet identified patient needs, and involves relevant disciplines and the patient and family. The care plan process review should also ensure that patient needs are identified; realistic, measurable care objectives are established; appropriate disciplines are responsible for performing essential functions; an expected time frame for achieving the goals and the anticipated disposition are proposed; and contingency plans exist for handling potential significant condition changes. Also, there should be evidence that the care plans are updated when significant condition changes occur.

Care plan reviews may also be used to assess gaps or inconsistencies in service provision by comparing the tasks (specific procedures or responsibilities) identified in or implied by the care plan to records of their actual provision. For example, any vital sign monitoring or attempts at weaning from a ventilator must be done as indicated.

Data Sources.   Patient care plans and related documentation (for example, progress notes relating family discussions) are sources for this care review. The responsibilities identified in the care plan should be matched to treatment records.

Problem Management

Effective problem management includes two major components: optimal practice and risk management. Problem management process review should ensure that responsibilities for performing these functions are identified, and that various conditions are managed according to accepted medical protocols and guidelines. Problem management that does not fall within such guidelines may be acceptable, but should be supported by adequate documentation. Some system should exist to identify and address practices or processes that are clearly inappropriate or substandard. There should also be identifiable reasons for not managing certain problems, for example, when an abnormality or potential problem is not clinically relevant or should not be managed due to advance directives, excessive risk, or because treatment is unlikely to improve care outcomes.

Data Sources.   Selected patient records should be reviewed for evidence of how identified problems were addressed. Wherever possible, this should be matched to appropriate standards, critical pathways, policies, protocols, and practice guidelines. Cases should be reviewed for whether predictable problems were anticipated and preventive measures were taken—especially where acute condition changes occurred during the stay, or where the treatment course had to be interrupted or the outcome was not as anticipated.

Patient Monitoring

Monitoring is the basis for adjusting the care plan and treatment and for discharge planning. Various phases of monitoring may be assigned to one specific discipline or sometimes may be interdisciplinary. Quality reviews of patient monitoring processes should ensure that the responsibilities for monitoring are assigned appropriately and carried out consistently.

Data Sources.   Patient record documentation (progress notes, vital signs, and other similar records) should reflect ongoing monitoring of each patient in essential areas. When unexpected problems occur, the treatment plan is interrupted unexpectedly, or complications result in substantial additional illness or treatment, it is important to review the monitoring processes to demonstrate that such outcomes resulted from the condition rather than from lapses in care.

Completion of Treatment Course

Numerous processes are involved in discharging and transferring patients. Some of these relate to the decision to discharge, some to the preparation for discharge, and some to the actual physical process of discharge. Each step should involve both the providers (sending and receiving facilities and practitioners) and the recipients (patients, families, and payers) of care.

A process review should ensure that appropriate criteria and processes were used to determine the appropriate time for patient discharge, and that the discharge was consistent with the care objectives, the length of stay was appropriate, significant interruptions of the treatment course were unavoidable, and the patient and family were appropriately involved in the planning.

Discharge processes should also be assessed for their support of care continuity. Additionally, processes should be examined for the factors that inhibit such goals, for example, if discharge is held up by the lack of adequate documentation or the failure to notify a receiving facility of some equipment or supply needs.

Data Sources.   The discharge process may be reviewed by examining related documentation for individual cases (for example, care plan meetings), and through feedback from staff, patients, and families. The quality of each program's support as a transferring site could be assessed in part by asking referral sources to assess the program's performance as a sending facility.

Patient/Family Education and Training

Patients and families should be helped to become more effective participants in the care. The exact impact of these educational efforts on patient and family behavior, and on the outcomes of an episode of illness, are hard to measure. However, the underlying presumption, based on some empirical evidence, is that effective patient and family participation helps make the care more effective and efficient, and respects patients' rights. A review should also assess the efficiency of the processes of providing the information and education.

Data Sources.   Cases should be reviewed for evidence of whether patients were informed about their condition, prognosis, treatments, continuing care, and care options. The effectiveness of such processes may be assessed by comparing patient and family understanding of the condition, treatments, care options, and follow-up needs, and assessing their ability to perform specific tasks such as changing dressings, before and after such instruction.

Follow-Up

A subacute care stay should achieve certain objectives. Care outcomes represent the impact on the patient, and process outcomes concern the means by which the care was delivered and supported.

Care processes and outcomes should be reviewed for each stay (Table 10–18, p. 348). Follow-up process review should attempt to identify the obstacles to efficient performance of tasks associated with the care. Problems and concerns raised by care providers or recipients during the stay should be identified and addressed as part of a quality improvement program. The costs of care and length of stay should be reviewed to see if they were justified or were increased by process or performance problems.

The program should consider and act upon the results of those reviews. Over time, there should be some measurable improvements in the processes of care, or verification that they are optimal, as a result of applying these principles. This can be assessed by analyzing the same elements in the care of subsequent patients.

Data Sources.   The two most important data sources for follow-up process assessment are the staff and the patients.

Patient Satisfaction.   Patient satisfaction evaluation is a critical component of any subacute program, reflecting outcomes of both care and care processes as they impact the patient and family. The questions must be specific enough so that the answers are relevant and useful (for example, see Figure 10–1). The findings of such surveys should be considered by the program or service (subacute, acute, long-term care, or the like) and by the whole organization or network.

Staff Satisfaction.   If patient and family satisfaction reflect results, then staff satisfaction helps measure the success of the processes underlying the care. Because care recipients and payers have little interest in the behind-the-scenes influences on processes, their satisfaction with the care or the results of their stay does not necessarily reflect the efficiency and support of the program for those giving the care. A relevant quality improvement program should seek to improve the efficiency and effectiveness of those providing the care and those who support them. Figure 10–2 gives an example of such a survey. Generic processes (that is, those related to the operation of the organization or program) should also be assessed periodically. For example, Figure 10–3 suggests survey questions to evaluate the effectiveness of communications processes, based on the principles discussed in Chapter 9.

IMPROVING PERFORMANCE AND OUTCOMES

Using Quality Assessment Information to Improve the Program

Quality-related findings should be used to improve all aspects of, and participants in, the program, from governance to direct care delivery. Undoubtedly, a balance is needed between the time and money spent delivering the care and that spent changing systems and processes. A pertinent quality management and improvement system addresses all of these issues—not all at once, but systematically and persistently. It coordinates the people, processes, reviews of care, data analyses, and applications of the analyses to improve the care. Eventually, all care- and support-related processes should be assessed for possible barriers and sources of improvement.

Care outcome assessments reflect past and current performance. Assessing the process helps provide information about whether performance can be sustained or improved, and about how processes may affect outcomes. Performance improvement in a complex system must be based upon both individual and systems development.

A Vital Investment.   Health care facility and program managers and staff may tend to shortchange quality programs. Unfortunately, some programs have failed to use adequate standards and quality assessment and improvement processes. Or, they may use such standards and processes only for some of those in the program, for example, for those delivering the care but not for those in support services, management, or governance.

In the past, many organizations were lax in addressing these weaknesses because reimbursement continued to flow in despite unresolved problems with the care, the support systems, or the management. Not recognizing the value of

FIGURE 10–1   PATIENT/FAMILY SATISFACTION SURVEY FOR A SUBACUTE PROGRAM

Item	Minimal Performance	Optimal Performance	Score
To what extent were the processes of care explained from preadmission through discharge?	None of the processes that were to occur before, during, and after the stay were explained to me (us).	All of the processes that were to occur before, during, and after the stay were explained to me (us).	Minimal Optimal 0 1 2 3 4 5 6 7 8 9 10
Were your questions and concerns during your stay addressed to your satisfaction?	No one tried to address any of my (our) questions and concerns during the stay.	Someone always tried to address my (our) questions and concerns during the stay.	Minimal Optimal 0 1 2 3 4 5 6 7 8 9 10
Were the objectives of care, and of this overall stay, explained to your satisfaction?	The objectives were not explained at all.	The objectives were explained so that I (we) understood fully.	Minimal Optimal 0 1 2 3 4 5 6 7 8 9 10
To what extent did you find the staff to be helpful and courteous?	The staff were almost never helpful and courteous.	The staff were always helpful and courteous.	Minimal Optimal 0 1 2 3 4 5 6 7 8 9 10
To what extent were the physician(s) providing your care responsive to your questions and concerns?	The physician(s) was (were) not attentive and not helpful.	The physician(s) was (were) very attentive and helpful.	Minimal Optimal 0 1 2 3 4 5 6 7 8 9 10
How would you rate the overall value of the care you received during your stay?	The care did not seem to me (us) to be what it should have been, in any way.	The care seemed to me (us) as good as one could reasonably anticipate in any setting.	Minimal Optimal 0 1 2 3 4 5 6 7 8 9 10
How would you rate the overall value of the service you received during your stay?	The overall service quality during this stay was uniformly poor.	The overall service quality during this stay was outstanding.	Minimal Optimal 0 1 2 3 4 5 6 7 8 9 10
To what extent do you believe that the outcome of your care was the best that could have been achieved in the situation?	The results of this stay were much worse than they should have been.	The results of this stay were the best that could possibly be attained anywhere.	Minimal Optimal 0 1 2 3 4 5 6 7 8 9 10
To what extent did the care meet your overall expectations?	Much worse than expected.	Much better than expected.	Minimal Optimal 0 1 2 3 4 5 6 7 8 9 10
To what extent did the outcome meet your overall expectations?	It was substantially less than what I (we) expected.	It met or exceeded my (our) expectations.	Minimal Optimal 0 1 2 3 4 5 6 7 8 9 10

Suggested scoring: evaluate above 10 items from 0 (worst case) to 10 (best case); add total score:_____

- 85+   : Superior performance highly pertinent to needs of this subacute patient
- 75–84 : Very good performance with some room for improvements in some areas
- 60–74 : Good performance with more than minimal improvement needed in some performance areas
- 50–59 : Borderline performance needing significant improvement in a number of areas
- < 50   : Should have detailed review to address overall performance for this patient's stay

FIGURE 10–2   STAFF/PRACTITIONER SATISFACTION SURVEY FOR A SUBACUTE PROGRAM

Item	Minimal Performance	Optimal Performance	Score
To what extent are you able to perform your job appropriately, effectively and efficiently during a patient's stay?	I am almost never able to do my job as efficiently and effectively as possible.	I am always able to do my job as efficiently and effectively as possible.	Minimal Optimal 0 1 2 3 4 5 6 7 8 9 10
To what extent were essential supplies and equipment available, adequate, and usable?	Essential supplies and equipment were almost always unavailable and rarely trouble-free.	Essential supplies and equipment were always available and trouble-free.	Minimal Optimal 0 1 2 3 4 5 6 7 8 9 10
To what extent are the patients appropriate for this setting and for the kinds of care that you are expected to deliver?	None of the patients are appropriate for this setting, or need the care that is being offered.	The patients are all appropriate for this setting, and need the care that is being offered.	Minimal Optimal 0 1 2 3 4 5 6 7 8 9 10
To what extent does this organization help you accomplish the objectives of providing or supporting the care?	The organization is never helpful or supportive.	The organization is always very helpful and supportive.	Minimal Optimal 0 1 2 3 4 5 6 7 8 9 10
To what extent are the other direct care staff and practitioners collaborative and supportive?	Other staff and practitioners are rarely collaborative and supportive.	Other staff and practitioners are consistently collaborative and supportive.	Minimal Optimal 0 1 2 3 4 5 6 7 8 9 10
To what extent are the management and support staff collaborative and supportive?	Management and support staff are rarely collaborative and supportive.	Management and support staff are consistently collaborative and supportive.	Minimal Optimal 0 1 2 3 4 5 6 7 8 9 10
How would you rate the quality of the information and communications you received?	The information and communications are rarely accurate, timely, or reliable.	The information and communications are routinely accurate, timely, and reliable.	Minimal Optimal 0 1 2 3 4 5 6 7 8 9 10
To what extent does this program avoid causing problems and complications in its patients?	The program often causes or contributes to problems and complications in the patients.	The program consistently avoids causing problems and complications in the patients.	Minimal Optimal 0 1 2 3 4 5 6 7 8 9 10
How would you rate the overall value of the care delivered to the patients treated in this program?	The care rarely appears to help achieve desired outcomes, and rarely seems to be of value to the patients and families.	The care consistently appears to contribute to desired outcomes, and appears to be of great value to the patients and families.	Minimal Optimal 0 1 2 3 4 5 6 7 8 9 10
How satisfied overall are you to be participating in delivering care or service in this program?	Very dissatisfied.	Very satisfied.	

Use of this instrument: rate each of the above items from 0 (minimal) to 10 (optimal).

FIGURE 10–3   STAFF/PRACTITIONER COMMUNICATIONS SURVEY FOR A SUBACUTE PROGRAM

Item	Score
To what extent do other staff and management with whom I try to communicate generally acknowledge what I wish to say?	Rarely Always 0 1 2 3 4 5 6 7 8 9 10
How willingly do those with whom I try to communicate accept additional information that I may try to present to clarify the communication or support the conclusion?	Not at all Totally 0 1 2 3 4 5 6 7 8 9 10
How well do those who try to communicate with me attempt to clarify whether I understand?	Not at all Totally 0 1 2 3 4 5 6 7 8 9 10
If I do not understand and ask for clarification, to what extent do those who try to communicate with me make additional effort to try to explain?	Rarely Always 0 1 2 3 4 5 6 7 8 9 10
To what extent do people try to explain the basis for their recommendations or conclusions?	Rarely Always 0 1 2 3 4 5 6 7 8 9 10
To what extent do we try to improve acknowledgment and understanding before trying to reach agreements?	Rarely Always 0 1 2 3 4 5 6 7 8 9 10
To what extent do we try to validate the information that is communicated?	Rarely Always 0 1 2 3 4 5 6 7 8 9 10
How well do we succeed at *not* personalizing disagreements (not viewing them as one person against another but as one set of ideas in contrast to another set)?	Not at all Totally 0 1 2 3 4 5 6 7 8 9 10
How well do we distinguish reaching agreement about facts from agreeing on the conclusions based on those facts?	Not at all Totally 0 1 2 3 4 5 6 7 8 9 10
Overall, to what extent do our overall communications systems and processes successfully support effective performance?	Rarely Always 0 1 2 3 4 5 6 7 8 9 10

efficient process and satisfied staff, some owners and managers justify minimal efforts to improve systems, and demand that their staff keep the beds filled and simply deliver the care.

Unlike systems and process readjustments, care delivery generates revenues directly. But things that impede practitioner performance will inhibit efficient care delivery, and things that enhance performance will help accomplish it. For example, an effectively designed computerized database and reporting system can allow the data collected while delivering the care to be used to analyze and improve the care, and also help analyze costs and collect reimbursements. Potential examples of obstacles include inadequate information or information systems, time-consuming barriers to effective communication, individual or departmental territorial and control squabbles, or difficulty in obtaining adequate supplies and having functioning equipment.

Tables 10–19 to 10–22, pp. 349–351, contain examples of structural and process issues where indicators should be developed to evaluate the program, the care, and the support systems.

Process Standardization

One objective of quality improvement activities generally is to standardize processes better to reduce undesirable individual variation while still maintaining adequate flexibility. This is helpful both to achieving care outcomes and to enable more meaningful comparison of them. Therefore, programs should try to standardize processes whenever excessive process variation may pose problems. This is not the same as restricting treatment options.

Two approaches to process standardization have been critical pathways and clinical practice guidelines (CPGs). Critical pathways are attempts to provide a roadmap of the overall care and service. For example, a knee replacement patient should have certain assessments on day 1, certain tests on day 3, and should be making a certain level of progress by day 7 (see Figure 9–2, p. 274).

CPGs are an attempt to provide guidance for "best practices" or appropriate performance to manage specific conditions or circumstances. For example, the Agency for Health Care Policy and Research (AHCPR) has produced a number of guidelines, including those for managing depression, pressure ulcers, and heart failure. They give practitioners (primarily physicians) a core approach to managing common conditions while still allowing them the flexibility to choose from a broad array of options at specific steps. But these guidelines are limited because they do not always recognize the variations relevant to different levels of care.

There is still ample resistance to the use of such guidelines. Concerns include the alleged limitations on flexibility for practitioners and the possibility of their use in legal actions. However, well-designed guidelines allow for variance that is appropriately explained and demonstrated to be in the patient's best interests. Both critical pathways and CPGs have an important place in quality assessment and improvement activities, especially in areas such as improving care efficiency, preventing iatrogenic illness, reducing risk, and evaluating the effectiveness of assessment, problem identification, problem management, and monitoring processes. Despite limitations, such guidelines are becoming more widely used, especially as studies gradually demonstrate which treatment protocols have more or less value in managing various conditions (Grimshaw & Russell, 1993).

SUBACUTE ACCREDITATION AND QUALITY STANDARDS

Many subacute programs are seeking accreditation from recognized agencies and organizations to demonstrate their level of compliance with standards or because of third-party insurer or state licensure requirements. The principal sources of accreditation for subacute programs are the Joint Commission on Accreditation of Healthcare Organizations (JCAHO) and the Commission on Accreditation of Rehabilitation Facilities (CARF). Both of these subacute accreditation programs began in 1995, and their standards and survey protocols are published and available to any interested parties.

JCAHO Subacute Accreditation

The JCAHO is an Illinois-based organization governed by a consortium of several major health care provider associations, including the American Hospital Association (AHA) and the American Medical Association. It offers voluntary accreditation surveys for a number of health-related programs including long-term care organizations, hospitals, nonhospital psychiatric and substance abuse organizations, home care and ambulatory care organizations, and health care networks. Its accreditation may be granted unconditionally or provisionally, with various levels of commendation or recommendations. An accreditation award is valid for 3 years unless revoked for specified reasons.

The subacute accreditation standards evolved from both the long-term care and hospital standards, reinterpreted to be more relevant to subacute care patients and care objectives. Many of these requirements represent core standards; that is, they are common to all levels and varieties of health care organizations. The standards are organized to encourage and reflect a functional rather than a discipline- or department-specific approach to providing care. The two main sections are patient- or resident-focused functions (patient/resident rights and organizational ethics, continuum of care, and patient/resident assessment, care and treatment, and education), and organization functions (improving organization performance, leadership, managing the environment of care, human resources, information management, and infection surveillance and control).

Overall, the JCAHO accreditation process and standards—including those for subacute care—have shifted from a heavy structure and process orientation to one emphasizing the impact of processes on care outcomes, and expecting a facility- and program-wide quality effort to improve both the efficacy and efficiency of care. Surveyors are guided to use quality indicators to assess actual organization performance, including the roles of leadership, practitioners, and other staff. They are also directed to focus on evidence of the organization's efforts to systematically identify and address areas for improvement, including important functions and work processes.

CARF Accreditation

CARF is an Arizona-based organization representing the principal accreditation source for rehabilitation providers. It is also sponsored by a consortium of organizations including the AHA, American Academy of Physical Medicine and Rehabilitation, and American Physical Therapy Association. CARF accredits various categories or types of rehabilitation programs, such as comprehensive inpatient rehabilitation, brain injury, chronic pain management, and spinal cord injury.

The core CARF principles require accredited organizations to promote basic human rights, health, and dignity; to incorporate the wishes and opinions of those served; to provide services designed to enhance the independence, self-sufficiency, and productivity of persons served; and to provide coordinated, individualized, goal-oriented services leading to desired outcomes. Providers are expected to have systems for measuring outcomes and using the results of those measurements in planning programs and services.

The CARF standards are divided into several sections: promoting organizational quality (organization philosophy and mission, governance, structure and management, fiscal management, planning, personnel, and physical plant and transportation); promoting program quality (patient rights, intake management, orientation, individual program planning, discharge planning, and medical records); outcome measurement and management (program evaluation, assessing service quality, analysis and utilization of information); and general and specific program standards (medical and occupational rehabilitation, brain injury, and so on; CARF, 1995).

Advantages and Limitations of Accreditation Programs

All subacute programs should provide appropriate and efficient care and should meet some quality standards. The difficult part is how much these survey results reflect compliance with standards and, in turn, how much compliance ensures appropriate care and service.

All parties (including government agencies, insurers, facilities, and patients) should have a clear understanding of the scope and limitations of accreditation programs. On the positive side, the evolution of standards has supported changes in the health care industry, including an essential focus on improving systems and processes. Standards also shift the focus away from government regulation and toward voluntary compliance. Licensure requirements, which are state-specific, grant organizations the right to operate facilities based on meeting certain general and some specific requirements. Accreditation programs provide many more specific expectations for the structure, processes, and expected results of the performance of individuals and organizations.

On the other hand, standards may explain in detail what is expected of various participants but still usually do not reveal how to achieve those expectations appropriately or efficiently. Accreditation visits only occur every several years, and are usually announced. Despite some recent progress, some surveys may still focus more on the potential for appropriate performance than on the actual performance and results. Progress in examining outcomes and holding programs to explicit quality indicators is still slow. It is also expensive for programs to have to comply with several different accreditation programs, especially when many of the standards are redundant. More, or more stringent, standards do not necessarily lead to better service value or quality. Standards related to organizational quality, physical plant management, patient rights, and care processes can and should be consolidated and made uniform for the various accrediting agencies.

Also, some current standards are of dubious value. For instance, some of the detailed structure and process requirements of the CARF standards may be contrary to desired flexibility and cost reduction in a managed care environment. For example, CARF standards (CARF, 1995) require that rehabilitation beds should be in a designated area and used for the purpose of providing a rehabilitation program (p. 91-5.A), despite the evidence that many rehabilitation patients have mixed medical and functional problems and the fact that other arrangements may work equally well. Specific CARF program standards require full-time social workers, physical and occupational therapists, psychologists, and other disciplines (p. 96-5.B), despite the lack of evidence that such structural requirements are better than the part-time or "as needed" participation of such individuals. Also, the CARF standards require medical directors for each specific program (pain management, spinal cord injury, etc.) who are either physiatrists or have special training or experience in the various areas (p. 87-5.A). However, this requirement fails to distinguish the administrative and clinical facets of medical direction. There are other possible arrangements such as a single medical director for an entire subacute medical or rehabilitation program, supported by various specialists as needed.

Furthermore (as explained in Chapter 3) the CARF criteria for dividing medical rehabilitation into acute and subacute are inconsistent with the changing roles of hospitals and the capabilities of alternative sites in providing services for those with less than a high degree of instability. CARF standards should recognize more clearly that rehabilitation is a service and not a level of care, and that classifying individuals based on their level of rehabilitation services is not comparable to doing so based on their acuity. They should also reflect more clearly the growing body of evidence that other things besides therapies may be equally or more relevant to the improvement of rehabilitation patients (Bernardini et al, 1995).

Ultimately, no one approach to overseeing and improving quality is sufficient. No program or agency should assume or claim that accreditation is sufficient evidence of desired performance. Compliance with accreditation standards must be combined with internal systems that enable effective problem solving, communication, and rational analysis and open discussion among all players. Like regulations, accreditation standards should be consolidated and made more compatible with empirical evidence wherever possible. The use of professional standards, practice guidelines, and protocols is important to reduce undesirable individual variation. Further development of efforts to demonstrate and improve care quality is needed based on the multiple dimensions of factors influencing outcomes in subacute patients. The factors most likely to be relevant appear to be defined already, but their exact contribution remains to be specified. Professional organizations have responsibilities to address performance problems of their disciplines, and the entire health care industry must assume the responsibility to upgrade the performance of health care management and governance.

REFERENCES

Aptaker RL, Roth EJ, Reichhardt G, et al. Serum albumin level as a predictor of geriatric stroke rehabilitation outcome. *Arch Phys Med Rehabil.* 1994; 75(1):80–84.

Bernardini B, Meinecke C, Pagani M, et al. Comorbidity and adverse clinical events in the rehabilitation of older adults after hip fracture. *J Am Geriatr Soc.* 1995; 43:894–898.

Chong DK. Measurement of instrumental activities of daily living in stroke. *Stroke.* 1995; 26(6):1119–1122.

Cohen HJ, et al. Predictors of two-year post-hospitalization mortality among elderly veterans in a study evaluating a geriatric consultation team. *J Am Geriatr Soc.* 1992; 40:1231–1235.

Commission on Accreditation of Rehabilitation Facilities (CARF). *Standards Manual and Interpretive Guidelines for Medical Rehabilitation.* Tucson: CARF; 1995.

Esteban A, Frutos F, Tobin MJ, et al. A comparison of four methods of weaning patients from mechanical ventilation. Spanish Lung Failure Collaborative Group. *N Engl J Med.* 1995; 332:345–350.

Falconer JA, Naughton BJ, Dunlop DD, et al. Predicting stroke inpatient rehabilitation outcome using a classification tree approach. *Arch Phys Med Rehabil.* 1994; 75(6):619–625.

Greenfield S, Apolone G, McNeil BJ, et al. The importance of co-existent disease in the occurrence of postoperative complications and one-year recovery in patients undergoing total hip replacement: Comorbidity and outcomes after hip replacement. *Med Care.* 1993; 31(2):141–154.

Grimshaw JM, Russell IT. Effect of clinical guidelines on medical practice: A systematic review of rigorous evaluations. *Lancet.* 1993; 342:1317–1322.

Iezzoni LI, Daley J. A description and clinical assessment of the Computerized Severity Index. *QRB Qual Rev Bull.* 1992; 18(2):44–52.

Incalzi AR, Capparella O, Gemma A, et al. A simple method of recognizing geriatric patients at risk for death and disability. *J Am Geriatr Soc.* 1992; 40:34–38.

Kidd D, Stewart G, Baldry J, et al. The Functional Independence Measure: A comparative validity and reliability study. *Disabil Rehabil.* 1995; 17(1):10–14.

Lefevre F, Feinglass J, Potts S, et al. Iatrogenic complications in high-risk, elderly patients. *Arch Intern Med.* 1992; 152(10):2074–2080.

Lichtenstein MJ, Federspiel CF, Schaffner W. Factors associated with early demise of nursing home residents: A case control study. *J Am Geriatr Soc.* 1985; 33:315–319.

Narain P, Rubenstein LZ, Wieland GD, et al. Predictors of immediate and 6-month outcomes in hospitalized elderly patients. *J Am Geriatr Soc.* 1988; 36:775–783.

Niskanen M, Kari A, Nikki P, et al. Acute physiology and chronic health evaluation (APACHE II) and Glasgow coma scores as predictors of outcome from intensive care after cardiac arrest. *Crit Care Med.* 1991; 19(12):1465–1473.

Prescott PA, Ryan JW, Soeken KL, et al. The Patient Intensity for Nursing Index: A validity assessment. *Res Nurs Health.* 1991; 14(3):213–221.

Rosenthal GE, Halloran EJ, Kiley M, et al. Predictive validity of the Nursing Severity Index in patients with musculoskeletal disease. *J Clin Epidemiol.* 1995; 48(2):179–188.

Rosenthal GE, Halloran EJ, Kiley M, et al. Development and validation of the Nursing Severity Index. A new method for measuring severity of illness using nursing diagnoses. *Med Care.* 1992; 30(12):1127–1141.

Rosko MD. DRGs and severity of illness measures: An analysis of patient classification systems. *J Med Syst.* 1988; 12(4):257–274.

Schyve P. Outcomes as performance measures. In: *Using Practice Guidelines to Evaluate Quality of Care.* U.S. Department of Health and Human Services, Agency for Health Care Policy and Research, AHCPR pub. no. 95-0046; 1995.

Soeken KL, Prescott PA. Patient intensity for nursing index: The measurement model. *Res Nurs Health.* 1991; 14(4):297–304.

Teasdale G, Jennett B. Assessment of coma and impaired consciousness. *Lancet.* July 13, 1974:81–83.

Thomas JW, Ashcraft ML. Measuring severity of illness: Six severity systems and their ability to explain cost variations. *Inquiry.* 1991; 28(1):39–55.

Wallace JI, Schwartz RS, LaCroix AZ, et al. Involuntary weight loss in older outpatients: Incidence and clinical significance. *J Am Geriatr Soc*. 1995; 43:329–337.

FOR FURTHER READING

Elwood PM. Outcomes management: A technology of patient experience. *N Engl J Med*. 1988; 318:1549–1556.

Epstein AM. The outcomes movement: Will it get us where we want to go? *N Engl J Med*. 1990; 323:266–270.

Evans RL, Connis RT, Hendricks RD, et al. Multidisciplinary rehabilitation versus medical care: A meta-analysis. *Soc Sci Med*. 1995; 40(12):1699–1706.

Green J, Wintfeld N, Sharkey P, et al. The importance of severity of illness in assessing hospital mortality. *JAMA*. 1990; 263(2):241–246.

Greenfield S. The state of outcome research: Are we on target? *N Engl J Med*. 1989; 320:1142–1143.

Institute of Medicine. Effectiveness and outcomes in health care: Proceedings of an invitational conference by the Institute of Medicine. Heitkoff KA, Lohr KN, eds. Washington, DC: National Academy Press; 1992.

Joint Commission on Accreditation of Healthcare Organizations. Primer on Indicator Development and Application: Measuring Quality in Health Care. JCAI-10. Oakbrook Terrace, IL: JCAHO; 1990.

Keith RA, Wilson DB, Gutierrez P. Acute and subacute rehabilitation for stroke: A comparison. *Arch Phys Med Rehabil*. 1995; 76(6):495–500.

Lohr KN. Outcome measurement: Concepts and questions. *Inquiry*. 1988; 25:37–50.

Sager MA, Rudberg MA, Jalaluddin MS, et al. Hospital admission risk profile (HARP): Identifying older patients at risk for functional decline following acute medical illness and hospitalization. *J Am Geriatr Soc*. 1996; 44:251–257.

Sandrick K. Networks and numbers: Is accreditation slow to change with the times? *Hosp Health Netw*. 1995;69(11):54,56,58.

Schroeder SA. Outcome assessment 70 years later: Are we ready? *N Engl J Med*. 1987; 316:160–162.

Tirlov AR, Ware JE, Greenfield S, et al. The medical outcomes study: An application of methods for monitoring the results of medical care. *JAMA*. 1989; 262:925–930.

TABLE 10–1   CATEGORIES OF CRITERIA FOR HEALTH CARE QUALITY

Category	Explanation
Accomplishment of care	Degree to which care achieves desired or projected outcomes
Appropriateness of care	Degree to which care received matches the patient's needs
Accessibility of care	Degree to which a patient can obtain needed care or service
Timeliness of care	Degree to which care is made available to a patient when it is needed
Effectiveness of care	Degree to which care is rendered correctly, consistent with the current state of knowledge
Efficiency of care	Degree to which care received has the desired effect with a minimum of possible effort, expense, or waste
Continuity of care	Degree to which care needed by the patient is coordinated effectively among practitioners and across organizations and time
Respectfulness of care	Degree to which care is given with consideration of a patient's participation, wishes, interests, privacy, and rights
Safety of care environment	Freedom of the patient care environment from hazard or danger either to the patient or to those providing the care

Adapted with permission from Joint Commission on Accreditation of Healthcare Organizations (JCAHO). *Comprehensive Accreditation Manual for Long-Term Care* (1996 edition). Oakbrook Terrace, IL: JCAHO; 1995:69.

TABLE 10–2   WAYS TO CATEGORIZE INDIVIDUALS TO HELP ASSESS OUTCOMES

Category	Approaches
Evaluate patients with specific conditions	Determine the usual course (including variations) of the illness or condition (e.g., knee replacement, chronic renal failure, left-sided stroke), and the impact of current interventions.
Identify individuals who are at risk for poor outcomes (e.g., death, skin breakdown, medication complications)	Assess impact of various risk factors (e.g., functional status, coma, number of medications) on outcomes.
Assess the impact of various interventions	Determine which interventions (e.g., turning and positioning, specialized beds, skin care, drug regimen review) may reduce the incidence and severity of complications.
Evaluate outcomes of patients receiving treatment from a specific health care organization or practitioner	Assess the effectiveness and appropriateness of an organization's or practitioner's care.
Evaluate outcomes for a defined population (geographic area, age group, etc.)	Assess effect of health care delivery system, population's lifestyle (e.g., diet), and environmental factors (e.g., environmental pollution) on population's health status, disability, and incidence and prevalence of disease.

Adapted from Schyve P. Outcomes as performance measures. In: *Using Practice Guidelines to Evaluate Quality of Care*. U.S. Department of Health and Human Services, Agency for Health Care Policy and Research, AHCPR pub. no. 95-0046;1995:28.

TABLE 10–3   CHARACTERISTICS OF SUBACUTE CARE PATIENTS AND PROCESSES INFLUENCING QUALITY INDICATOR DEVELOPMENT

Patients

- A patient's current status is the cumulative result of multiple dimensions of acute and chronic problems, and other nonmedical factors (family situation, mood and cognition, etc.).
- Outcomes may be less than full recovery, despite appropriate care.
- Patient outcomes often require management of much more than just the primary problem or condition necessitating admission.
- Secondary and tertiary prevention of additional problems are often major components of patient need.
- Some potential complications in these patients may result from the site, practitioners, or treatment, not the underlying illnesses.

Processes

- Multiple processes are involved in care.
- It may be difficult to separate the degree to which individual factors contribute to the overall result.
- Care recipients should ultimately be satisfied with both the results and with the processes that led to those results.
- Inconsistent process performance creates potential risk, and may negatively affect outcome.
- Care processes include many tasks that involve support beyond the direct care provision.
- Efficiency of care depends partially on the support processes.

Practitioners

- Depending on the task, various levels of knowledge and skill are needed for providing treatments, monitoring, assessment, and selecting treatments.
- The roles of individuals and disciplines may differ from their roles in other settings, even if they are treating the same conditions as elsewhere.
- Care outcomes are rarely attributable to any one individual or discipline.

External Influences

- External factors such as regulation and reimbursement influence the scope, frequency, or types of treatments given.
- Efficiency is increasingly considered as important as effectiveness.
- External requirements are often divergent, or of unclear origin or purpose.
- Only some care processes are directly related to achieving outcomes; others are oriented principally to other issues such as reimbursement and regulatory compliance.

| TABLE 10–4 | POSSIBLE OBJECTIVES OF SUBACUTE CARE |

General Objective	Examples
Relieve discomfort	• Relieve physical discomfort, such as pain or paresthesia • Relieve psychological discomfort, such as depression
Stabilize condition	• Prevent further general deterioration • Reduce scope and frequency of any fluctuations in condition
Restore or maintain function affected by disease	• Physical function, such as locomotion, vision, or activities of daily living, including feeding and toileting • Psychological function, such as memory, cognition, or mood • Social function, such as interpersonal relations or communication • Role function, such as that of a parent, student, or worker
Cure an illness or condition	• Treat infection • Continue treatment of cancer
Prevent illness, disability, or death; or retard progression of disease	• Primary prevention of additional illness (anticoagulation for patient with atrial fibrillation) • Secondary prevention of complications (manage hypertension, prevent serious skin wound infections) • Tertiary prevention of further functional decline due to irreversible condition (chronic renal failure)

Adapted from Schyve P. Outcomes as performance measures. In: *Using Practice Guidelines to Evaluate Quality of Care*. U.S. Department of Health and Human Services, Agency for Health Care Policy and Research, AHCPR pub. no. 95-0046; 1995:27.

| TABLE 10–5 | TEMPORAL RELATIONSHIP OF SUBACUTE OUTCOMES |

Time Frame	Discussion	Examples
Immediate	• Emerge during or immediately after a step or specific procedure in the care process • Frequently can be attributed to the specific activity during which they occurred or that immediately preceded them • Relevant to specific procedures and processes in subacute care, but not to the overall care	• Bleeding from a complication during a surgical procedure • Adverse drug–drug interaction after administration of a medication • Improved blood pressure from IV infusion
Intermediate	• Occur by the time an episode of care is completed • Can usually be associated with the procedures and other activities during that episode	• Ability to breathe without a ventilator after a stay for weaning and general care of a ventilator-dependent patient
Long-term	• Ultimate outcomes of the treatment for a particular disease or condition • Of special interest to health services and clinical researchers, health policy-makers, and population health authorities as well as to patients	• Five-year survival rate for cancer patient • Maintenance of functional status and relative freedom from pain 1 year after knee replacement

Adapted from Schyve P. Outcomes as performance measures. In: *Using Practice Guidelines to Evaluate Quality of Care*. U.S. Department of Health and Human Services, Agency for Health Care Policy and Research, AHCPR pub. no. 95-0046; 1995:29.

TABLE 10–6   FACTORS THAT MAY INFLUENCE PATIENT OUTCOMES

	Questions	Supporting Evidence
Patient Characteristics		
• Normal biological variations among patients (e.g., those associated with sex and age)	• Does an individual's age, gender, or other demographic factor influence the outcome of a given illness or injury?	• Older age is a risk factor for decline and death, but responses to illness vary widely within the same age group.
• Underlying problems/medical diagnoses	• Do certain underlying conditions significantly influence outcomes?	• Those with certain underlying problems and a higher collective burden of underlying disease are at greater risk for dying and may need more care for a longer time to achieve the same care objective. • Those with more secondary medical problems may recover less fully and have more functional impairments.
• Severity of illness	• Does the initial severity of an illness influence the results of care, length of stay, or eventual recovery? • Are certain patients less likely to improve, or more likely to die, no matter what or where the care is given?	• Individuals with a greater cumulative burden of multidimensional problems have a higher risk of dying from an acute illness. • Individuals with a greater cumulative burden of multidimensional problems are likely to stay longer, and their care is likely to cost more to achieve the same care objective. • Individuals with greater physiological instability are at higher risk for dying.
• Lifestyle/personal factors	• Do lifestyle, socioeconomic level, education, occupation, environment, home, family situation, or other personal factors influence outcomes?	• Smoking, alcohol consumption, exercise, and environment all may influence the onset and severity of an illness. • Socioeconomic factors are associated with the frequency of obtaining medical care, the risk of getting various illnesses, and the likelihood of complying with a medical treatment regimen. • The availability of adequate social support systems influences an individual's discharge destination. • Adequacy of financial resources is a predictor of favorable outcome in stroke patients (Falconer et al, 1994).
• Functional status	• Does a person's functional level at the onset of treatment influence and/or help predict the outcomes of care?	• Functional status at the start of a course of treatment is a useful predictor of morbidity, functional improvement, mortality, and risk of complications. • Toilet management, bladder management, and toilet transfer are predictors of favorable outcome in stroke patients (Falconer et al, 1994). • IADL function is a predictor of the potential for home discharge.

TABLE 10–6   FACTORS THAT MAY INFLUENCE PATIENT OUTCOMES (CONTINUED)

	Questions	Supporting Evidence
• Level of neurological functioning	• Does the level of impairment of consciousness have any relationship to outcome or resource use?	• Those with impaired levels of consciousness are at a higher risk for dying and for complications of their treatments. • Those with impaired levels of consciousness require more care overall, but not necessarily more highly skilled nursing care.
• Cognitive status	• Does the degree of cognitive impairment have any relationship to outcome or resource use?	• To the extent that cognitive impairment affects a person's function, it may also influence outcomes.
• Other factors	• What other factors may impact outcomes?	• Total number of medications relates to risk of iatrogenic illness and mortality. • Nutritional impairment is a risk factor for death and complications.
• Patient preferences and consent	• Do patient preferences or consent either for a specific treatment intervention or for lack of interventions have an impact on outcomes?	• Patient preferences may affect outcome if they lead to a requested or undesired limitation on assessment, treatment, and transfer.
Site/Program Characteristics • Physical characteristics	• Do a health care facility's size, location, or other characteristics influence the outcomes of care or the cost of delivering care?	• No consistent relationships have been demonstrated.
• Licensure/accreditation	• Do licensure requirements or accreditation status influence or help predict the outcomes of care?	• Licensure/accreditation status may reflect a site's capability to support care provision. • No clear links between specific aspects of licensure or accreditation and outcomes have been demonstrated.
• Staffing	• Do levels of staffing influence the outcomes of care? • Do credentials, degrees, or certificates affect care outcomes? • Do level of knowledge and skills relevant to performing care processes affect care outcomes?	• Staffing levels may be correlated with ability to deliver care safely and effectively. • Staffing and staff characteristics may relate to the occurrence of nosocomial/iatrogenic illness. • Participation of more highly skilled individuals may improve some short-term outcomes.
• Systems and processes	• To what extent do the processes of care influence the outcomes and costs of care? • Do a program's systems and processes for governance, management, clinical care, and support services affect outcomes?	• Systems and processes influence performance; performance may influence outcome where it affects proper performance of care-related processes. • The consistency, effectiveness, and efficiency of care processes (assessment, monitoring, treatment, follow-

(continued)

TABLE 10–6   FACTORS THAT MAY INFLUENCE PATIENT OUTCOMES (CONTINUED)

	Questions	Supporting Evidence
		up) may influence the timely implementation of treatment and other important interventions. • Care processes may influence the occurrence of nosocomial and iatrogenic complications.
Practitioner Characteristics • Current level of knowledge and skills	• Do practitioners' level of knowledge and skills (based on education and experience) affect outcomes?	• Knowledge and skills may affect outcomes when they impact treatment or evaluation decisions.
• Performance	• Does practitioner performance (both technical and interpersonal skills) influence outcome?	• Practitioner performance may affect the safety of care and the occurrence of potentially preventable complications. • Practitioner provision of guidance, support, or information may influence the decisions and performance of other care providers, patients, or families.
• Provision of treatments and services	• What treatments, services, and aspects of care are essential to the outcome, and which could be optional?	• The relationships between frequency and types of services and outcomes remains ill defined for many therapies.
External Influences/Incentives • Facility reimbursement	• Does the level or methodology of facility reimbursement influence the outcomes of care?	• Various reimbursement methodologies may result in different approaches to care provision and the quantity and frequency of certain services.
• Practitioner reimbursement	• Does the level or methodology of practitioner reimbursement influence the outcomes of care?	• Various reimbursement methodologies may result in different approaches to care provision and the quantity and frequency of certain services.
• Community-related factors	• Does the structure of a community's health care system (e.g., whether it is integrated to provide continuity of care across provider organizations and clinicians, across organizations, and through time) influence outcome? • Do the amount and allocation of health care resources in the community (e.g., financial resources available for health care, allocation of resources between preventive and treatment services) affect outcomes?	• The structure and availability of programs and services may impact efficiency. • The relationship between service availability and effective utilization remains ill defined. • Some preventive services influence overall public health. • It is unclear whether more resources or services result in significantly improved overall morbidity and mortality, although they may help in selected individual cases.

TABLE 10–7   PATIENT-RELATED FINDINGS IN SUBACUTE CARE THAT MAY HELP PREDICT RISK AND OUTCOMES

Outcome	Likelihood Increased By
Risk of short-term mortality	• Higher overall severity-of-illness score • Presence of the following problems: depression, bowel incontinence, urinary incontinence, altered level of consciousness, impaired life support systems, impaired verbal communications • Low Glasgow Coma Scale score (i.e., impaired level of consciousness) • Low ADL score (i.e., high dependency level) • Presence of diagnosis of neoplastic or cardiovascular diseases • Greater number of prescription medications • Involuntary weight loss > 4% of body weight • Cholesterol < 120 or albumin < 2.5
Risk of longer-term mortality	• Protein–energy undernutrition (1-year postdischarge mortality)
Risk of iatrogenic illness	• Low Glasgow Coma Scale score • Greater number of prescription medications
Risk of subsequent physical dependency	• Low ADL score • Diagnosis of neoplastic or cardiovascular diseases
Likely discharge disposition	• Total problem-based severity-of-illness score (Rosenthal, 1995) • Combined score of nursing severity/dependency/complexity scale (Prescott, 1991) • Level of IADL function
Amount of care resources needed	• Higher total problem-based severity-of-illness score (Rosenthal, 1995) • Greater ADL dependency • Presence of second- or third-degree burns, open wound or skin lesions, explicit terminal prognosis, hemiplegia or quadriplegia, vomiting, and septicemia • Complexity of nursing skills involved in the care

TABLE 10–8   GROUPING SUBACUTE PATIENTS BASED ON THE COMBINED IMPACT OF ACUTE ILLNESS AND COEXISTING PROBLEMS

Acuity of Medical Problem

Impact of Coexisting Conditions	Low	Moderate	High
None	Group 1	Group 1	
Minimal impairment		Group 2	Group 2
Moderate impairment			Group 2
Severe/global impairment		Group 3	Group 3

TABLE 10–9   VARIATION IN LIKELY OUTCOMES FOR DIFFERENT PATIENT GROUPS IN TABLE 10–8

Outcomes	Group 1	Group 2	Group 3
Likelihood of recovery from acute illness (return to at least baseline status)	+++	++	+
Risk of complications/iatrogenic illness	+	++	+++
Likely length of stay for same primary diagnosis	+	++	+++
Resource use (nursing and total staff time)	+	++	+++
Likelihood of residual functional impairments	+	++	+++

+, low; ++, moderate; +++, high.

TABLE 10–10   SUMMARY OF CORE PATIENT-RELATED DATA IN ALL PROGRAMS

- Vital signs
- Nutrition measures: height, weight, albumin, cholesterol, hematocrit
- Medical diagnoses
- Problems (nursing diagnoses)
- Assessment of neurological/cognitive function
- Severity of illness (acuity) score
- Goals of care
- Limits on medical interventions and other care
- ADL status/IADL status

TABLE 10–11   COMMON VARIATIONS AMONG SUBACUTE SITES

- Case mix
- Licensure categories
- Governance/ownership
- Frequency and intensity of services
- Nurse staffing
- Physician organization and staffing
- Approach to handling patient complications and acute condition changes

TABLE 10–12   EXAMPLES OF USING CLINICALLY RELEVANT DATA TO IMPROVE CARE

Assessment Component	Potential Uses of the Information for Care
Vital signs	• Indicate relative stability and possible need for transfer.
Level of consciousness	• A patient with impaired consciousness should be considered at higher risk for developing complications, particularly related to medications and treatments, which should help focus preventive efforts. • A program that accepts a lot of patients with high levels of impaired consciousness may need to adjust its staffing (especially LPNs/nursing assistants).
Cognitive status	• Staffing planning may be helped by taking into account the number of patients with cognitive impairment. • More cognitively impaired patients may need closer scrutiny to predict and identify possibly preventable complications.
Mood and behavior problems	• Staffing planning may be helped by taking into account the number of patients with mood and behavior impairment. • Evidence of persistent mood alteration, problem behaviors, verbal expressions of distress, demonstrated signs of mental stress, delusions/hallucinations should trigger additional assessment.
Physical functioning (ADLs)	• Staffing (especially, nursing assistants) planning may be helped by taking into account the number of patients with ADL impairments, contractures, and a toileting plan. • Those with greater ADL dependency needs should be monitored closely for possible occurrence of complications of care.
Practical functioning (IADLs)	• Individuals with greater IADL dependency may need more vigorous placement efforts and arrangement of appropriate support to enable discharge when their treatment course is completed.
Other physical problems	• Staffing planning may be influenced by the number of patients with pressure ulcers, burns, or using specialized beds for wound care. • Patients with physical and lab evidence of mild to moderate undernutrition should receive vigorous nutrition/hydration support. • Patients with evidence of severe undernutrition are at higher risk for dying.
Rehabilitative/ restorative nursing services	• Staffing planning may be helped by taking into account the number of patients receiving splint/ brace/prosthesis assistance, exercise/conditioning program, or training and skill practice.
Medications	• Medications should be monitored for possibly preventable complications and side effects (quality and risk management indicator).

TABLE 10–13	STEPS TO CREATING THE FOUNDATION FOR AN EFFICIENT QUALITY ASSESSMENT PROGRAM

- Identify the program's care-related and support processes.
- Define the patient database.
- Select criteria for evaluating patients and coding information.
- Format the information appropriately so that it can be computerized and used to provide the care.
- Assess patients in all applicable dimensions (physiological, functional, and overall).
- Monitor and measure relevant information on admission, on discharge, and periodically during the stay.
- Use the data to determine patient progress and help make effective care-related decisions.
- Set up computer-based reports and queries to analyze the care for individual patients and for various groups of the collective patient population.
- Use the results of data analysis to establish internal benchmarks and look for ways to improve quality.
- Use the results of data analysis to compare program performance to appropriate benchmarks.
- Compare results over time to look for areas of improvement and areas needing further refinement.

TABLE 10–14	VARIOUS WAYS TO COMPENSATE FOR FACTORS INFLUENCING OUTCOMES

Category	Examples	Limitations
• Select patients by ensuring that other factors that affect the outcomes are held constant.	• Compare outcomes of ventilator care or stroke management by similar levels of severity of illness (acuity).	• Large number of factors that would have to be held constant by this method may make it impractical to control for all of them.
• Stratify selection of patients whose outcomes are measured so that they are studied in groups in which the other factors that affect the outcomes are held constant.	• Measure outcomes separately for acute myocardial infarction patients with and without a specific comorbidity, such as diabetes.	• Large number of factors need to be controlled. • Patients may need to be stratified into many groups, and each group may be too small to study statistically.
• Measure changes in health outcomes to adjust for varying levels of severity of illness among patients.	• Measure the difference between the patient's baseline health status and the health status after intervention.	• By itself, does not include additional relevant factors.
• Statistically adjust rates of outcomes for groups of patients in which the other factors that affect outcomes are not constant, so that they are made to act as if they are constant.	• If low ADL function is known to predict higher mortality for certain subacute patients, then adjust the observed survival rates of provider organizations or clinicians whose subacute patients have uncommonly high ADL dependency scores.	• Such statistical adjustment must usually be combined with stratifying data collection, subject selection, and/or measurement of changes from baseline.

Adapted from Schyve P. Outcomes as performance measures. In: *Using Practice Guidelines to Evaluate Quality of Care.* U.S. Department of Health and Human Services, Agency for Health Care Policy and Research, AHCPR pub. no. 95-0046; 1995: 31.

TABLE 10–15	EXAMPLES OF DATA ELEMENTS USED TO MEASURE OUTCOMES FOR VARIOUS SPECIFIC PROGRAMS OR SERVICES

Pain Management
- Patient ID #
- Attending physician ID #
- Date treatment initiated
- Pain scale—worst, least, and current pain
- Duration of pain
- Frequency of pain
- Pain interference with walking, sitting, and standing

Wound Treatment
- Patient ID #
- Attending physician ID #
- Total number of wounds
- Wound site
- Wound surface area by length and width
- Type of wound
- Stage of wound
- Perimeter involved by induration and erythema

Data elements provided by Formations in Health Care, Inc., a Medirisk Co., as used in the Formations[SM] National Outcomes System.

TABLE 10–16	THE VARIOUS CATEGORIES OF PROCESS AND THEIR RELATIONSHIP TO CARE

Area	Rationale
• Processes directly related to giving the care (assessment, monitoring, problem identification, etc.)	• These are both the result and the proximate stage for practitioner performance; they must be done to provide the care; how they are done may affect care consistency and effectiveness; there are several ways to accomplish similar ends.
• Processes related to operating the facility (accounting, maintenance, plant management, etc.)	• These are most likely to indirectly affect the efficiency, safety, and consistency of practitioner performance.
• Processes related to supporting the care (admissions, medical records, etc.)	• These are most likely to directly affect practitioner performance.
• Processes that cross all these boundaries (communications, problem solving, planning, etc.)	• These must be performed effectively to enable both effective facility operations and care provision.

TABLE 10–17	POSSIBLE REASONS FOR DISCHARGE FROM A SUBACUTE PROGRAM

- Condition improved to point where level of care no longer needed
- Individual no longer able to benefit from programs and services at this level of care
- Condition required acute hospital admission
- Condition required admission to another health care facility
- No longer qualified by payer
- Left against medical advice
- Individual expired

TABLE 10–18	ITEMS FOR CARE AND PROCESS OUTCOMES ASSESSMENTS AFTER A PATIENT'S SUBACUTE STAY

Area	Specific Issues
Review of outcomes	**For Stay** - Achieved versus predicted result - Occurrence of complications of illness - Occurrence of iatrogenic/nosocomial conditions - Assessment of unanticipated transfers (e.g., hospital) **Subsequent** - Longer-term functional levels - Rehospitalization - Recurrence of condition that was treated during stay
Review of problems/concerns	- Problems/concerns raised by patient and family - Issues raised by staff - Issues raised by payers, other outsiders

TABLE 10–19	EXAMPLES OF AREAS FOR DEVELOPING SUBACUTE STRUCTURAL QUALITY INDICATORS

Physical Plant
- Enough space is available for patients, delivery of treatments and therapies, meals, staff conferencing, etc.

Equipment and Supplies
- Adequate, operational equipment and supplies are available to provide specific treatments and perform necessary procedures.

Staffing
- Enough properly trained, licensed, and skilled individuals are available to perform care-related processes.
- Enough properly trained primary care physicians and consultants are available to provide direct care and support others who are providing care.
- Consultants are available in relevant specialties.

Care Management (CM) System
- CM system exists to coordinate development and implementation of patient care treatment plans and continuous monitoring of patient status or progress; mechanism to detect, report, and manage side effects and complications of medications, illnesses, and treatments; consistent process to decide when a patient can or should be discharged to another level of care; mechanism to provide patient and family instruction for all services.

Supplementary Arrangements
- Program has service coordination with other care sites.
- Program has transfer agreements with an acute-care hospital and procedures for immediate transfer of patients who require services that cannot be provided in the subacute facility or unit.

Policies and Procedures
- Program has policies, procedures, and protocols for all programs and services provided, consistent with generally accepted professional practice standards.

TABLE 10–20	EXAMPLES OF AREAS FOR DEVELOPING SUBACUTE PROCESS QUALITY INDICATORS

Patient Selection
- Systematic process is used to decide whether subacute is optimal site in terms of patient need and cost of care.
- Documentation indicates why subacute care was needed, or why other alternatives were not appropriate or were not used.

Admission
- Preadmission screening and admission decisions follow relevant policies and procedures.
- Systematic process is used to establish likely prognosis and care objectives at the time of accepting the patient, and again at the time of admission.
- Analysis is made of patients not accepted into the program.
- Appropriate mechanism is used to handle patients who are worse than expected, or who do not meet admission criteria on further assessment.

Assessment
- Systematic process is used to identify and define the nature, severity, scope, intensity, and duration of all significant medical, psychosocial, and functional problems.
- Severity of illness (acuity) level is documented for each patient.

(continued)

TABLE 10–20   EXAMPLES OF AREAS FOR DEVELOPING SUBACUTE PROCESS QUALITY INDICATORS (CONTINUED)

- Causes of problems are identified and described appropriately.
- Functional limitations caused by illness or disability are defined and described accurately and completely.

Monitoring

- Vital signs are monitored as required and are documented consistently.
- Effects of illness are described accurately and completely.
- Exacerbations and complications of illness are recognized in a timely fashion and accurately described.
- New onset of additional illnesses are recognized in a timely fashion and accurately described.

Treatment of Primary Problems

- Appropriate treatments are selected based on protocols and guidelines.
- Treatments are given correctly, consistently, and in a timely fashion.
- Effectiveness of treatments is assessed and described.
- Monitoring for complications of treatments is done in each patient.
- Timely and appropriate interventions are made in case of complications.
- Scope and duration of treatments are assessed reasonably and explained adequately.

Preparation for Subsequent Care

- Appropriate arrangements are made for postcare placement.
- Appropriate information and communication is provided to support continuation of care and treatments.
- Relevant instructions and information are given to the patient and family.
- Scope of patient and family understanding of information is evaluated.

TABLE 10–21   EXAMPLES OF AREAS FOR DEVELOPING SERVICE-SPECIFIC CLINICAL PROCESS QUALITY INDICATORS

Cardiac Care

- Cases of patients returned to the hospital because of recurrent cardiac instability.
- Management of patients developing acute arrhythmias while on the subacute unit.
- Appropriate recognition and management of any side effects or complications of medication regimen.
- Appropriate use of rehabilitation therapies, including appropriate cardiac precautions.

Oncology

- Essential psychosocial support provided for patient and family.
- Adverse side effects of chemotherapy identified and managed effectively.
- Evaluation of pain and provision of pain relief done consistently.

Orthopedics

- Monitoring done for complications and side effects of fractures and surgery.
- Management of casts, braces, traction done correctly.

Respiratory Services

- Blood oxygenation measured by pulse oximetry or blood gases upon admission for anyone admitted with borderline pO_2 or pCO_2 on discharge from hospital, and for any significant or prolonged change in symptoms or condition.

TABLE 10–21	EXAMPLES OF AREAS FOR DEVELOPING SERVICE-SPECIFIC CLINICAL PROCESS QUALITY INDICATORS (CONTINUED)

- An outcome less than anticipated (death, return to hospital) can be reasonably explained by the information in the progress notes describing the clinical course.
- Nurse and physician progress notes document patient progress on ventilator.
- Weaning from ventilator done appropriately and clinical justification exists for those who cannot be weaned.
- Nutrition and hydration status are assessed and managed aggressively in all patients.

Stroke

- Complications, such as poststroke depression, are identified and managed effectively.
- Functional evaluation and rehabilitation therapies are started in a timely fashion.
- Functional recovery is compared to that predicted for the type of stroke and acuity level.

Wound Care

- Mobility limitations imposed by care plan (e.g., bed rest) are managed.
- Positive and negative changes in wounds are recorded and reported promptly and accurately.
- Skin grafts are managed appropriately, and graft failures are due to medical factors.
- Proper equipment (air-fluidized beds, etc.) is available and used.
- Proper procedures are followed to manage wound infections.
- Nutrition and hydration status are assessed and managed aggressively in all patients.

TABLE 10–22	EXAMPLES OF ORGANIZATION-WIDE SYSTEMS AND PROCESS AREAS FOR DEVELOPING QUALITY INDICATORS

Human Resources

- Is there a means to assess general and discipline-specific staff knowledge and skills?
- How often do staff receive performance-related feedback and what does it include?
- Are appropriate individuals and disciplines included in giving and receiving relevant feedback?
- How does the program select and train staff and management for the unit?

Business

- How does the facility establish its costs of care in dealing with managed care organizations?
- What does the marketing staff tell or promise potential patients and referral sources?

Care and Care Support

- How efficiently does the program handle the rapid patient turnover and multiple daily admissions?
- How does the program promote and practice early intervention, prevention, and risk-management activities?
- How does the program control waste?
- What preventive maintenance programs for equipment are utilized?
- How does the program promote appropriate patient and family expectations?
- How does the program help assess and improve staff skills and performance in problem analysis and management?

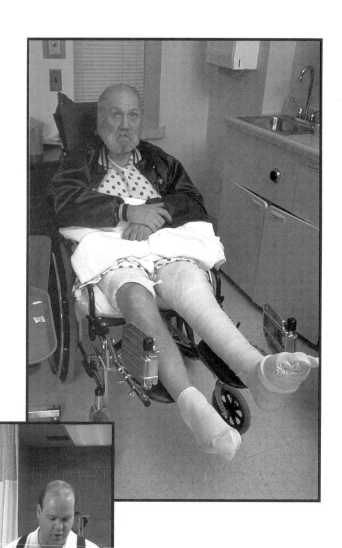

SUBACUTE CARE PATIENT CASES

*T*his book has discussed the subject of subacute care. A case-oriented approach helps test the value of a subject-oriented discussion. The definitions, categories, criteria, and principles should be relevant to specific cases, and the cases should effectively illustrate those definitions, categories, criteria, and principles. This chapter presents nine different subacute cases in depth, and summarizes the principles that those cases represent regarding subacute patients, their service needs, and subacute care.

All nine cases in this chapter are based on actual patients who have received care in subacute programs. Although all names have been modified, most of the other information is presented unmodified. Both individually and collectively, these cases illustrate a number of important principles about subacute care and subacute patients. These principles are summarized in boldface below. The format for presenting the cases—explained in Table 11–1, pp. 357–358—incorporates many of the concepts (problem identification, care objectives, interdisciplinary participants, and so on) that have been discussed in earlier chapters. This format might also be a useful way to provide a subacute discharge summary.

Characteristics and Problems of Subacute Patients

The subacute patients in these cases span the age spectrum from young to very old. Prior to the events that brought them to a subacute program, their level of health and function ranged from totally independent and leading fully functional lives in the community, to totally dependent and receiving daily institutional support.

Subacute programs are typically defined and marketed by their services (wound management, ventilator care, postoperative care). Despite that approach, only some subacute care is defined primarily by the treatment, specifically, when the objective is to complete a defined treatment course (antibiotics, chemotherapy, dialysis, and so on).

These subacute patients are all distinguished by the need for problem management. They had between 6 and 19 identifiable problems. All of them had multidimensional problems. That is, they included at least one significant *health-related* (for example, infection, injury potential) or *nutritional and metabolic* (such as fluid volume deficit, skin impairment, altered nutrition) problem; plus others related to *urinary and fecal elimination* (urinary incontinence or other altered urinary elimination pattern, constipation or diarrhea, for example); *activity and exercise* (for example, activity intolerance, ineffective breathing pattern or impaired gas exchange, impaired mobility, self-care deficit); or *psychosocial status* (for example, depression, altered family process, ineffective individual coping).

All of these individuals had some problems caused by one or several diagnoses. The same diagnosis caused different problems in different individuals, and the same problems in different individuals resulted from a variety of diagnoses. **Therefore, the improvement and ultimate discharge of most subacute patients depends on managing the problems in all relevant dimensions, not just the health-related ones.**

Many subacute patients are admitted with almost the same scope of problems as when they were in the hospital, except for being more stable. For the hospital referrals, the subacute care program continued treatments for problems that had already been addressed, initiated management of others that had only been identified, and defined others that had not yet been recognized.

Hospital care tends to focus on controlling life-threatening instability, defining major causes of the instability, determining the scope of damage, and initiating direct interventions to achieve physical improvement. Subacute care emphasizes ongoing management of causes (treat infection, provide adequate nutrition and hydration, adjust medications) and aggressive management of consequences of illness and injury, including functional impairment and comfort. Much of the overall improvement results from the patient's own pace of recovery aided by the management of the scope of his or her medical and non-medical problems.

Subacute patients have multiple diagnoses. Not all of those diagnoses are resolved fully during the subacute stay. Their diagnoses alone do not appear to predict the outcomes or duration of their stay. Some of these subacute patients achieved only marginally improved overall status, but they all had some of their problems addressed. Most of them required 15 to 40 days to have their major problems managed enough to achieve a desired status, enabling transfer elsewhere. Furthermore, although functional measurements may indicate attainment of some care objectives, it is hard to separate out the impact of individual services as the cause of those improvements.

New-onset problems arising during a subacute stay tend to be either mostly predictable (infections, seizures, bleeding, medication side effects) or they can be handled with a few basic, low technology interventions. Although appropriate diagnostic support (lab, radiology) is needed, there can be a delay while the patient or the specimen is transported, or the equipment is brought in. Patients who are highly unstable as a result of their primary condition or new-onset problems are usually not well placed in a subacute program.

Additionally, these subacute patients were discharged from the subacute setting with many of the same underlying medical conditions with which they were admitted (except for infections). Therefore, a subacute program only cures some medical conditions. Instead, it manages the complications and problems caused by the diagnoses while the body attempts to regain some balance or to heal itself.

Service Needs of Subacute Patients

As a result of their multidimensional problems, these subacute patients all had significant service needs. Some were medically related (assessment, monitoring, medical or nursing treatments or procedures); but many others were physical function-related (ADL support and restoration) or psychosocial function-related (management of disruptions of behavior, mood, cognition, or social and family situations).

None of these subacute patients had a significant need for complex or frequent diagnostics because almost all major diagnoses had been established prior to their subacute transfer. But all these patients needed more than isolated or occasional monitoring and treatment to address their problems, determine the progress of their conditions, define their response to various treatments, recognize the onset of new problems or complications of existing ones, and identify possible complications associated with the care and treatments.

Meeting the service needs of subacute patients requires skills and treatments that involve many different individuals from many different disciplines. All of these subacute patients had problems benefitting from the collaboration of those of several disciplines, often repeated during all or most of their stay. As a rule, individuals with a higher severity of illness (SOI) level received more services involving more disciplines during their stay. More than in the acute setting, all relevant disciplines contribute to the achievement of various objectives, and none of them can achieve the desired objectives alone. The program must be able to access these individuals and disciplines repeatedly, in a timely fashion, and sometimes in a specific sequence, to resolve multiple problems. **One strength of subacute programs is their ability to apply a broad in-**

terdisciplinary approach to manage multiple problems that result from one or several causes.

Care Objectives and Outcomes of Subacute Patients

Care objectives are essential for all subacute patients. They include not only expectations for overall improvement in status, but also problem-specific objectives. **Subacute care objectives are a mixture of disease resolution, functional improvement, and prevention. Primary, secondary, and tertiary prevention are major aspects of subacute care and care outcomes.**

General care goals for subacute patients may include improvement to or beyond status prior to current episode of illness, improvement but less than previous status, stabilization (prevention of further decline), or progressive decline or death. Specific care objectives relate to management of individual problems (for example, improve nutritional status, resolve infection, retrain in activities of daily living). Subacute care may handle a patient's problems and thereby improve his or her status, or may manage the problems yet do little or nothing for overall status.

For all of these patients, length of stay depended in part on how the care objectives were defined. Problem-specific care objectives differed from overall status-related care objectives. As happened with some of these patients, these objectives (and therefore the length of stay) may be influenced by several factors, including the patient's current social situation and the insurer. More than in acute care, each patient's psychosocial situation played a role in the services received, length of stay, discharge potential, and the ultimate discharge site.

TABLE 11–1   GENERAL EXPLANATION OF FORMAT FOR CASE PRESENTATIONS

Item	Description
	Preadmission Selection and Preparation
Referral source/reasons	• What was the source of referral to subacute program? • What was the reason for referral? • What was the clinical course that led to need for referral?
Anticipated treatments/ services	• At the time of referral, what treatments and services were anticipated to be needed in the subacute program?
Anticipated care outcome	*Practitioners* • At the time of referral, what did the care providers anticipate to be the likely outcome of the stay in the subacute program? *Patient/Family* • At the time of referral, what did the patient and/or family anticipate to be the likely outcome of the stay in the subacute program?
Significant decision makers	• Who is (are) the significant decision maker(s) for this individual?
Limits on medical care/ directives	• What, if any, limits have been placed on the degree, scope, frequency, or type of medical interventions based on advance directives or other discussions or statements of patient wishes?
Financial status/insurance coverage	• Who is paying for the subacute stay?
	Postadmission Care Management
Significant findings on assessment	*Physical Status* • On initial postadmission examination, what were the significant physical findings? *Functional Status* • On initial postadmission assessment, what was the individual's functional status? *Decision-Making Capacity* • On initial postadmission examination, what was the individual's capacity to make health-care decisions? *Psychosocial Information* • At the time of admission, what was the individual's pertinent social and personal situation?
Medical diagnoses	*Primary* • What was the primary medical diagnosis leading to the current status or recent need for inpatient medical and nursing care? *Secondary* • What were the coexisting medical conditions that were not necessarily related to the current situation or the principal reason for admission, but could be relevant to the care?
Identified problems	• What problems (as opposed to diagnoses) were identified in this individual?
Risk/acuity assessment	*Other High-Risk Factors* • What other major risk factors did the individual present?
Care objectives/plan	*General* • What were the overall care goals for the individual's stay? *Problem-Related* • What were the care objectives for specific medical diagnoses and other problems?
Principal care providers	• Who were the principal care providers involved in the care of this individual and what were their major roles during the stay?

(continued)

Table 11–1   General Explanation of Format for Case Presentations (Continued)

Item	Description
Treatment course	*Management of Known/New-Onset Problems* • How were the known problems, and those that arose during the stay, managed? *Changes in Care Objectives During Stay* • What, if any, changes occurred in the care goals and objectives during the stay? *Significant Interruptions in Treatment Plan* • What, if any, interruptions of the treatment plan occurred during the stay?
Patient/family education provided	• What information and training was provided to patients and families during the stay?
Discharge	*Site* • To where was the person discharged? *Resources/Services/Follow-Up* • What postdischarge services, resources, and follow-up care were arranged? *Problems* • What problems had to be faced in planning or actually executing the discharge?
Follow-up of patient status	• What is known about the individual's subsequent course?
Postdischarge quality review	*Outcomes* • How did the person's severity of illness (acuity level) change by the end of the stay based on a problem-oriented acuity scale (as described in Chapter 7)? • To what extent did the individual achieve his or her predicted outcome (based on practitioner expectations)? • What was the individual's length of stay? • Were any complications of illness that occurred during the stay identified and handled appropriately? • Did any iatrogenic/nosocomial conditions occur during the patient's stay? • Did the individual have to be transferred unexpectedly out of the program before the anticipated completion of the treatment course? *Programmatic Issues* • Were any significant problems or concerns raised by the patient and family during the stay that need to be addressed? • Were any significant problems or concerns raised by the staff about the care, the support, equipment, supplies, etc. during the stay that need to be addressed? • Were any significant problems or concerns raised by the payers during the stay that caused or might have caused a problem or that now need to be addressed?

CASE 1:	BEVERLY, AGE 69

Item	Discussion
	Preadmission Selection and Preparation
Referral source/reasons	• Acute hospital • Widely metastatic squamous cell lung cancer/Laminectomy 6 weeks prior to referral/Severe back pain even after laminectomy/Also severely deconditioned and dependent in bed-to-chair transfers and ambulation
Anticipated treatments/ services	• Pain management • Rehabilitative and restorative care
Anticipated care outcome	*Practitioners* • Improvement but less than previous status *Patient/Family* • Improvement but less than previous status (patient expectation) • Improvement to or beyond status prior to current episode of illness (family expectation)
Significant decision makers	• Patient is primary decision maker
Limits on medical care/ directives	• Patient decided to receive comfort measures only • Patient requested help in discussing this decision with the family
Financial status/insurance coverage	• Private indemnity insurance (through husband's employer)
	Postadmission Care Management
Significant findings on assessment	*Physical Status* • R-sided lower extremity paresis/General weakness/Signs of undernutrition *Functional Status* • Limited mobility *Decision-Making Capacity* • Intact *Psychosocial Information* • Lives in a ranch style home with her husband of 50 years/Only son died 5 years ago/Many supportive friends/Husband works part-time/Part-time hired help for heavy housework/ Husband still not accepting of her diagnosis
Medical diagnoses	*Primary* • Carcinoma of lung, squamous cell, with widespread metastases *Secondary* • Laminectomy 6 weeks prior to admission • Right thoracotomy 4 months prior to admission • Coronary artery disease (CAD), severe, with an implantable defibrillator • Chronic obstructive pulmonary disease (COPD), severe
Identified problems	**Group 1. Overall Health** • Risk for injury (weak/deconditioned) • Prolonged disease/disability (cancer, COPD) **Group 2. Nutrition and Metabolism** • Altered nutrition (poor appetite, signs of malnutrition) • Potential skin impairment (malnourished, limited mobility) **Group 3. Urinary and Fecal Elimination** • Urinary incontinence **Group 4. Activity and Exercise** • Activity intolerance (severe deconditioning, CAD, COPD, recent thoracotomy and lobectomy) • Ineffective breathing pattern (COPD, cancer of lung)

(*continued*)

Case 1:	Beverly, Age 69 (Continued)

Item	Discussion
	• Impaired gas exchange (COPD) • Decreased cardiac output • Altered health maintenance (severe deconditioning) • Impaired mobility (severe back pain, paresis of the right lower extremity) • Self-care deficit **Group 5. Psychosocial Concerns** • Depression (situational) • Altered family process (patient needs to support and help husband)
Risk/acuity assessment	*Severity of Illness Score (NSI)* • 14 *Other High-Risk Factors* • Falls
Care objectives/plan	*General* • Improvement to status prior to current episode of illness • Discharge to enable dying at home *Problem-Related* • Control pain and nausea • Improve nutritional status • Prevent injury • Improve incontinence • Improve endurance, mobility, and activity intolerance • Minimize dependency and need for ADL support • Manage depression • Support family situation (help husband accept her diagnosis, ensure support for husband after her death)
Principal care providers	• Physician involvement to assess the pain and nausea • Social work to begin to counsel and facilitate the husband's understanding and acceptance of the patient's prognosis and future needs • Spiritual care provider to work with the patient and her husband regarding their grief over the patient's illness, as well as the rekindling of the grief over their only son's death • Clinical pharmacist to educate the nursing staff, patient, and family concerning the use of a subcutaneous morphine pump and the continuous use of prochlorperazine • Physical therapy daily for endurance training, transfers, ambulation, and use of assistive devices • Occupational therapy for ADL activities and for energy-conservation techniques • Nursing to monitor the pain and nausea control • Neurology consultation for evaluation of increasing weakness in the right leg • Nutritional consultation to try to stimulate patient's appetite and counsel the husband about nutritional needs of the dying person • Evaluation of the home to determine durable medical equipment needed when the patient is discharged • Coordination by the discharge planners with insurance company and a home care agency to provide hospice care and to continue the rehabilitative services begun in the subacute unit
Treatment course	**Management of Known/New-Onset Problems** • Begun on subcutaneous morphine pump with good pain control/Patient felt pump interfered with ability to ambulate/Trial of fentanyl patch begun with the use of immediate release morphine for breakthrough pain or air hunger with excellent results/Prochlorperazine was added on a regular basis to her regimen and the nausea was eliminated

CASE 1:	BEVERLY, AGE 69 (CONTINUED)

Item	Discussion
	• Once symptoms were under better control, she participated in rehabilitation program/Was transferring with minimal assistance and beginning to ambulate when she developed increasing weakness in her right leg/Begun on dexamethasone, and weakness resolved/At time of discharge she was able to transfer to chair independently and was walking with a walker with supervision
	Changes in Care Objectives During Stay • None
	Significant Interruptions in Treatment Plan • None
Patient/family education provided	• Medications: Purpose of fentanyl, proper usage, potential problems • Likely progressive decline and death • Arrangements for follow-up services
Discharge	*Site* • Home
	Resources/Services/Follow-Up • Home care agency for in-home therapy and medication management/Social worker visits to help with the expected deterioration in the patient's health/Possible subsequent evaluation for hospice care
	Problems • None related to discharge
Follow-up of patient status	• Patient's death anticipated
Postdischarge quality review	*Outcomes* • Change in acuity score from 14 on admission to 7 on discharge • Achieved predicted outcome • Length of stay: 13 days • Complications of illness (R leg weakness due to tumor compression) identified and handled appropriately • No iatrogenic/nosocomial conditions • No unanticipated transfers
	Programmatic Issues • No significant problems/concerns raised by patient and family • No significant issues raised by staff • No significant issues raised by payers

CASE 2:   ALAN, AGE 52

Item	Description
	Preadmission Selection and Preparation
Referral source/reasons	• Acute hospital • Patient on disability for past 15 years since first coronary artery bypass graft (CABG)/Since then, increasing problems with ambulation and lower extremity pain/Began having crescendo angina 5 months prior to his transfer to the subacute unit/Underwent repeat CABG, which was complicated by an episode of adult respiratory distress syndrome (ARDS)/Spent 2 months in the intensive care unit on a ventilator/Acquired multiple pressure ulcers while in hospital/Needed transfer for multiple problems
Anticipated treatments/ services	• Weaning from ventilator • Management of pressure ulcers, general deconditioning, brittle diabetes, severe pain, undernutrition, severe and continuous diarrhea which contaminated the wound, gastroparesis, arrhythmias
Anticipated care outcome	*Practitioners* • Improvement but less than previous status *Patient/Family* • Improvement to or beyond status prior to current episode of illness (expected independence in all ADLs and return to previous limited ambulatory status)
Significant decision makers	• Patient is primary decision maker
Limits on medical care/ directives	• Do Not Resuscitate
Financial status/insurance coverage	• Medicaid
	Postadmission Care Management
Significant findings on assessment	*Physical Status* • Large grade 4 sacral pressure sore with bone visible, measuring 15.4 × 9 × 4.6 × 5.3 cm, and one on the left hip (4.3 × 3.7 × 2.0 cm), with significant necrosis of both wounds *Functional Status* • Dependent in all ADLs *Decision-Making Capacity* • Intact *Psychosocial Information* • Married
Medical diagnoses	*Primary* • Multiple pressure ulcers *Secondary* • Coronary artery disease (CAD), severe, with arrhythmias • Malnutrition • Peripheral vascular disease • Peripheral neuropathy • Chronic renal failure • Osteomyelitis • Diabetes mellitus, brittle, with frequent episodes of hypoglycemia • Hypothyroidism • Respiratory failure
Identified problems	**Group 1. Overall Health** • Infection/contagion (infected pressure ulcers) • Prolonged disease/disability (long history of disability from coronary artery disease)

CASE 2:	ALAN, AGE 52 (CONTINUED)

Item	Description
	• Instability (needing ventilatory support, brittle diabetes with fluctuating blood sugar levels) • Impaired life-support systems (unable to breathe without ventilatory support) **Group 2. Nutrition and Metabolism** • Altered nutrition (poor oral intake, evidence of malnutrition) • Skin impairment (multiple pressure ulcers) **Group 3. Urinary and Fecal Elimination** • Other altered urinary elimination pattern (chronic renal failure) • Diarrhea • Bowel incontinence **Group 4. Activity and Exercise** • Ineffective airway clearance • Ineffective breathing pattern • Impaired gas exchange • Decreased cardiac output (CAD with continued episodes of chest pain, arrhythmias) • Altered health maintenance (severe pain in back and lower extremities requiring IV Dilaudid/ Noncompliance with insulin regimen) • Self-care deficit (dependent in all ADLs) **Group 5. Psychosocial Concerns** • Altered family processes (financial problems, prolonged chronic and acute illness) • Depression • Impaired verbal communication (on ventilator) • Ineffective individual coping
Risk/acuity assessment	*Severity of Illness Score (NSI)* • 19 *Other High-Risk Factors* • Further skin breakdown
Care objectives/plan	*General* • Improvement but less than previous status *Problem-Related* • Initiate healing of pressure sores • Improve nutritional status • Wean from ventilator • Reduce back and leg pain and discomfort secondary to the pressure sore and the diabetic neuropathy • Control nausea, vomiting, and diarrhea • Reduce number of medications and medication complications • Improve depression and overall coping ability • Resolve osteomyelitis • Manage hypothyroidism effectively • Improve deconditioning and reduce contractures • Improve family functioning
Principal care providers	• Physician assessment and debridement (surgical and mechanical) of the large sacral pressure sore • Nutritionist to assess the nutritional deficits and to develop a gastrostomy and oral feeding regimen • Respiratory therapist and physicians (primary MD and pulmonary consultant) to assess and develop a weaning strategy • Physician evaluation of back and leg pain and the management of the patient's discomfort secondary to the pressure sore and the diabetic neuropathy

(continued)

CASE 2:   ALAN, AGE 52 (CONTINUED)

Item	Description
	• Pharmacist to provide education and coordination of the subcutaneous pump for pain management/Provide information for alternative therapeutic methods for pain management (capsaicin cream for diabetic peripheral neuropathy, etc.)
	• Evaluation by the nursing staff, physician, pharmacist, nutritionist, and gastroenterologist regarding nausea, vomiting, and diarrhea
	• Physician and pharmacist review of admission medications to see if some current medications were contributing to patient problems and could be discontinued
	• Psychiatric evaluation of the patient's depression and inappropriate management of the antidiabetic regimen
	• Evaluation of the osteomyelitis and determination of time course needed for intravenous antibiotics
	• Endocrinologist consult to monitor patient with long history of hypothyroidism who was also now on amiodarone (known side effect of causing hypothyroidism)
	• Follow-up by cardiology and nephrology
	• Nursing assessment and care of the Hickman catheter site
	• Physical and occupational therapy to begin bedside work daily to improve deconditioning and decrease the contractures which were developing secondary to prolonged bed rest
	• Social work intervention to investigate the possible placement options for rehabilitation once the medical problems were stable and the pressure sore was healed sufficiently to allow time in a wheelchair
	• Family counseling to help deal with the many issues with this chronically ill father and husband, and to help with financial issues resulting from inability to return to work
	• Activities therapist to provide activities
Treatment course	*Management of Known/New-Onset Problems*
	• Patient-controlled subcutaneous pump started for pain control, thereby reducing conflicts that had existed between patient and staff in acute hospital and earlier on subacute unit
	• When pain controlled, patient became more open to suggestions regarding management of discomfort caused by his diabetic neuropathy and his need for dietary and medication compliance
	• Careful monitoring of caloric intake and blood sugar levels indicated the need for only a sliding scale/Extreme variations of blood sugar, which had been significant problem on admission, were rapidly controlled
	• Patient and family reeducated regarding diet to control brittle diabetes
	• Pressure ulcer was debrided at the bedside/Infectious disease consultants recommended at least 6 weeks of antibiotics until bone no longer visible/Antibiotics discontinued after 6 weeks and Hickman catheter was removed
	• Patient's prealbumin level rose from 9.0 (normal 24 to 40) to 22 with oral feedings during the day and the use of the gastrostomy tube at night
	• Diarrhea resolved with the treatment of *Clostridium difficile* and discontinuation of casanthrone and lactulose
	• Gastroparesis continued to be a problem despite many attempts to improve it with cisapride, metaclopromide, and erythromycin
	• With improvement in nutritional status and overall condition, patient was easily weaned from the ventilator/Tracheostomy was removed at discharge
	• Thyroid functions checked routinely, given history of hypothyroidism and use of amiodarone/Synthroid adjusted according to hormone blood levels
	• The pressure sore continued slow improvement/Decision made not to do a flap because of recent myocardial infarction and risk due to patient's overall status and multiple problems/Continuation of Clinitron bed therapy and aggressive wound care was elected
	• Patient continued on physical therapy and occupational therapy to strengthen and preserve function while the sores were healing

Case 2:	Alan, Age 52 (Continued)

Item	Description
	Changes in Care Objectives During Stay • None *Significant Interruptions in Treatment Plan* • None
Patient/family education provided	• Procedures for managing pain medications • Dietary and medication management of diabetes • Likely longer-term outcomes and residual deficits • Plan for follow-up rehabilitation
Discharge	*Site* • Transfer to long-term care facility to complete therapy to the pressure sore once the infection was controlled and the sore had begun to heal *Resources/Services/Follow-Up* • Plan to return the patient to the subacute unit for aggressive physical therapy once able to sit in a wheelchair *Problems* • None related to discharge
Follow-up of patient status	• Current treatment in nursing facility to enable continued healing of pressure ulcer • Reduced pain • Breathing without ventilatory support • Better compliance with treatment regimen
Postdischarge quality review	*Outcomes* • Change in acuity score from 19 on admission to 10 on discharge • Achieved predicted result • Length of stay: 58 days • Correction of iatrogenic/nosocomial conditions from hospital stay • No new iatrogenic/nosocomial conditions occurred during subacute stay *Programmatic Issues* • No problems/concerns raised by patient and family • No issues raised by staff • No issues raised by payers, other outsiders

CASE 3:   CYNTHIA, AGE 60

Item	Description
	Preadmission Selection and Preparation
Referral source/reasons	• Acute hospital • Need for continuing care 2 weeks after surgical drainage of an epidural abscess
Anticipated treatments/ services	• Complete 6-week course of IV antibiotics • Improve patient's functional status • Surgical wound care and removal of sutures at day 14
Anticipated care outcome	*Practitioners* • Improvement to or beyond status prior to current episode of illness *Patient/Family* • Improvement to or beyond status prior to current episode of illness
Significant decision makers	• Patient is primary decision maker
Limits on medical care/ directives	• No limits
Financial status/insurance coverage	• Managed care organization
	Postadmission Care Management
Significant findings on assessment	*Physical Status* • Paraparesis *Functional Status* • Deficits in ADLs and IADLs *Decision-making Capacity* • Intact *Psychosocial Information* • Special education teacher for elementary school age children/Divorced mother of two grown sons/Lives alone in her own two-story home/Bathroom is on second floor (up 15 steps)
Medical diagnoses	*Primary* • Epidural abscess *Secondary* • Wolfe–Parkinson–White (WPW) syndrome • Angina • Hypertension • Degenerative joint disease • History of bilateral radical mastectomies • History of peptic ulcer disease • Low back pain, severe • Anxiety, severe
Identified problems	**Group 1. Overall Health** • Infection/contagion (epidural abscess) • Prolonged disease/disability (degenerative joint disease, angina) • Instability (recurrent fever, central nervous system infection) **Group 2. Nutrition and Metabolism** • Altered body temperature (epidural abscess) **Group 3. Urinary and Fecal Elimination** • Other altered urinary elimination pattern (in-dwelling Foley catheter) **Group 4. Activity and Exercise** • Activity intolerance (angina) • Impaired mobility (severe low back pain)

CASE 3:	CYNTHIA, AGE 60 (CONTINUED)

Item	Description
	• Self-care deficit (ADL and IADL dependent) **Group 5. Psychosocial Concerns** • Social isolation (lives alone) • Ineffective individual coping (severe anxiety)
Risk/acuity assessment	*Severity of Illness Score (NSI)* • 10 *Other High-Risk Factors* • None
Care objectives/plan	*General* • Improvement to or beyond status prior to current episode of illness *Problem-Related* • Determine etiology of persistent fevers • Complete treatment of epidural abscess • Monitor for neurological complications of abscess • Control persistent low back pain • Monitor for cardiovascular decompensation • Improve urinary continence • Heal surgical wound • Improve mobility, ambulation, and ADL functional status
Principal care providers	• Infectious disease consultation to help determine etiology of persistent fevers despite consistently negative fever workups • Close monitoring of neurologic status of patient's lower extremities by the primary care physician and the nursing staff • Continuation of the IV antibiotics needed to complete the 6 week treatment of the epidural abscess • Treatment and investigation of the persistent low back pain, which continued to incapacitate this woman even though the abscess had been debrided • Monitoring by the staff regarding patient's cardiovascular status, given history of angina and WPW syndrome • Attending physician to determine whether urinary continence could be achieved now that the acute neurological problem had been resolved • Attending physician to monitor wound and remove sutures • Physical therapy to help the patient resume ambulation, given mild but persistent paraplegia • Occupational therapy to improve ADL status • Continuous contact by physician with the patient's Health Maintenance Organization (HMO) regarding the patient's status and approval for consultations and investigations
Treatment course	*Management of Known/New-Onset Problems* • Remained febrile and began to have urinary retention during first week of admission/Blood and urine cultures repeatedly negative • After prolonged discussions with HMO, permission granted to repeat magnetic resonance imaging of spine, which revealed continued collection of fluid in epidural space • After consultation with neurosurgeon and infectious disease consultation, change in antibiotics made/Fever resolved and there was improved ability to participate in rehabilitation therapies • Shortly after completion of antibiotic course and shortly before her discharge, experienced change in mental status with increased confusion/Only lab abnormalities were minimal elevation of white blood cells and 28% bands/Valium and Tylenol #3 discontinued/Stool assay positive for *C. difficile*/Treated with oral metronidazole with resolution of fever and confusion *Changes in Care Objectives During Stay* • None

(continued)

Case 3:	Cynthia, Age 60 (Continued)

Item	Description
	Significant Interruptions in Treatment Plan • Persistence of abscess necessitating treatment change • Late-stage confusion due to *C. difficile* infection
Patient/family education provided	• Medications: purpose of each, proper usage, potential problems • Possibilities for new or recurrent problems • Likely longer-term outcomes and residual deficits • Anticipated course (improvement, stabilization, complications) • Appointments for follow-up care
Discharge	*Site* • Home *Resources/Services/Follow-Up* • Visiting Nurse Association follow-up for additional physical therapy and occupational therapy *Problems* • None related to discharge
Follow-up of patient status	• Remains at home
Postdischarge quality review	*Outcomes* • Change in acuity score from 10 on admission to 4 on discharge • Achieved predicted result • Length of stay: 57 days • Occurrence of complications of primary illness and new-onset condition • No iatrogenic/nosocomial conditions *Programmatic Issues* • No problems/concerns raised by patient and family • No issues raised by staff • Problem with payer reluctance to authorize additional testing and length of stay despite evident complications

Case 4:	Andrew, Age 85

Item	Description
	Preadmission Selection and Preparation
Referral source/reasons	• Acute hospital • Patient had fallen and been found after 48 hours on the floor of apartment/Admitted to hospital/On hospital admission, creatine phosphokinase (CPK) 4874; severely dehydrated; severe generalized weakness; new R facial weakness; several pressure sores/Rehydrated; renal function and CPK monitored until danger of acute renal failure secondary to rhabdomyolysis no longer present
Anticipated treatments/ services	• Care of pressure sores • Improve ability to ambulate and perform ADLs • Safety teaching • Control of gout • Management of hypertension
Anticipated care outcome	*Practitioners* • Improvement to or beyond status prior to current episode of illness *Patient/Family* • Unknown/unclear

CASE 4:   ANDREW, AGE 85 (CONTINUED)

Item	Description
Significant decision makers	• Patient has partial decision-making capacity
Limits on medical care/directives	• Do Not Resuscitate
Financial status/insurance coverage	• Medicare
Significant findings on assessment	**Postadmission Care Management** *Physical Status* • R facial droop; Grade II pressure sores on R knee and elbow *Functional Status* • Dependent in some ADLs *Decision-Making Capacity* • Impaired *Psychosocial Information* • Lives alone in handicapped-accessible senior citizen apartment/Attends Senior Day Care Center three times a week/Estranged from both his divorced wife and only son/Two nieces keep in touch with him
Medical diagnoses	*Primary* • Rhabdomyolysis *Secondary* • Cerebrovascular accident, L sided, new onset • Paranoid schizophrenia • Dementia • Hypertension • Gout
Identified problems	**Group 1. Overall Health** • Potential for injury (recurrent falls, dementia) • Prolonged disease/disability **Group 2. Nutrition and Metabolism** • Fluid volume deficit • Altered nutrition • Potential skin impairment **Group 3. Urinary and Fecal Elimination** • Other altered urinary elimination pattern (potential renal impairment from rhabdomyolysis, gout) **Group 4. Activity and Exercise** • Activity intolerance • Altered health maintenance • Impaired mobility • Self-care deficit **Group 5. Psychosocial Concerns** • Social isolation • Ineffective individual coping
Risk/acuity assessment	*Severity of Illness Score (NSI)* • 12 *Other High-Risk Factors* • Falls • Cognitive/behavioral status alteration
Care objectives/plan	*General* • Improvement to or beyond status prior to current episode of illness *Problem-Related* • Care of pressure sores

(continued)

CASE 4:	ANDREW, AGE 85 (CONTINUED)

Item	Description
	• Improve ability to ambulate and perform ADLs • Safety teaching • Control of gout • Management of hypertension
Principal care providers	• Careful medical monitoring of renal functioning and CPK level • Medical management of generalized gout which flared on the admission to the subacute unit • Nursing treatment of grade 2 pressure sore on right elbow and knee with Duoderm • Physical therapy twice a day for ambulation, transfers, and safety with a walker • Occupational therapy daily for ADL training • Social worker to coordinate between family, staff of the senior apartment building, and the day care center for improved care on discharge • Social worker to help obtain Lifeline service • Psychiatry consultation to monitor and assist in care of schizophrenia • Consultation with neurologist and clinical pharmacologist regarding the use of prophylaxis against future cerebrovascular accidents in face of risk of gout and patient history of falls
Treatment course	*Management of Known/New-Onset Problems* • Renal function remained stable • Myopathy and gout both resolved • Pressure sores on right elbow and knee resolved • Patient became independent with a walker on level surfaces • R facial droop resolved • Became independent with light meal preparation, but it was felt that his mental status made cooking unsafe without supervision • Placed on Ticlid as stroke prophylaxis *Changes in Care Objectives During Stay* • None *Significant Interruptions in Treatment Plan* • None
Patient/family education provided	• Possibilities for new or recurrent problems • Likely longer-term outcomes and residual deficits • Appointments for follow-up care • Precautions to prevent high-risk complications such as falls
Discharge	*Site* • Apartment *Resources/Services/Follow-Up* • Arrangements for participation in assisted living program with all meals provided in the apartment complex/Stove in apartment disabled/Lifeline rented, to be worn whenever he is in his apartment/Patient also returned to participate in Senior Day Care Center 5 days a week *Problems* • None related to discharge
Follow-up of patient status	• Functional status maintained
Postdischarge quality review	*Outcomes* • Change in acuity score from 12 on admission to 6 on discharge • Achieved predicted result • Length of stay: 12 days • Recurrent complications managed appropriately • Iatrogenic/nosocomial conditions anticipated and prevented *Programmatic Issues* • No problems/concerns raised by patient and family • No issues raised by staff • No issues raised by payers, other outsiders

CASE 5:   RONALD, AGE 45

Item	Description
	Preadmission Selection and Preparation
Referral source/reasons	• Acute hospital • Hospitalized with symptoms of weakness and shortness of breath/Found to have staphylococcal subacute bacterial endocarditis, probably from toe wound/Begun on intravenous antibiotics/ Transferred to subacute for continuing treatment
Anticipated treatments/ services	• Four weeks of additional IV antibiotics • Treatment of foot ulcer • Management of diabetes
Anticipated care outcome	*Practitioners* • Improvement to or beyond status prior to current episode of illness *Patient/Family* • Unknown/unclear
Significant decision makers	• Patient is primary decision maker
Limits on medical care/ directives	• No limits
Financial status/insurance coverage	• Managed care organization (HMO from job)
	Postadmission Care Management
Significant findings on assessment	*Physical Status* • Grade II/VI systolic heart murmur/Amputated L first toe/Stump with grade III ulcers with necrosis/Poor pedal pulses/Hickman catheter in place *Functional Status* • Able to perform ADLs and IADLs/Restricted by non-weight-bearing status *Decision-Making Capacity* • Not cognitively impaired, but history of poor judgment *Psychosocial Information* • 45 y.o. disabled prison guard/Divorced and lives alone/History of alcohol abuse/Son who occasionally lives with him is known to be a drug abuser
Medical diagnoses	*Primary* • Subacute bacterial endocarditis (SBE) *Secondary* • Diabetes mellitus, insulin dependent • Necrotic ulcer, left great toe • History of alcohol abuse
Identified problems	**Group 1. Overall Health** • Infection/contagion (SBE) • Prolonged disease/disability (alcoholism) **Group 2. Nutrition and Metabolism** • Altered nutrition • Skin impairment (ulcers) **Group 3. Urinary and Fecal Elimination** • None **Group 4. Activity and Exercise** • Activity intolerance (SBE) • Altered health maintenance (alcoholism/noncompliance with diabetes management)

(continued)

CASE 5:   RONALD, AGE 45 (CONTINUED)

Item	Description
	Group 5. Psychosocial Concerns • Social isolation • Ineffective individual coping
Risk/acuity assessment	*Severity of Illness Score (NSI)* • 8 *Other High-Risk Factors* • None
Care objectives/plan	*General* • Improvement to or beyond status prior to current episode of illness *Problem-Related* • Resolve subacute endocarditis • Heal necrotic foot ulcer • Address patient's substance abuse and noncompliance issues
Principal care providers	• Physician management of antibiotics for treatment of subacute endocarditis • Nursing (wound care team) provision of wound care for lesion on foot, including use of enzymatic preparations and wet-to-dry dressing to necrotic areas • Dietitian and nurse reeducation regarding diabetes management • Physical therapy to improve ambulation and teach use of assistive devices
Treatment course	*Management of Known/New-Onset Problems* • Endocarditis resolved with 4 weeks of antibiotics/Central line removed • Toe wound healed well at time of discharge *Changes in Care Objectives During Stay* • None *Significant Interruptions in Treatment Plan* • None
Patient/family education provided	• Diabetes management compliance • Appointments for follow-up care
Discharge	*Site* • Home *Resources/Services/Follow-Up* • HMO for primary care/HMO refused other referrals, including visiting nurses and outpatient physical therapy *Problems* • None related to discharge
Follow-up of patient status	• Functional status achieved
Postdischarge quality review	*Outcomes* • Change in acuity score from 8 on admission to 5 on discharge • Achieved predicted result • Length of stay: 28 days • No occurrence of complications of illness • No occurrence of iatrogenic/nosocomial conditions • No unanticipated transfers out of program *Programmatic Issues* • No problems/concerns raised by patient and family • No issues raised by staff • Issues raised by payer: During stay, third-party payer refused psychiatric consultation regarding alcoholism and patient noncompliance problem/Also did not allow 24 to 48 hours of monitoring after completion of antibiotic course to ensure that symptoms would not recur

CASE 6: ALICIA, AGE 89

Item	Description
	Preadmission Selection and Preparation
Referral source/reasons	• Primary care physician (direct admission) • Patient found on office assessment to be dehydrated, probably from diarrhea/Referred for primary treatment instead of to hospital
Anticipated treatments/ services	• Rehydration • Management of diarrhea • Improvement of general deconditioning
Anticipated care outcome	*Practitioners* • Improvement to or beyond status prior to current episode of illness *Patient/Family* • Unknown/unclear
Significant decision makers	• Patient lacks decision-making capacity • Family member is primary decision maker (once located)
Limits on medical care/ directives	• No limits
Financial status/insurance coverage	• Medicare
	Postadmission Care Management
Significant findings on assessment	*Physical Status* • Dehydrated/Disoriented/Decreased hearing/Mildly paranoid *Functional Status* • Dependent in some ADLs and IADLs (cooking, bathing, medication administration) *Decision-Making Capacity* • Absent *Psychosocial Information* • Lives alone in senior highrise, participates in assisted living program (three meals a day and an aide to provide personal assistance once a day; light housekeeping provided weekly)/Nephew controls patient's finances
Medical diagnoses	*Primary* • Dehydration secondary to diarrhea *Secondary* • Cerebrovascular accident, old • Dementia • Degenerative joint disease • Paranoia, mild
Identified problems	**Group 1. Overall Health** • None **Group 2. Nutrition and Metabolism** • Fluid volume deficit (diarrhea) • Risk for impaired skin integrity **Group 3. Urinary and Fecal Elimination** • Diarrhea **Group 4. Activity and Exercise** • Activity intolerance (fluid volume deficit) • Altered health maintenance (dementia) • Impaired mobility • Self-care deficit

(continued)

CASE 6:   ALICIA, AGE 89 (CONTINUED)

Item	Description
	Group 5. Psychosocial Concerns • None
Risk/acuity assessment	*Severity of Illness Score (NSI)* • 7 *Other High-Risk Factors* • None
Care objectives/plan	*General* • Improvement to or beyond status prior to current episode of illness *Problem-Related* • Rehydration • Control of diarrhea • Improvement of endurance and function
Principal care providers	• Physician and nurse management of intravenous rehydration • Nurse application of barrier cream to the sacrum to prevent skin breakdown • Socialization activities to avoid catastrophic reaction in this demented woman • Rehabilitation services to improve ADL status and endurance
Treatment course	*Management of Known/New-Onset Problems* • Fluid balance restored with intravenous hydration/IV discontinued • Diarrhea resolved after 48 hours; no bacterial etiology • Skin integrity maintained • Patient became more functional in ambulation/Used walker instead of a cane *Changes in Care Objectives During Stay* • None *Significant Interruptions in Treatment Plan* • None
Patient/family education provided	• Appointments for follow-up care
Discharge	*Site* • Back to senior living apartment *Resources/Services/Follow-Up* • Followed by a home care agency for 3 weeks after discharge *Problems* • None related to discharge
Follow-up of patient status	• Functional status achieved
Postdischarge quality review	*Outcomes* • Change in acuity score from 7 on admission to 2 on discharge • Achieved predicted result • Length of stay: 9 days • No complications of illness • Iatrogenic/nosocomial conditions successfully prevented *Programmatic Issues* • No problems/concerns raised by patient and family • No issues raised by staff • No issues raised by payers, other outsiders

CASE 7:   ROSEMARY, AGE 29

Item	Description
	Preadmission Selection and Preparation
Referral source/reasons	• Acute hospital • Patient post-pancreas and kidney transplant/While hospitalized, became severely deconditioned and experienced decreased appetite with nausea/Bedside therapy initiated with minimal progress/Transferred to subacute program
Anticipated treatments/ services	• Improvement in ADL function and endurance • Improved blood pressure control • Safety teaching • Management of depression
Anticipated care outcome	*Practitioners* • Improvement to or beyond status prior to current episode of illness *Patient/Family* • Improvement to or beyond status prior to current episode of illness
Significant decision makers	• Patient is primary decision maker
Limits on medical care/ directives	• No limits
Financial status/insurance coverage	• Managed care organization
	Postadmission Care Management
Significant findings on assessment	*Physical Status* • Deconditioned/Fluctuating blood pressure/Poor vision/Depressed *Functional Status* • At least partially dependent in 3 ADLs *Decision-Making Capacity* • Intact *Psychosocial Information* • Previously lived with a roommate and had worked as a second-grade school teacher/Parents both living/Patient planned to return to parents' row home, which included 13 steps to second floor bathroom
Medical diagnoses	*Primary* • Post-pancreas and kidney transplant *Secondary* • Diabetic neuropathy • Diabetes mellitus, insulin dependent • Hypertension • Orthostatic hypotension • Depression
Identified problems	**Group 1. Overall Health** • Risk for injury (legally blind, orthostatic hypotension) • Prolonged disease/disability (pancreatic/kidney transplant) **Group 2. Nutrition and Metabolism** • Altered nutrition **Group 3. Urinary and Fecal Elimination** • Altered urinary elimination (postdialysis) **Group 4. Activity and Exercise** • Activity intolerance (weak, deconditioning) • Impaired mobility (orthostatic hypotension) • Self-care deficit (ADL dependencies) **Group 5. Psychosocial Concerns** • Social isolation (diminished recreational and social skills) • Depression

(*continued*)

CASE 7:   ROSEMARY, AGE 29 (CONTINUED)

Item	Description
Risk/acuity assessment	*Severity of Illness Score (NSI)* • 9 *Other High-Risk Factors* • None
Care objectives/plan	*General* • Improvement to or beyond status prior to current episode of illness *Problem-Related* • Stabilize blood pressure • Improve appetite and nutritional status • Improve ADL function and reduce dependency • Improve recreational and social skills • Compensate for poor vision • Elevate mood (depression related to chronic illness)
Principal care providers	• Physical therapy two times daily for ambulation, transfer, and stair training • Occupational therapy two times daily for ADL activities, transfer training, strengthening, and homemaking activities • Nursing intervention to monitor organ rejection, blood pressure, and investigational drugs • Coordination of lab work with referring hospital • Dietary counseling to provide education on dietary restrictions • Therapeutic recreation to facilitate community reentry and development of leisure activities • Family counseling and discharge planning assistance • Initiation of vocational rehabilitation • Psychological counseling for depression • Follow-up with endocrinologist and nephrologist
Treatment course	*Management of Known/New-Onset Problems* • Became independent with transfers and ambulated with a cane on level surfaces/ Independent in light meal preparation/Blood pressure stabilized/Appetite improved as nausea resolved *Changes in Care Objectives During Stay* • None *Significant Interruptions in Treatment Plan* • None
Patient/family education provided	• Safe transfers and ambulation • Possibilities for new or recurrent problems • Appointments for follow-up care by transplantation team
Discharge	*Site* • Discharged to her parent's home *Resources/Services/Follow-Up* • Referred to the Commission for the Blind for follow-up training *Problems* • None related to discharge
Follow-up of patient status	• Functional status achieved
Postdischarge quality review	*Outcomes* • Change in acuity score from 9 on admission to 4 on discharge • Achieved predicted result • Length of stay: 22 days • No occurrence of complications of illness • No occurrence of iatrogenic/nosocomial conditions *Programmatic Issues* • No problems/concerns raised by patient and family • No issues raised by staff • No issues raised by payers, other outsiders

CASE 8:   MONICA, AGE 52

Item	Description
	Preadmission Selection and Preparation
Referral source/reasons	• Acute hospital • Admitted to hospital with sepsis from salmonella infection/During lengthy stay, experienced multiple complications including surgery for aortic aneurysm and secondary spinal cord infarction causing paraparesis/Complicated postoperative course with respiratory and urinary problems/Developed neurogenic bladder/Acquired stage III sacral decubitus and multiple lower extremity joint contractures
Anticipated treatments/services	• Improve ADL functional status • Manage neurogenic bladder/Prevent complications of chronic catheter • Improve sacral ulcer
Anticipated care outcome	*Practitioners* • Improvement but less than previous status *Patient/Family* • Improvement but less than previous status
Significant decision makers	• Patient is primary decision maker
Limits on medical care/directives	• Do Not Resuscitate
Financial status/insurance coverage	• Managed care organization
	Postadmission Care Management
Significant findings on assessment	*Physical Status* • Generally debilitated/Paraparetic/Lower extremity contractures/Indwelling urinary catheter/Stage III 4 x 6 cm sacral pressure ulcer/Healed abdominal scar from aneurysm surgery *Functional Status* • Dependent in all ADLs *Decision-Making Capacity* • Mildly impaired *Psychosocial Information* • Lives with her husband, who works full-time/One daughter in home/Lives in a ranch-style home
Medical diagnoses	*Primary* • Spinal cord infarction with paraparesis *Secondary* • Recent abdominal aortic aneurysm repair • Sacral ulcer, stage III • Neurogenic bladder
Identified problems	**Group 1. Overall Health** • Potential for injury (immobility) **Group 2. Nutrition and Metabolism** • Altered nutrition • Impaired skin integrity (pressure ulcer) **Group 3. Urinary and Fecal Elimination** • Other altered urinary elimination pattern (neurogenic bladder with Foley catheter) **Group 4. Activity and Exercise** • Activity intolerance (general debilitation) • Impaired mobility (bedbound) • Self-care deficit (dependent in ADLs)

(continued)

CASE 8:   MONICA, AGE 52 (CONTINUED)

Item	Description
	Group 5. Psychosocial Concerns • Depression • Altered family processes (patient's prolonged illness) • Ineffective individual coping • Family coping: potential for growth (family involvement in care)
Risk/acuity assessment	*Severity of Illness Score (NSI)* • 11 *Other High-Risk Factors* • None
Care objectives/plan	*General* • Improvement but less than previous status *Problem-Related* • Improve transfers, wheelchair mobility, strength and endurance • Progress toward wound healing • Manage depression and recent social isolation • Bowel and bladder retraining program and urology consultation • Individualized patient and family counseling focusing on reintegration into the family unit • Medication exploration to decrease pain and frequency of spasms • Dietary evaluation and follow through to promote skin healing
Principal care providers	• Physical therapy two times daily for transfer training, wheelchair independence, range of motion, standing tolerance, and upper extremity strengthening • Physician titration of pain medications • Occupational therapy two times daily to improve ability to assist in lower extremity care, homemaking skills, and vocational training • Nursing and physical therapy jointly providing wound care • Community reintegration program utilizing past leisure interests and expanding into new opportunities • Bowel and bladder retraining program and urology consultation • Individualized patient and family counseling focusing on reintegration into the family unit • Medication exploration to decrease pain and frequency of spasms • Dietary evaluation and follow-through to promote skin healing
Treatment course	*Management of Known/New-Onset Problems* • Became independent in wheelchair management • Substantial but not total wound healing/Dressing changes to continue at home with visiting nurse • Fever due to bacteremia from chronic bacteriuria resolved with injectable cephalosporin • Pain symptoms improved using TENS unit supplemented by nonnarcotic analgesics *Changes in Care Objectives During Stay* • None *Significant Interruptions in Treatment Plan* • None
Patient/family education provided	• Procedures for managing catheter, dressings • Medications: purpose of each, proper usage, potential problems • Possibilities for new or recurrent problems • Likely longer-term outcomes and residual deficits • Appointments for follow-up care • Precautions to prevent high-risk complications such as falls, wound site infection, dehydration
Discharge	*Site* • Home

CASE 8:   MONICA, AGE 52 (CONTINUED)

Item	Description
	Resources/Services/Follow-Up • Husband trained to assist with her personal care/Became active in wheelchair bowling league in community *Problems* • None related to discharge
Follow-up of patient status	• Functional status achieved • Recurrence of condition that was corrected during stay
Postdischarge quality review	*Outcomes* • Change in acuity score from 11 on admission to 5 on discharge • Achieved predicted result • Length of stay: 30 days • Complication of illness (urinary tract tract infection) handled appropriately • No occurrence of iatrogenic/nosocomial conditions *Programmatic Issues* • No problems/concerns raised by patient and family • No issues raised by staff • No issues raised by payers, other outsiders

CASE 9:   HARVEY, AGE 36

Item	Description
	Preadmission Selection and Preparation
Referral source/ reasons	• Acute hospital • Hospitalized for 8 days after motor vehicle accident with extensive open and closed injuries, including traumatic brain injury/Developed wound on left heel/Jaw wired, preventing adequate oral intake
Anticipated treatments/services	• Rehabilitative care to assist recovery • Management of multiple medical and postoperative problems
Anticipated care outcome	*Practitioners* • Improvement but less than previous status *Patient/Family* • Improvement to or beyond status prior to current episode of illness
Significant decision makers	• Patient has partial decision-making capacity • Family member is primary decision maker
Limits on medical care/directives	• No limits
Financial status/ insurance coverage	• Private indemnity insurance
	Postadmission Care Management
Significant findings on assessment	*Physical Status* • Alert, fluctuating levels of consciousness/Tracheostomy in place/Patient able to communicate but not speak/Infected operative wound on head/Cast on L leg/Grade III ulcer 2 x 1.4 cm on L heel *Functional Status* • Dependent in bathing, dressing, grooming, ambulation

(continued)

CASE 9:   HARVEY, AGE 36 (CONTINUED)

Item	Description
	Decision-Making Capacity • Partially impaired by accident *Psychosocial Information* • Worked as a landscaper prior to accident/Wife works full-time/One small child in the home/ Lives in ranch-style home with two steps to enter
Medical diagnoses	*Primary* • Multiple trauma secondary to motor vehicle accident *Secondary* • Fracture, left acetabulum • Fracture, left femur • Open fracture, left patella • Fracture, left maxilla • Left heel wound • Left lower extremity wound • Open traumatic brain injury
Identified problems	**Group 1. Overall Health** • Infection/contagion risk (scalp wound, tracheostomy, heel wound) **Group 2. Nutrition and Metabolism** • Altered nutrition (poor oral intake, recent major trauma) • Impaired skin integrity (heel ulcer) **Group 3. Urinary and Fecal Elimination** • Urinary incontinence (occasional) • Constipation (due to immobility and pain medications) **Group 4. Activity and Exercise** • Activity intolerance (multiple injuries, pain) • Ineffective airway clearance (tracheostomy) • Impaired mobility (immobility, multiple injuries, pain) • Self-care deficit (multiple ADL dependencies) **Group 5. Psychosocial Concerns** • Depression (due to major trauma) • Altered family processes (small child, wife works, stress of prolonged hospitalization) • Impaired verbal communication (tracheostomy)
Risk/acuity assessment	*Severity of Illness Score (NSI)* • 12 *Other High-Risk Factors* • None identified
Care objectives/plan	*General* • Improvement but less than previous status *Problem-Related* • Manage pain so that it can be controlled on oral or cutaneous medications • Family recognition of lengthy recovery process and some likely permanent disability • Improve endurance, transfers, ambulation, ADL function • Healing of pressure sore on heel and other wounds • Weaning from tracheostomy • Monitoring for complications of head injury • Improve nutritional status, moving towards adequate oral intake
Principal care providers	• Physician involvement to assess and manage the pain • Social work to counsel family and help them accept patient's diagnosis and future needs • Pharmacist to educate the nursing staff, patient and family about use of subcutaneous morphine pump • Physical therapy daily for endurance training, transfers, ambulation, and use of assistive devices • Occupational therapy to improve ADL function

CASE 9:   HARVEY, AGE 36 (CONTINUED)

Item	Description
	• Nursing to monitor the pain control • Nursing treatment of grade III pressure sore on heel and scalp incision wound • Nursing management of tracheostomy • Physician assessment and debridement (surgical and mechanical) of heel pressure sore • Neurology consultation for follow-up of head injury • Activities therapist to engage patient in rehabilitative activities • Nutritionist to assess the nutritional deficits and develop tube-feeding regimen • Physical therapy/occupational therapy evaluation of the home to determine durable medical equipment needed when the patient is discharged
Treatment course	*Management of Known/New-Onset Problems* • Intense pain persisted, requiring frequent adjustment of dosages/Gradually stabilized and subsided/At discharge, using fentanyl patch with occasional oral supplementation • Wife had difficulty accepting seriousness of injuries, managing with job and small child/Some improvement with social worker counseling and arrangement for child day care • Endurance gradually improved/Able to transfer from bed to chair with minimal assist/Short-distance ambulation with assistance and walker/Able to assist with some ADLs • Healing of pressure sore on heel • Small grade 2 pressure ulcer developed on R heel/Treated with topical medication and dressings/Healed after 13 days • Gradual weaning from tracheostomy/Discontinued just prior to discharge • Several episodes of possible seizures/Transferred to emergency room/Repeat CT scan done with no new findings/Begun on diphenylhydantoin • When jaw wiring removed, able to increase oral intake/Tube feedings tapered and then discontinued/Feeding tube removed prior to discharge • Scalp incision wound healed with local treatment and dressings *Changes in Care Objectives During Stay* • None *Significant Interruptions in Treatment Plan* • Emergency room transfer for evaluation of possible seizures
Patient/family education provided	• Procedures for managing dressings, walker, pain medications • Possibilities for recurrent seizures • Likely longer-term outcomes and residual deficits • Anticipated course of slow improvement, likely residual deficits • Appointments for follow-up care • Precautions to prevent falls
Discharge	*Site* • Home *Resources/Services/Follow-Up* • Outpatient rehabilitation/Neurologist/Surgeon to follow up on fractures *Problems* • None related to discharge
Follow-up of patient status	• Improved functional status maintained • Rehospitalization avoided
Postdischarge quality review	*Outcomes* • Change in acuity score from 12 on admission to 4 on discharge • Achieved predicted result, except for more improvement in self-care than expected • Length of stay: 27 days • Complications of illness (seizures) managed appropriately • Nosocomial condition (R heel ulcer) developed during stay, managed promptly • Unanticipated transfers (to ER) considered appropriate *Programmatic Issues* • No problems/concerns raised by patient and family • Issue raised by staff: adequacy of staffing to manage skin care • No issues raised by payers, other outsiders

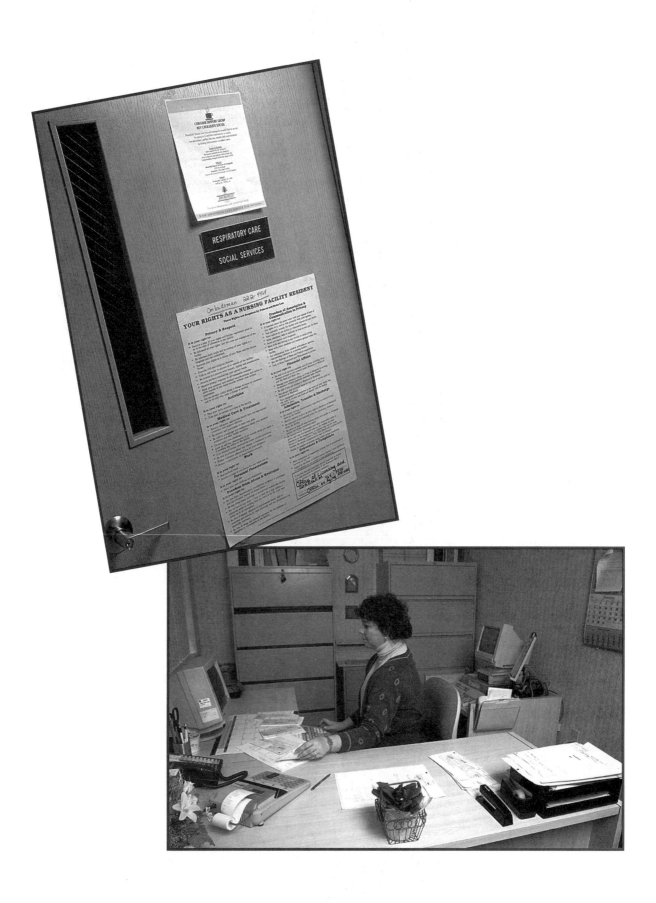

Public Policy, Reimbursement, and Regulatory Implications

*T*he American health care system is undergoing major changes while other countries wrestle with many similar health care and public policy issues, although with different systems. The debates over subacute care have helped highlight some of these conceptual, structural, and operational issues. They have pointed out advances in disease management, the weaknesses of an uncoordinated delivery system, the many potential areas for systems realignment and improvements, and the substantial current misunderstanding about alternative forms of care, especially that portion of the spectrum of care between the outpatient and the hospital environments. Certain things about the health care system overall should be reassessed and revamped to create a truly coordinated, cost-effective approach to delivering health care services. These renovations are also important if subacute care is to fulfill its promise and purpose.

This chapter will explore the public policy, reimbursement, and regulatory implications of transitional care, and the implications of changes in the health care system for that level of care. In the process, it will summarize many points that have been made throughout the book.

The emerging interest in subacute care has coincided with other major changes in the organization, reimbursement, and delivery of health care services in the United States. To date, its development has been driven principally by economic forces. Competing interests have fought legislative and regulatory battles over the rights to deliver this care.

Many practitioners and regulatory agencies, and some insurers, have been skeptical about all of this. Questions frequently asked about subacute care are who are the subacute patients; is there a distinct level of care; and if so, how should that level of care be regulated or reimbursed?

For several reasons, a more intimate understanding of the characteristics and value of the middle of the health care spectrum, including transitional care, should help create a better coordinated, more cost-effective health care system. First, these transitional care settings are potentially beneficial for many individuals. Second, many of the principles underlying transitional care can help address issues relevant to the whole health care system (Table 12–1, p. 396). Therefore, the following discussion summarizes how subacute care fits from a care standpoint in a modern health care system, and considers some of the relevant systems issues.

UNDERSTANDING SUBACUTE CARE

Although subacute care is not a new form of health care, it does meet a legitimate need. It is a package of various treatments and related services (Chapter 5) provided to individuals with complex collections of problems and other service needs (Chapter 2) by an identifiable collection of individuals (Chapter 6) participating in a specific series of processes for a limited time to address both the causes and consequences of illness and injury to try to achieve certain care objectives (Chapter 7). Subacute sites must be able to manage patient needs by providing systems (Chapters 8 and 9) that enable practitioners and support staff to consistently and efficiently perform those care processes to achieve those outcomes.

Subacute care may serve a variety of individuals with a broad spectrum of conditions. There is no "average" episode of subacute care. However, there are typical episodes for some categories of patients with common characteristics (for example, those with a left-sided stroke or those who have had hip replacement surgery, with comparable severity of illness and levels of comorbidity). The cases in Chapter 11 illustrate some of this variety.

But subacute care cannot be distinguished from other care just by the treatments rendered (IVs, ventilators, wound care, and so on). Any of these treatments could be rendered elsewhere. For example, rehabilitation therapies, nursing services, dialysis, and ventilator care may be provided in nursing facilities or in people's homes. Because many patients are similar to those in skilled nursing facilities (SNFs) or hospitals, subacute care is best viewed as a program rather than a place. Even while health care is shifting out of traditional sites and into noninstitutional settings, logistical and financial limits to the ability to provide multidimensional care in the home or in ambulatory settings persist.

IMPLICATIONS OF SUBACUTE CARE FOR A MODERNIZED HEALTH CARE SYSTEM
A Shifting to Problem-Oriented Management

This book has pointed out that effective subacute care centers on managing problems, not just diseases. This principle of problem-oriented management, which is also common in long-term care and other care of the chronically ill, is beneficial across the entire health care spectrum, including hospital-based care. Whether functioning independently or as part of an integrated delivery system, various service sites and practitioners must coordinate their care of individuals around the core of their problems, even though they may each handle various aspects of service (problem definition, cause identification, cause management, consequence management, and the like). The successful management of underlying problems frequently influences the outcomes of episodes of illness or injury, regardless of the principal reason for an admission or other health care intervention.

It is essential to move away from an approach to health care where roles are so rigidly defined that known risks are not addressed and likely problems are not sought or managed in various settings because they are considered to be irrelevant to that setting. For example, nutritional status is a common risk factor in all settings, and undernutrition is common in many of those with serious illness (Sullivan et al, 1995). One recent study found that stroke patients admitted to a rehabilitation service had a very high prevalence of malnutrition. Early and ongoing detection and treatment of malnutrition were recommended during rehabilitation of stroke patients both on the service and at follow-up (Finestone et al, 1995). Therefore, managing nutritional status is as much a part of the care of patients receiving rehabilitative therapies as assessing functional status should be part of the care of those receiving mainly medical treatments.

Another study found that protocols in place on a rehabilitation unit resulted in earlier detection and management of stroke-related problems and prevention of potentially life-threatening complications compared to similar patients on a general medical unit (Kalra et al, 1995). Therefore, those same protocols should be utilized on general medical units and not just considered to be relevant to rehabilitation units.

For these and other reasons, a case management approach should be beneficial by coordinating care around people's problems and arranging appropriate combinations of services and support to identify and address both causes and consequences. But for this to succeed, case managers must be more than gatekeepers (that is, dedicated to minimizing services and controlling costs of care). They must understand that problems have multidimensional causes and know how to assemble the individuals and resources to define those problems and identify causes.

Focusing on More Effective Management of Common, Recurrent Problems

Subacute care provides evidence that little things can often make a big difference, and that problems often worsen unnecessarily when the little things are overlooked. A revamped health care system should more effectively address the common problems identified repeatedly for several decades in the medical and health services literature, but all too often ignored or excused. Examples include failures of patient compliance with medications and treatments; inadequate efforts or lack of success in addressing reasons for such noncompliance; overtreatment of those with advance directives and incurable conditions despite wishes to the contrary; failure to address risks for developing iatrogenic or nosocomial conditions; and insufficient attention to the known risks and complications of medications.

Although some of these problems can be addressed by specific disciplines or practitioners, others will require broader social initiatives or pressure. For instance, the medical profession has so far been only partially successful in getting physician cooperation in discussing ethical issues and honoring patient's wishes. Although physicians may often be unsuccessful in obtaining patient compliance, community-based interventions for home-bound individuals may be more successful. Because a relatively few medications appear to be the source of a large portion of medication-related complications and hospitalizations, a combined public and professional effort might be able to address this, whereas professional efforts alone have been only partially successful.

Thus, the entire health care system should divert its attention more toward dealing with the many comparatively little things that could make a significant difference in results. It does not make sense to continue to have to deny resources for potentially useful care while money is being wasted on preventable problems.

Better Understanding the Relevance of Medical Care

A changing future requires a more realistic, balanced appraisal of the positive and negative affects of medical care on health, and promotion of the benefits. Subacute care points out the multiple dimensions of causes of illness and the important difference between managing causes and handling consequences. Modern medicine's successes are well known. They include increased survival with hereditary, congenital, or acquired illnesses; wider availability of tools to help make diagnoses, allowing physicians to be more efficient and to lower the risks for patients; and a broader spectrum of treatments, many of which are more effective and carry fewer complications.

But many factors that affect health and wellness are largely unrelated to scientific, medical, or technical interventions. Our conceptions of the determinants of health change periodically. Sometimes socioeconomic factors have predominated in policy-making, and at other times the emphasis has been largely on identifying the causes of disease and treating the sick. Public policy and resource allocation are strongly affected by definitions of health and illness and by accepted theories about the determinants of health (Frank & Mustard, 1994).

Figure 12–1 illustrates the various possible relationships between a person's physical well-being (optimal bodily structure and function) and overall functioning both as an individual and as part of a social group. For instance, developmental deformities or cancer may have a major impact on organ function, and therefore on personal or social function. Personally satisfying habits like smoking or drug use may damage bodily structure and function or be socially undesirable. Social function or status clearly affect personal well-being, which can affect bodily function and eventually structure.

Clearly, health-related services may have many different effects on personal function and its social consequences. The services may partially or completely address the causes of problems, and addressing the causes may or may not address the consequences.

Medical technology can correct many gross imbalances in physiological or anatomic function, and can even stabilize those with terminal and end-stage conditions. But technology is markedly effective only for some problems, marginally effective for others, ineffective for others, and may cause more problems than it helps resolve in still others. Intermediate- and long-term recovery are often decidedly labor-intensive, relatively low-technology processes.

Many individuals who survive serious illness and injury still have significant long-term consequences. For example, many of those with multiple chronic con-

FIGURE 12–1   THE MUTUAL INFLUENCES OF PHYSICAL STRUCTURE AND FUNCTION AND
PERSONAL AND SOCIAL FUNCTION

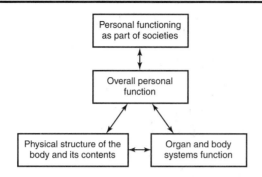

ditions have recurrent episodes of illness despite repeated medical interventions. Those with end-stage conditions may be kept alive despite general organ systems failure, but die anyway with little functional improvement. Many infants who survive birth defects and many severely injured accident survivors require extensive care for their entire lives. Aggressive medical treatments and medications often cause significant complications and side effects that require a whole additional set of interventions. Some abnormalities or diseases are better left untreated.

Therefore, the value of subacute care must be appreciated relative to broader definitions of health and its determinants. Many subacute patients improve substantially or totally. For others, reduction of long-term dependency, secondary and tertiary prevention, and prompt recognition and management of significant intercurrent illness are worthy accomplishments when primary prevention or cure is impossible.

Therefore, public policy will need to rethink these issues of defining health and determining valuable services, including the desirable balance between paying to treat causes and paying to prevent problems or to manage consequences.

Understanding and Differentiating the Phases of Illness and Treatment

Subacute care points out that there are different phases of sickness and different kinds of severity of illness. Some health care programs, and many health care practitioners, are involved principally in managing discrete conditions in otherwise healthy individuals where there is a more or less direct relationship between managing the cause and fixing the problem. But subacute and long-term care demonstrate that this is very different from managing those with multidimensional problems whose consequences are cumulative. The health care system must not be defined or organized from just one perspective. Payers and providers must recognize these different phases, and the issues and approaches that are common to all of them and unique to each of them. Subacute care also emphasizes that the disease-oriented approach to categorizing the patient population or to designing reimbursement approaches may not be the proper model to use throughout the health care system (see Chapter 2).

Recognizing the Different Kinds of Sickness.   The instability of those with high-acuity conditions relates mainly to their risk of dying or of having serious complications of their primary illness. Other levels of care also may manage those with instability, but instead of the immediately life-threatening variety, it is instability due to frequent new-onset intermittent illnesses (such as fevers or gastrointestinal bleeding) and increased risk due to collections of underlying deficits and disabilities (cognitive impairment, decreased mobility, and so on). That is why disease-based or physiologically based severity of illness (SOI) scales useful in hospitals have little relevance to assessing subacute patients (see Chapter 10).

Integrating Health Management into Everyday Life

Subacute care must often deal with individuals who are overwhelmed and frightened by major illnesses with potentially ominous implications and by complex care provided in imposing institutional settings. Many individuals have little or no understanding of what is happening to them or why they wound up where they are. They are often asked to make decisions based on little firm understanding of the underlying issues or choices. They are substantially or wholly dependent on strangers of unknown competence and intention.

Over the past few decades, individuals became increasingly dependent on health care professionals to manage almost all aspects of their health and illness. But such dependencies tend to reduce incentives for people to take more responsibility for preventing problems, influencing the consequences of illness, or controlling the costs of care.

For all of these reasons, a revamped health care system should strive to better integrate health maintenance and illness management into everyday life. Health care provision and decision making is likely to be more effective and less costly when individuals participate more intelligently. Laymen should be able to understand a lot about health care and health care decision making. Their first real exposure to the health care system and to medical decision making should not await a major personal or family crisis.

Making informed, responsible decisions is an acquired skill. Public policy and education at all levels should educate people to consider health and health care as a routine part of their everyday lives—just as managing mental health problems has become much more integrated into everyday social institutions and much less the exclusive domain of psychiatrists and other professionals. Learning how to take personal responsibility for health and understanding the framework for making health care decisions should be a core component of everyone's ongoing education.

Education and training are also major responsibilities of settings that deal with complex illness and injury. For various reasons discussed in earlier chapters, subacute programs may be ideal sites to provide patient and family education, especially because declining hospital stays rarely afford the luxury of time for such initiatives. Nevertheless, every level of care has a role in such efforts (for example, in discussing the likely course of illness or ethical issues), and the discussions of many of these issues should be coordinated across care settings.

Changing the Roles of Various Providers

Like other components of the health care system, subacute programs have assumed many functions—for example, providing rehabilitative and medical services—formerly done elsewhere. Practitioner roles are also shifting; for instance, primary care physicians may do more things formerly done by specialists; nurse practitioners may assume some physician functions; and nursing assistants are doing things that nurses once did.

These changing roles should be recognized and validated when they can maintain or improve the effectiveness and efficiency of care. Practitioners and provider organizations must be prepared to adjust their roles, programs, and services as needed. Past performance or contribution does not necessarily ensure a future role.

Accumulating evidence continues to call into question long-standing assumptions that have limited those role shifts in the past. For instance, there is evidence that subacute rehabilitation outcomes for stroke patients compare favorably to those in more costly hospital-based rehabilitation units, and that the two populations may be largely comparable (Keith et al, 1995). The reasons for these and other similar findings deserve closer attention and better comprehension (see Chapters 2 and 10).

Recognizing Equal Value for Different Roles

Because the factors that influence health and illness are so diverse, no one discipline or profession can possibly dominate health care. Various care sites and practitioners play important but different roles. All roles that help achieve the overall objectives of effective, efficient service are equally valid. For example, subacute care, ambulatory care, and long-term care providers are as important as hospitals to the overall system. Subacute practitioners and other support staff should be just as respected for their knowledge and skills as those at any other level of care. Surgeons performing technically complex operations are intrinsically no more important than primary care physicians, and practitioners who successfully prevent problems and the complications of incurable conditions are as valuable as those who cure acute illness.

Recognizing That Organization-Based Care Has Some Unique Influences

This book has tried to explain why complex multidimensional care like subacute care is influenced by certain factors that may not be as relevant in other settings, and that may not be readily apparent to practitioners or to the public as patients. Delivering such care is affected by intricate social interactions among diverse individuals and disciplines, and the time and energy that these individuals must spend dealing with one another instead of being directed toward the care of patients.

Despite the growing body of literature confirming these important issues, they are still often misunderstood or ignored. They must now be fully acknowledged because they represent some of the root causes of quality and cost problems in the health care system. Many of them could be readily corrected.

Along these lines, the systems of governance and management of health care organizations must be substantially overhauled. Qualifications for selection to health care organization governing bodies should be upgraded. These individuals must recognize the relationship between their attitudes and actions and the performance of those providing the care. They should have certain responsibilities and relevant knowledge of modern health care and of what they oversee. They must understand how they or their decision making may be among the root causes of their own organization's problems. Also, the real expertise of various professionals needs to be clarified. For example, physicians sitting on health care organization boards of directors may know much about treating disease, but little about the details of giving care in specific programs or settings such as long-term care or subacute care.

Revamping Practitioner Education and Training

Subacute care points out the important roles of health care practitioners as advisors, educators, and communicators. Yet it is handicapped by a scarcity of individuals—especially physicians—with such skills. Health professional education has been changing, but more change is still needed. Much of this education and training has focused heavily on teaching technical skills, while being weaker in cultivating other vital abilities, such as communicating effectively and learning how to define problems (not just diagnoses) precisely. Other practitioners in nonmedical fields should become more capable of recognizing situations where biological problems may affect social and personal function, so that they may help ensure that all relevant services are provided.

For example, some physicians have difficulty communicating information effectively, may have trouble defining or recognizing the nonmedical causes of health-related problems, may not appreciate the variable impact of health care services on health, or may not understand or acknowledge reasons why patients may not absorb, understand, or be able to assess properly some or all of what they are told.

Health care professional education and training programs need to teach proper conceptual models, and they need more faculty to serve as role models who can reinforce the right approaches and attitudes, not just convey the right technical skills. The idea of rivalry and competition within the profession must be diminished. But for this to happen, academic settings must develop their own systems of performance evaluation and feedback that value such attributes. For instance, medical academia has long focused on well-trained specialists and researchers. Many of these individuals know little about transitional or long-term care, and therefore could not readily teach or explain much about the value of these practitioners or the great importance of these levels of care.

Subacute care also shows the importance of effective decision-making processes in which all parties distinguish between having major input into decision making and having the authority to make final decisions. Physicians cannot equate input from other disciplines in the decision-making process with intrusion upon their prerogatives. All health care practitioners must be helped to understand the proper team models because these are not intuitively obvious. They must learn to move away from the idea of asserting control through exercise of authority.

These principles also apply to the training of all management and professional disciplines involved in health care and its organizations. As explained throughout this book, much of the health care system has been handicapped by power-based decision making in which those in authority positions (administrators, board members, department heads, practitioners, nursing unit managers, and the like) may make or veto decisions based primarily on personal perspectives and political considerations instead of on objective data. Unfortunately, power-based decision making (whether by practitioners, managers, owners, or others) impedes effective problem solving.

Physicians must also learn to take related nonmedical issues, such as ethical decision making, seriously instead of considering them to be unscientific matters to be shunted off on nurses, social workers, or administrators. Every physician needs to learn how to distinguish the likely impact of treatments on bodily function from their likely consequences for overall personal and social function. They must also learn not to express their displeasure about things by impeding others from doing what they need to do (for example, by refusing to authorize desired medical orders).

Subacute care points out the importance of practicing professions in context, and having the judgment and skill to match knowledge to each situation to solve real problems. In a new health care era, the application of knowledge must be considered at least as important as discovering new knowledge.

A new generation of health care managers must understand the general principles of medical decision making, the processes of service delivery, and the roles of various practitioners. They need to learn to serve as effective referees and coaches and to address the factors that influence performance and ultimately may influence the care outcomes.

Subacute care also points out the importance of practitioners who can vary their roles depending on the occasion or the setting. Thus, all health care professionals need a broader education about the different kinds of illness and levels of care. Many of them may spend their entire careers just treating discrete conditions in otherwise well individuals. But they should all understand the basic differences between these situations and managing those with chronic illnesses, comorbidities, and frequent fluctuations in condition.

Physicians and nurses should also learn how to anticipate, prevent, identify, and manage iatrogenic conditions—especially those related to medications. These are an all too common source of potentially preventable complications leading to more expensive care.

REGULATIONS AND QUALITY STANDARDS IN SUBACUTE CARE

Regulatory Issues

Governments do not deliver care, but they influence care delivery by establishing rules and providing incentives, principally through laws, regulations, and reimbursement. The acknowledged limits to the capacity to spend public money on health care implies the need for rational public policy to try to get the most out of available resources.

Licensure. Licensure is one way for government to influence care quality and cost. Many state governments are trying to identify their appropriate roles in licensing and regulating subacute care. In some states, various interests have fought major political battles over the rights to convert beds or the licensure or reimbursement of facilities to provide subacute care.

In the future, licensure categories should be consistent with shifting care delivery. Traditional hospital, nursing facility, and other licensure categories no longer fit the circumstances of care being delivered in these settings or within health networks. Care networks cross institutional boundaries.

These categories should become less focused on sites and more oriented to levels of care based on what is needed to provide a level of service to individuals with relevant characteristics and needs. Organizations and networks should be licensed or accredited for each level of service that they can provide, such as high-acuity care, moderate- or low-acuity care, care for high-level chronic illness or disability, and so on. Regardless of the relative roles of licensure and accreditation, regulations and standards must be coordinated better to reduce requirements of unproven benefit and duplicate standards that require demonstrating the same competencies repeatedly.

Licensure and accreditation should be based both on core requirements (those essential to all levels of care) and care-specific requirements (those needed for a particular level of care). For instance, risk-management programs and information-management systems are relevant to all levels of care, and housekeeping or plant-management capabilities are relevant only to inpatient programs or some residential care settings. Assessment capabilities are relevant to all programs managing those with complex illness, although expectations for having the equipment and staffing needed to manage ventilator patients are only relevant to those who provide such care. The capacity to manage one level of care or acuity should not be assumed to imply the capacity for providing other levels of service.

Certain licensure categories may need to be adjusted or may no longer be needed in an era of health care networks and managed care. For example, many states have separately licensed psychiatric, rehabilitation, long-term care, and cancer hospitals. The fact that these settings principally provide subacute care has only added to the confusion about their capabilities and roles in a changing environment.

Responsibility in Establishing and Using Standards

Society has usually relied on health care organizations and practitioners to establish standards of practice and to judge the value of various treatments and other interventions, but with inconsistent results. Traditionally, patients and payers have had a relatively limited basis for judging the value of the care and the soundness of its oversight.

Practitioner opinions about optimal selection and duration of treatment for a given condition and patient will often differ. Although flexibility is needed to accommodate legitimate differences in approach, a substantial amount of care can be agreed to by professional consensus on standards and guidelines, by standardizing various care-related processes, and by encouraging practitioners (through education, feedback, reimbursement, sanctions, and so on) to use practice guidelines as a starting point. Public policy should encourage the use of standards and guidelines to address long-standing problems such as medication-related illness.

As broadly interdisciplinary enterprises, subacute programs point out the importance of having appropriate performance expectations for all players. Such initiatives should transcend the traditional approach in which each participant defines and guards his or her own standards. Instead, all those whose performance may be influenced by others should have some say in what those others do. Thus, nurses and administrators should have input into expectations for physicians, physicians and administrators should influence standards for governing body members, and so on.

Reimbursement for Care

Important Principles

Because economic incentives heavily influence personal and social decision making, reimbursement methodologies necessarily affect care delivery, which in turn often influences outcomes. Imbalances in care provision have both caused and been exaggerated by imbalances in the reimbursement system, which has emphasized specialized, procedure-oriented, hospital-based, high-technology care.

Some argue that simply allowing market forces to function will correct the problems. But market forces alone have been inadequate to stem costs because the suppliers of service (practitioners and facilities) have often been the ones who also stimulated the demand or determined the need on behalf of the care recipients.

The means of reimbursing health care are shifting rapidly away from fee-for-service and toward managed care. Many states are trying to shift their Medicaid programs to managed care. Advocates of managed care suggest that this approach will provide more of the desired incentives and help correct the health care system's problems.

But no payment methodology by itself can correct the problems of health care or necessarily ensure desired results. Managing costs is not the same as managing care. The effects of cost controls can range from more appropriate utilization to highly imprudent limitations that later result in the need for even more expensive care. Managed care is not likely to effectively address the problems of access and quality without recognizing the various kinds and phases of illness and optimal approaches to determining placement, and without allowing some flexibility for those situations where spending additional money at one point may reduce the need for more expensive care subsequently. Therefore, quality standards (both for outcomes and for processes) must evolve simultaneously.

Paying for Value.   Traditionally, health care has often been valued for its own sake, that is, with little regard for whether it accomplishes desired objectives. Increasingly, accountability requires a different emphasis on more objective assessments of performance and results. In a modern health care system, care should have value to be reimbursable. Further effort is needed to define what constitutes value, but any criteria should consider what the care accomplishes for personal and social function, not just what it does for bodily structure or function.

Options for Subacute Reimbursement

Even under managed care, there will still be different ways of reimbursing various components of the health care system. For example, a subacute program may be reimbursed by a negotiated all-inclusive rate for caring for patients within that program's network, or by a negotiated per-diem rate under contract to care for patients of another organization needing that level of care. Some capitated subacute programs are even beginning to act as both payers and providers, subcapitating other subacute sites to provide care over a region.

Shifting trends in reimbursement methodologies will also influence the use of subacute care settings. They may be used less if treatments and other related services can be delivered elsewhere with equal effectiveness but at less cost. Or, they may be used more if their potential to manage other situations is recognized more fully. Sometimes, the short-term costs of subacute care may be justified if the care can improve on intermediate- or longer-term outcomes by achieving clinical stability and promoting preventive efforts (Evans et al, 1995).

For example, subacute settings may be valuable for assessing and managing community-dwelling individuals who have new-onset incontinence, an abrupt change in their level of activities of daily living (ADL) function, or significant but relatively uncomplicated pneumonia. Such individuals may need some evaluation of causes; the controlled, monitored initiation and adjustment of treatment; close but not continuous monitoring of their responses to treatment; and management of the functional and psychosocial complications of their illness. Under Medicare, the ability to use SNFs for such care has been limited by policies requiring 3 days of acute hospitalization to qualify for Skilled benefits.

Whatever the arrangement, the objectives of the stay must be clearly defined. For example, in caring for a patient referred from another source, a subacute program may be expected to treat an acute condition, manage coexisting problems, and provide short-term rehabilitation. But the same program as part of a comprehensive network may be expected to provide only a brief period of treatment for a similar patient, and to then discharge the patient for continued in-home or outpatient care.

Prospective Payment.   A prospective payment system (PPS) provides a predetermined rate for care, rather than a payment based on the cost of giving the care. As discussed previously, the diagnosis related group (DRG)–based PPS for hospitals does not apply readily to long-term or to subacute care.

Some states have developed distinct reimbursement rates for specific categories of subacute patients (for example, ventilator or wound-care patients). A Case-Mix Demonstration Project has attempted to settle the cost versus rate issue by using a rate-based, state- or area-specific national payment plan for Medicaid and Medicare beneficiaries in long-term and skilled settings (Fries et al, 1994). RUGs-III (the latest version as of 1996) represents a way to categorize SNF patients and nursing facility (NF) residents based upon their intensity of service, functionality, and certain additional problems. It promotes the principle of the same work value for equal care for equal needs, but allows for differential reimbursement because of regional differences in labor costs.

A Clinical Basis for Subacute Reimbursement.   Possible ways to reimburse for subacute care are (1) by case mix/acuity, (2) by treatments and services provided, or (3) by average cost per patient. An "average" payment system would only work well if the patients in each category have comparable characteristics and likely outcomes. Spreading the cost across all such patients would not accurately reflect the case mix.

Some form of prospective payment system for subacute care based on case mix and adjusted for acuity is likely to make more sense. Under a case-mix/acuity approach, a prospective rate would be based on relevant patient characteristics and service needs, including comorbidities and level of medical stability. As the acuity level declined during their stay, the payment would be adjusted accordingly.

Referring to the cases in Chapter 11 as examples, case 2 (with an acuity score of 19) requires more care and resources overall than case 6 (with an acuity score of 7). Therefore, the initial reimbursement for the care of the patient in case 2 should be higher than that for the care of the patient in case 6. But as the condition of each patient improves, the reimbursement would be adjusted downward in stages because fewer resources are needed to provide the care.

A Process Basis for Reimbursement.   When patients discharged from one setting are reevaluated by a whole new group of individuals at a new site, reimbursement may cover duplicate comprehensive assessment and testing, or the cost of managing problems that could have been treated at an earlier stage. For example, under the DRG system hospitals receive a fixed payment for a given episode of illness, regardless of how long the individual stays. As more alternative sites have become available for managing postacute care, hospitals have had an incentive to transfer patients elsewhere after briefly initiating treatment because they still receive the full DRG payment. This is a significant disadvantage of a piecemeal reimbursement system, and one reason that a single prospective payment is now being contemplated for managing an entire episode of illness.

Therefore, another possible approach to reimbursement in a changing environment would consider the relative contributions of various providers to achieving overall objectives. This could offer a more objective basis for dividing a capitated or a bundled payment for a single episode of illness among several care providers. Table 12–2, p. 397, illustrates examples of different levels of performance for various care processes, where a provider's performance may influence the ultimate success or cost of the overall care.

REFERENCES

Evans RL, Connis RT, Hendricks RD, Haselkorn JK. Multidisciplinary rehabilitation versus medical care: A meta-analysis. *Soc Sci Med*. 1995; 40:1699–1706.

Finestone HM, Greene-Finestone LS, Wilson ES, Teasell RW. Malnutrition in stroke patients on the rehabilitation service and at follow-up: Prevalence and predictors. *Arch Phys Med Rehabil*. 1995; 76:310–316.

Frank JW, Mustard J. The determinants of health from a historical perspective. *Daedalus*. 1994; 123;1–19.

Fries BE, Schneider DP, Foley WJ, et al. Refining a case-mix measure for nursing homes: Resource Utilization Groups (RUG-III). *Med Care*. 1994; 32:668–685.

Kalra L, Yu G, Wilson K, Roots P. Medical complications during stroke rehabilitation. *Stroke*. 1995; 26:990–994.

Keith RA, Wilson DB, Gutierrez P. Acute and subacute rehabilitation for stroke: A comparison. *Arch Phys Med Rehabil*. 1995; 76:495–500.

Sullivan DH, Walls RC, Bopp MM. Protein-energy undernutrition and the risk of mortality within one year of hospital discharge: A follow-up study. *J Am Geriatr Soc*. 1995; 43:507–512.

TABLE 12–1 EXAMPLES OF SUBACUTE CARE ISSUES RELEVANT TO PUBLIC POLICY AND BROADER HEALTH CARE SYSTEMS ISSUES

- Giving treatment versus achieving care objectives
- Having regulatory flexibility to give care at lowest cost sites
- Having the flexibility to give several levels of care at same site, or even at different times in the same licensed bed
- Roles and responsibilities of various practitioners
- Education and training required to provide effective care
- Licensure and certification categories for individuals and organizations
- Systems to enable consistent processes to achieve more consistent care
- Relationship of processes to outcomes
- Treating diseases versus managing problems
- Reimbursement methodologies to reflect care realities
- Subacute's place in a full continuum of care
- Risks of managed care without outcome expectations and quality standards

TABLE 12-2   EXAMPLES OF HOW VARIABLE LEVELS OF PERFORMANCE MIGHT RESULT IN DIFFERENTIAL REIMBURSEMENT

Process	Level 1	Level 2	Level 3	Comments
Assessment	No information about the individual relevant to proper definition of his or her problems has been collected	Some information has been collected	All significant information has been collected	The more detailed, pertinent assessment should be reimbursed more
Problem definition	None of the individual's problems and needs have been fully and accurately defined	Some of the problems and needs have been defined	All significant problems and needs have been fully and accurately defined	More reimbursement for more fully defining a person's problems
Achieving care objectives	Stabilization, prevention of further decline and death	Partial improvement below preillness level	Improvement to or beyond preillness level	Different level of reimbursement for different objectives
Management of known problems	Problem management focuses on single problem	Discrete problem management plus prevention of complications/iatrogenic conditions	Multidimensional problem management plus prevention	Greater reimbursement for broader problem-oriented focus

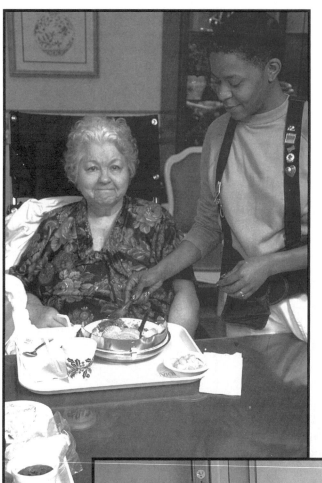
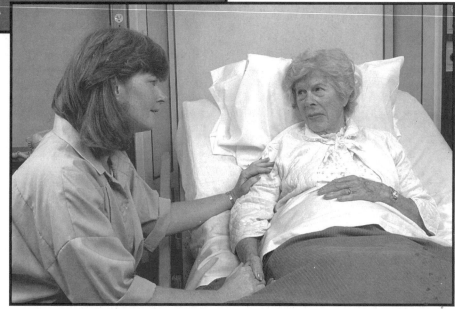

A FINAL WORD:
THE CHALLENGES OF CHANGE

*T*he most visible subject of this book is subacute care. But its more general themes have been change and balance. That is, subacute care will be most successful if provided within a framework of appropriate attitudes, systems, and processes. The purpose of this chapter is to suggest what that desirable broader framework might be.

Changing Human Nature or Changing Human Performance

Although the ultimate shape of health care reform is still unclear, individuals and organizations rush to position themselves for the future. Only some of them understand in depth what they are doing or why it should be done in a particular way. In the rush to survive, simple approaches that address common recurrent problems may be overlooked.

There are ways to achieve the desired improvement in performance of individuals and organizations. Currently, there is broad acknowledgement that health care delivery systems should change. This book has included discussions of desired major changes in the attitudes and performance of practitioners and other care providers, organizations, owners, management, and insurers.

There are several common reasons for successful and unsuccessful human efforts to effect change (Table 13–1, p. 404). Individuals and organizations often tend to retreat into familiar patterns (Table 13–2, p. 404). Human nature tends to emphasize self-interest. But although it is difficult to change human nature, it is possible to change performance, largely by changing what is considered to represent self-interest.

To change the performance of so many diverse individuals and organizations will require a substantial effort, including different expectations and incentives than in the past. Effective change also requires capitalizing on the strengths and addressing forthrightly the weaknesses of human behavior. Problems persist when the strengths are undermined and the weaknesses rationalized.

There is growing recognition that many old ways of doing things make it harder to enhance performance to meet future challenges. But only some of those who own, manage, or work in health care settings recognize the opportunities and appreciate how best to meet the challenges.

The Proper Balances

Effective, efficient care requires certain ingredients and balances. In cooking or baking, optimal results depend on having the proper balance of essential ingredients. When ingredients are missing, defective, or in the wrong proportions, the results may range from slightly off to horrendous. For example, even producing a simple product such as bread may be thrown off by the wrong amount of flour or salt, by the right amount of flour that is too old, or even by having all of the ingredients but mixing them in the wrong order.

As also discussed, the right balances are critical to successful health care at all levels from the societal level to the care of individual patients. Attaining optimum results from complex health care provided to people with complex problems requires the ingredients to be present in the right amounts—and sometimes in a specific order. Individual performance must be properly adjusted and coordinated. Some results can be attained without some of the ingredients, or with the right ingredients but in the wrong proportions. However, such results are likely to be less consistent, less predictable, less efficient, or less desirable.

For several decades, health care organizations have been driven by growth and expansion, or by vague notions of community service. Practitioners and providers have often demanded the right to decide on the value of their performances and the appropriateness of their methods. But the approach of having

many fiercely independent entities doing their own thing jointly is often unworkable.

Practitioners and interest groups must now think more in systems terms
and should be prepared to function in more collaborative environments.
Traditional perspectives and incentives have made it harder for many of them to
adapt to situations where a truly interdisciplinary approach is needed, as in subacute or long-term care. Health care organizations must concentrate on providing solid operational foundations that enable truly consistent, effective care, not
just the perception of it. Together individuals and organizations must address
the many lingering problems of service delivery (for example, high turnover of
key staff, poor systems, and inadequate management) and outcomes, such as
medication-related complications and need for recurrent inpatient care because
of inadequate follow-up. For any health care practitioner or organization, the
care should be considered the source of success for the business. Although in-
vestors and communities may risk their money in programs and facilities providing health care, the personal risks and social consequences of inadequate or
inappropriate care are equally or more important. Decisions about care provision that restrict service utilization so tightly that they inhibit reasonable outcomes will only tilt the balance farther away from the patients. Ironically, those
who recognize and achieve the proper balance of forces are likely to achieve desired clinical and business objectives.

Thus, as with many forms of health care, the subacute care equation applies
(Figure 13–1). A combination of knowledge, skills, and resources can achieve
some results. But attitudes and processes are the catalysts for successful outcomes; that is, their presence can enable more consistent achievement of a desired result for a given amount of individuals and resources. Conversely,
ineffective processes and improper conceptual frameworks inhibit results or increase the costs of attaining them.

The ultimate purpose of providing health-related services must be clarified
and reinforced. As the health care system changes, many providers (both organizations and practitioners) have focused on the business aspects: Who will reimburse them, how and how much will they be reimbursed, who will they work
with or for, or who will work for them? Although all these questions are important, a more central issue for health care reform is: What is the purpose of health
care, and how is that purpose best achieved?

Serious illnesses or injuries often cause significant physical or psychological
imbalances, which have both personal and social consequences. Achieving or
restoring proper individual physical and psychological balance yields both personal and public benefits. Consequently, things that help create, maintain, or restore appropriate balances are generally desirable.

Both providers and recipients may benefit from the delivery of care and services. Clearly, practitioners and organizations have several different primary
motivations for wanting to provide health care. These may include the desire to
help people recover from or cope with significant physical and psychological

FIGURE 13–1 THE SUBACUTE CARE EQUATION

$$\text{Knowledge} + \text{Skills} + \text{Resources} \xrightarrow[\text{Attitudes}]{\text{Process}} \text{Outcomes}$$

imbalance, the wish to achieve certain psychological and financial benefits (primarily power and money) for themselves, or some combination of these and other factors.

But ultimately, all care and services (not just health-related ones) succeed or fail based on what they do for the recipients. In all social relationships, individuals are both ends in themselves and a means to the ends of others. When an activity such as health care has broad individual and social implications, its impact depends heavily on the balance between these two perspectives.

The marketplace alone cannot create an effective health care system unless it is also governed by the right principles. If ill and dysfunctional individuals are viewed principally as an end in themselves—as people whose productive lives and well-being are disrupted by significant illness and injury—then health care becomes primarily a means to the end of helping them restore their lost balance. Its value is then determined more by what it does for the care recipients than for the care providers.

But if ill and dysfunctional people are viewed principally as a means to the ends of the providers or payers, then health care provision becomes a means to principally benefit those who provide or fund the services. If care and services benefit the providers or payers out of proportion to the patients, then they are likely to cost a lot relative to what they accomplish.

The fact that health care now costs a great deal, yet is often of questionable benefit, suggests the need to restore a better balance. Therefore, as with any health care service or treatment, subacute care should be evaluated principally for its benefits to the recipients of the care. It should be considered useful when it contributes significantly to achieving essential personal and social objectives. If it is not likely to do so, then it should not necessarily be provided just because it is available. Its financial (fill empty beds, maximize revenues, employ practitioners) and psychological (power, control, influence) benefits for providers are relevant but secondary.

The further development of subacute care should fit in with the need for a properly balanced health care system in which the components are aligned properly and operate together effectively. Each care site or program must be concerned about its impact on other providers and on the overall course of the care, not just short-term outcomes. For example, many significant secondary problems of subacute patients (for example, confusion, dehydration, medication side effects) are often at least somewhat related to earlier treatment deficits. A systematic approach to optimizing care would be more likely to prevent and resolve problems before they become too great. Greater preventive efforts could also lessen the impact of other acute problems, and thereby reduce the overall duration and costs of subacute care.

Identifying Common Interests

Therefore, both subacute care and the overall health care system could be improved by applying the same principles. Addressing a few root causes can help influence or improve many different issues or problems. Although some of those causes have to do with resources, many are related to attitudes, systems, and processes.

All health care programs in a community, like all the players in a subacute program, have certain common interests:

- A well-trained, competent, flexible work force
- Maximum feasible individualization and flexibility of care
- Pertinent, flexible external rules and requirements
- Financial viability
- Satisfaction of care recipients (patients and families), care providers, and payers
- Appropriate compliance with regulations and standards
- Minimal loss and legal liability

In a competitive, individualistic culture, only some people recognize or acknowledge that enhancing mutual interests promotes self-interest in the long run. However, there is a great difference between starting with a foundation of mutual interest, which then allows personal flexibility and competition, in contrast to a primarily individualistic approach, which is then supposed to find a common ground. The former approach provides a solid basis for flexible decision making and effective performance, and the latter tends to exacerbate confusion and conflict.

Ultimately, the key to all self-interest lies in having a solid foundation of effective performance based primarily on mutual interests and accountability. Only through this route can service be delivered both effectively and efficiently. These principles are the key to effective subacute care. They are also relevant to all social issues and systems.

TABLE 13–1 COMMON REASONS FOR PROBLEMS IN INITIATING OR ACCOMPLISHING CHANGE

- Belief that change puts one at a personal and competitive disadvantage because others will get ahead using established methods
- Reluctance to try new approaches; comfort with the familiar
- Inability or unwillingness to recognize inadequacy of old methods
- Fear of loss of control leads to retreat into authoritarian approach
- "Macro" and "micro" systems struggles for power and control; trying to keep out "intruders"
- Beneficiaries of traditional authority-based rule do not want to relinquish it
- Struggles between resisters and overreactors
- Struggles between the "haves" and the "have-nots"

TABLE 13–2 COMMON TACTICS FOR RESISTING ESSENTIAL CHANGE

- Asserting control through care or administrative decisions
- Denial of personal role or responsibility
- Blaming others
- Rationalizing existing systems and processes
- Claiming interference with essential functions
- Clinging to old ways in the hope that pressure to change will subside
- Deliberate actions or inaction to sabotage change

INDEX

Note: Page references to tables and figures are italicized.